KETO WOMEN over 50

600 TASTY EASY RECIPES TO LOSE WEIGHT NATURALLY AND QUICKLY AND SLOW DOWN AGING. INCLUDING SOME TIPS FOR BEGINNERS TO BE SUCCESSFUL

Suzanne Newton

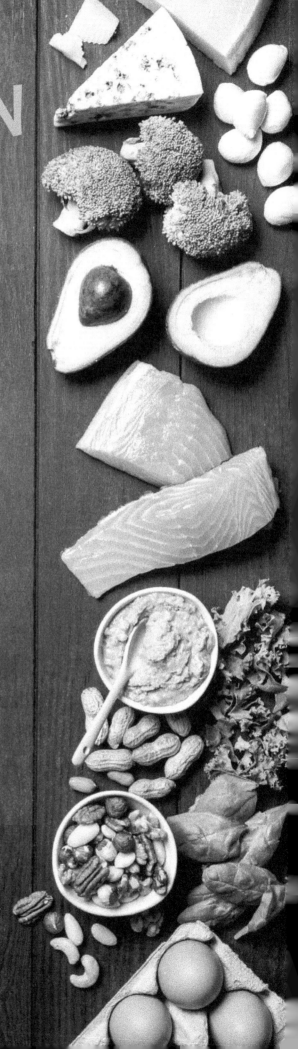

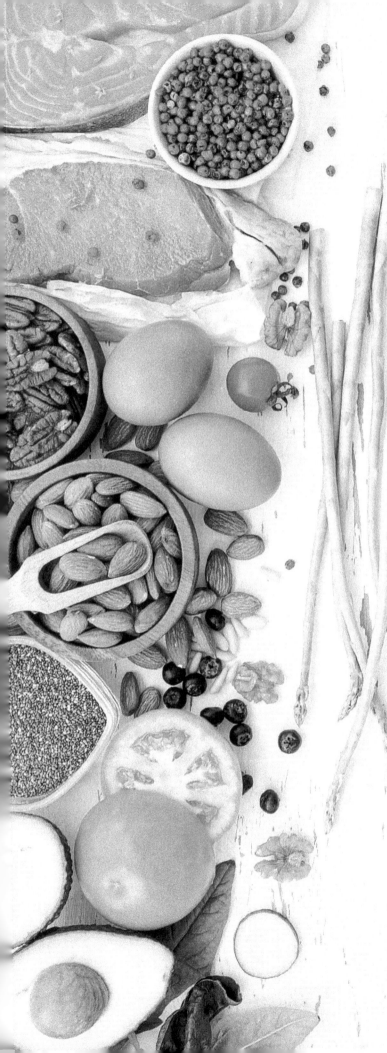

Copyright - 2020 - Suzanne Newton

All rights reserved.

The content contained within this book may not be reproduced, duplicated or transmitted without direct written permission from the author or the publisher.

Under no circumstances will any blame or legal responsibility be held against the publisher, or author, for any damages, reparation, or monetary loss due to the information contained within this book. Either directly or indirectly.

Legal Notice:

This book is copyright protected. This book is only for personal use. You cannot amend, distribute, sell, use, quote or paraphrase any part, or the content within this book, without the consent of the author or publisher.

Disclaimer Notice:

Please note the information contained within this document is for educational and entertainment purposes only. All effort has been executed to present accurate, up to date, and reliable, complete information. No warranties of any kind are declared or implied. Readers acknowledge that the author is not engaging in the rendering of legal, financial, medical or professional advice. The content within this book has been derived from various sources. Please consult a licensed professional before attempting any techniques outlined in this book.

By reading this document, the reader agrees that under no circumstances is the author responsible for any losses, direct or indirect, which are incurred as a result of the use of information contained within this document, including, but not limited to, - errors, omissions, or inaccuracies.

TABLE OF CONTENTS

Introduction	4
Chapter 1.	
What Is Keto And Why Is So Important For Your Health	6
Chapter 2.	
Benefit of Keto Diet for People Over 50	8
Chapter 3.	
Some Tips for Beginner to Achieve Keto Success	12
Chapter 4.	
What does the ketogenic diet mean to women after 50?	16
Chapter 5.	
What Keto Does to an over 50 Woman's Body	20
Chapter 6.	
How Can Ketogenic Diet Can Aid With the Sign and Symptoms of Ageing and Menopause	24
Chapter 7.	
Foods Allowed in Keto Diet	26
Chapter 8.	
Keto Grocery List	30
Chapter 9.	
Breakfast	34
Chapter 10.	
LUNCH	60
Chapter 11.	
Dinner	92
Chapter 12.	
Side Dishes	138
Chapter 13.	
Vegetables	154
Chapter 14.	
Poultry	180

Chapter 15. Beef	194
Chapter 16. Pork Recipes	206
Chapter 17. Lamb Recipes	212
Chapter 18. Seafoods	226
Chapter 19. Soup and Stew	246
Chapter 20. Bread	258
Chapter 21. Pancake and Muffins	266
Chapter 22. Basic Chaffles	272
Chapter 23. Smoothie and Drinks Recipes	282
Chapter 24. Appetizers	306
Chapter 25. Snacks	318
Chapter 26. Desserts	346
Conclusion	366

INTRODUCTION

Even before we talk about how to do keto – it's important to first consider why this particular diet works. What actually happens to your body to make you lose weight?

As you probably know, the body uses food as an energy source. Everything you eat is turned into energy, so that you can get up and do whatever you need to accomplish for the day. The main energy source is sugar so what happens is that you eat something, the body breaks it down into sugar, and the sugar is processed into energy. Typically, the "sugar" is taken directly from the food you eat so if you eat just the right amount of food, then your body is fueled for the whole day. If you eat too much, then the sugar is stored in your body – hence the accumulation of fat.

But what happens if you eat less food? This is where the Ketogenic Diet comes in. You see, the process of creating sugar from food is usually faster if the food happens to be rich in carbohydrates. Bread, rice, grain, pasta – all of these are carbohydrates and they're the easiest food types to turn into energy.

So the Ketogenic Diet is all about reducing the amount of carbohydrates you eat. Does this mean you won't get the kind of energy you need for the day? Of course not! It only means that now, your body has to find other possible sources of energy. Do you know where they will be getting that energy? Your stored body fat!

So here's the situation – you are eating less carbohydrates every day. To keep you energetic, the body breaks down the stored fat and turns them into molecules called ketone bodies. The process of turning the fat into ketone bodies is called "Ketosis" and obviously – this is where the name of the Ketogenic Diet comes from. The ketone bodies take the place of glucose in keeping you energetic. As long as you keep your carbohydrates reduced, the body will keep getting its energy from your body fat.

Sounds Simple, Right?

The Ketogenic Diet is often praised for its simplicity and when you look at it properly, the process is really straightforward. The Science behind the effectivity of the diet is also well-documented, and has been proven multiple times by different medical fields. For example, an article on Diet Review by Harvard provided a lengthy discussion on how the Ketogenic Diet works and why it is so effective for those who choose to use this diet.

But Fat Is the Enemy...Or Is It?

No — fat is NOT the enemy. Unfortunately, years of bad science told us that fat is something you have to avoid — but it's actually a very helpful thing for weight loss! Even before we move forward with this book, we'll have to discuss exactly what "healthy fats" are, and why they're actually the good guys. To do this, we need to make a distinction between the different kinds of fat. You've probably heard of them before and it is a little bit confusing at first. We'll try to go through them as simply as possible:

Saturated fat. This is the kind you want to avoid. They're also called "solid fat" because each molecule is packed with hydrogen atoms. Simply put, it's the kind of fat that can easily cause a blockage in your body. It can raise cholesterol levels and lead to heart problems or a stroke. Saturated fat is something you can find in meat, dairy products, and other processed food items. Now, you're probably wondering: isn't the Ketogenic Diet packed with saturated fat? The answer is: not necessarily. You'll find later in the recipes given that the Ketogenic Diet promotes primarily unsaturated fat or healthy fat. While there are definitely many meat recipes in the list, most of these recipes contain healthy fat sources.

Unsaturated Fat. These are the ones dubbed as healthy fat. They're the kind of fat you find in avocado, nuts, and other ingredients you usually find in Keto-friendly recipes. They're known to lower blood cholesterol and actually come in two types: polyunsaturated and monounsaturated. Both are good for your body but the benefits slightly vary, depending on what you're consuming.

Polyunsaturated fat. These are perhaps the best in the list. You know about omega-3 fatty acids right? They're often suggested for people who have heart problems and are recognized as the "healthy" kind of fat. Well, they fall under the category of polyunsaturated fat and are known for reducing risks of heart disease by as much as 19 percent. This is according to a study titled: Effects on coronary heart diseases of increased poly-unsaturated fat in lieu of saturated fat: systematic review & meta-analysis of randomized controlled tests. So where do you get these polyunsaturated fats? You can get them mostly from vegetable and seed oils. These are ingredients you can almost always find in Ketogenic Recipes such as olive oil, coconut oil, and more. If you need more convincing, you should also know that omega-3 fatty acids are actually a kind of polyunsaturated fats and you will find them in deep sea fish like tuna, herring, and salmon.

CHAPTER 1.
WHAT IS KETO AND WHY IS SO IMPORTANT FOR YOUR HEALTH

The health benefits of the Keto diet are not different for men or women, but the speed at which they are reached does differ. As mentioned, human bodies are a lot different when it comes to the ways that they are able to burn fats and lose weight. For example, by design women have at least 10% more body fat than men. No matter how fit you are, this is just an aspect of being a human that you must consider. Don't be hard on yourself if you notice that it seems like men can lose weight easier that's because they can! What women have in additional body fat, men typically have the same in muscle mass. This is why men tend to see faster external results, because that added muscle mass means that their metabolism rates are higher. That increased metabolism means that fat and energy get burned faster. When you are on Keto, though, the internal change is happening right away.

Your metabolism is unique, but it is also going to be slower than a man's by nature. Since muscle is able to burn more calories than fat, the weight just seems to fall off of men, giving them the ability to reach the opportunity for muscle growth quickly. This should not be something that holds you back from starting your Keto journey. As long as you are keeping these realistic bodily factors in mind, you won't be left wondering why it is taking you a little bit longer to start losing weight. This point will come for you, but it will take a little bit more of a process that you must be committed to following through with.

Another unique condition that a woman can experience but a man cannot be PCOS or Polycystic Ovary Syndrome; a hormonal imbalance that causes the development of cysts. These cysts can cause pain, interfere with normal reproductive function, and, in extreme and dangerous cases, burst. PCOS is actually very common among women, affecting up to 10% of the entire female population. Surprisingly, most women are not even aware that they have the condition. Around 70% of women have PCOS that is undiagnosed. This condition can cause a significant hormonal imbalance, therefore affecting your metabolism. It can also inevitably lead to weight gain, making it even harder to see results while following diet plans. In order to stay on top of your health, you must make sure that you are going to the gynecologist regularly.

Menopause is another reality that must be faced by women, especially as we age. Most women begin the process of menopause in their mid-40s. Men do not go through menopause, so they are spared from yet another condition that causes slower metabolism and weight gain. When you start menopause, it is easy to gain weight and lose muscle. Most women, once menopause begins, lose muscle at a much faster rate, and conversely gain weight, despite dieting and exercise regimens. Keto can, therefore, be the right diet plan for you. Regardless of what your body is doing naturally, via processes like menopause, your internal systems are still going to be making the switch from running on carbs to deriving energy from fats.

When the body begins to run on fats successfully, you have an automatic fuel reserving waiting to be burned. It will take some time for your body to do this, but when it does, you will actually be able to eat fewer calories and still feel just as full because your body knows to take energy from the fat that you already have. This will become automatic. It is, however, a process that requires some patience, but being aware of what is actually going on with your body can help you stay motivated while on Keto.

Because a Keto diet reduces the amount of sugar you are consuming, it naturally lowers the amount of insulin in your bloodstream. This can actually have amazing effects on any existing PCOS and fertility issues, as well as menopausal symptoms and conditions like pre-diabetes and Type 2 diabetes. Once your body adjusts to a Keto diet, you are overcoming the things that are naturally in place that can be preventing you from losing weight and getting healthy. Even if you placed your body on a strict diet, if it isn't getting rid of sugars properly, you likely aren't going to see the same results that you will when you try Keto. This is a big reason why Keto can be so beneficial for women.

You might not even realize that your hormones are not in balance until you experience a lifestyle that limits carbs and eliminates sugars. Keto is going to reset this balance for you, keeping your hormones at healthy levels. As a result of this, you will probably find yourself in a better general mood, and with much more energy to get through your days.

For people over 50, there are guidelines to follow when you start your Keto diet. As long as you are following the method properly and listening to what your body truly needs, you should have no more problems than men do while following the plan. What you will have are more obstacles to overcome, but you can do it. Remember that plenty of women successfully follow a Keto diet and see great results. Use these women as inspiration for how you anticipate your own journey to go. On the days when it seems impossible, remember what you have working against you, but more importantly what you have working for you. Your body is designed to go into ketogenesis more than it is designed to store fat by overeating carbs. Use this as a motivation to keep pushing you ahead. Keto is a valid option for you and the results will prove this, especially if you are over the age of 50.

CHAPTER 2.
BENEFIT OF KETO DIET FOR PEOPLE OVER 50

Benefits Ketogenic Diet

Reduction of cravings and appetite

Many people gain weight simply because they cannot control their cravings and appetite for caloric foods. The ketogenic diet helps eliminate these problems, but it does not mean that you will never be hungry or want to eat. You will feel hungry but only when you have to eat. Several studies have shown that the less carbohydrates you eat, the less you eat overall. Eating healthier foods that are high in fat helps reduce your appetite, as you lose more weight faster on a low-fat diet. The reason for this is that low carbohydrate diets help lower insulin levels, as your body does not need too much insulin to convert glycogen to glucose while eliminating excess water in your body. This diet helps you reduce visceral fat. In this way, you will get a slimmer look and shape. It is the most difficult fat to lose, as it surrounds the organs as it increases. High doses can cause inflammation and insulin resistance. Coconut oil can produce an immediate source of energy as it increases ketone levels in your body.

Reduction of risk of heart disease

Triglycerides, fat molecules in your body, have close links with heart disease. They are directly proportional as the more the number of triglycerides, the higher your chances of suffering from heart disease. You can reduce the number of free triglycerides in your body by reducing the number of carbohydrates, as is in the keto diets.

Reduces chances of having high blood pressure

Weight loss and blood pressure have a close connection; thus, since you are losing weight while on the keto diet, it will affect your blood pressure.

Fights type 2 diabetes

Type two diabetes develops as a result of insulin resistance. This is a result of having huge amounts of glucose in your system, with the keto diet this is not a possibility due to the low carbohydrate intake.

Increases the production of HDL

High-density lipoprotein is referred to as good cholesterol. It is responsible for caring calories to your liver, thus can be reused. High fat and low carbohydrate diets increase the production of HDL in your body, which also reduces your chances of getting a heart disease. Low-density lipoprotein is referred to as bad cholesterol.

Suppresses your appetite

It is a strange but true effect of the keto diet. It was thought that this was a result of the production of ketones but this was proven wrong as a study taken between people on a regular balanced diet and some on the keto diet and their appetites were generally the same. It, however, helps to suppress appetite as it is it has a higher fat content than many other diets. Food stays in the stomach for longer as fat and is digested slowly, thus provides a sense of fullness. On top of that, proteins promote the secretion cholecystokinin, which is a hormone that aids in regulating appetite. It is also believed that the ketogenic diet helps to suppress your appetite by continuous blunting of appetite. There is increased appetite in the initial stages of the diet, which decreases over time.

Changes in cholesterol levels

This is kind of on the fence between good and bad. This is because the ketogenic diet involves a high fat intake which makes people wonder about the effect on blood lipids and its potential to increase chances of heart disease and strokes, among others. Several major components play a lead role in determining this, which is: LDL, HDL, and blood triglyceride levels. Heart disease correlates with high levels of LDL and cholesterol. On the other hand, high levels of HDL are seen as protection from diseases caused by cholesterol levels. The impacts of the diet on cholesterol are not properly known. Some research has shown that there is no change in cholesterol levels while others have said that there is change. If you stay in deep ketosis for a very long period of time, your blood lipids will increase, but you will have to go through some negative effects of the ketogenic diet which will be corrected when the diet is over. If a person does not remain following the diet strictly for like ten years, he/she will not experience any cholesterol problems. It is difficult to differentiate the difference between diet and weight loss in general. The effect of the ketogenic diet on cholesterol has been boiled down to if you lose fat on the ketogenic diet then your cholesterol levels will go down, and if you don't lose fat, then your cholesterol levels will go up. Strangely, women have a larger cholesterol level addition than men, while both are on a diet. As there is no absolute conclusion on the effect of the ketogenic diet on cholesterol, you are advised to have your blood lipid levels constantly checked for any bad effects. Blood lipid levels should be checked before starting the diet and about eight weeks after starting. If repeated results show a worsening of lipid levels, then you should abandon the diet or substitute saturated fats with unsaturated fats.

Risk of a Ketogenic Diet

Low energy levels

When available, the body prefers to use carbohydrates for fuel as they burn more effectively than fats. General drop-in energy level is a concern raised by many dieters due to the lack of carbohydrates. Studies have shown that it causes orthostatic hypotension which causes lightheadedness. It has come to be known that these effects can be avoided by providing enough supplemental nutrients like sodium. Many of the symptoms can be prevented by providing 5 grams of sodium per day. Most times, fatigue disappears after a few weeks or even days, if fatigue doesn't disappear, then you should add a small number of carbohydrates to the diet as long as ketosis is maintained. The diet is not recommended when caring out high-intensity workouts, weight training, or high-intensity aerobic exercise as carbohydrates are an absolute requirement but are okay for low-intensity exercise.

Effects on the brain

It causes increased use of ketones by the brain. The increased use of ketones, among other reasons, result in the treating of childhood epilepsy. As a result of the changes that occur, the concern over the side effects, including permanent brain damage and short-term memory loss, has been raised. The origin of these concerns is difficult to understand. The brain is powered by ketones in the absence of glucose. Ketones are normal energy sources and not toxic as the brain creates enzymes, during fetal growth, that helps us use them. Epileptic children, though not the perfect examples, show some insight into the effects of the diet on the brain in the long term. There is no negative effect in terms of cognitive function. There is no assurance that the diet cannot have long term dietary effects, but no information proves that there are any negative effects. Some people feel they can concentrate more when on the ketogenic diet, while others feel nothing but fatigue. This is as a result of differences in individual physiology. There are very few studies that vaguely address the point on short term memory loss. This wore off with the continuation of the study.

Kidney stones and kidney damage

As a result of the increased workload from having to filter ketones, urea, and ammonia, as well as dehydration concerns of the potential for kidney damage or passing kidney stones have been raised. The high protein nature of the ketogenic diet raises the alarms of individuals who are concerned with potential kidney damage. There is very little information that points to any negative effects of the diet on kidney function or development of kidney stones. There is a low incidence of small kidney stones in epileptic children this may be as a result of the state of deliberate dehydration that the children are put at instead of the ketosis state itself. Some short term research shows no change in kidney function or increased incidents of kidney stones either after they are off the diet or after six months on a diet. There is no long term data on the effects of ketosis to kidney function; thus, no complete conclusions can be made. People with preexisting kidney issues are the only ones who get problems from high protein intake. From an unscientific point of view, one would expect increased incidents of this to happen to athletes who consume very high protein diets, but it has not happened. This suggests that high protein intake, under normal conditions, is not harmful to the kidneys. To limit the possibility of kidney stones, it is advised to drink a lot of water to maintain hydration. For people who are predisposed to kidney stones should have their kidney function should be monitored to ensure that no complications arise if they decide to follow through with the diet.

Constipation

A common side effect of the diet is reduced bowel movements and constipation. This arises from two different causes: lack of fiber and gastrointestinal absorption of foods. First, the lack of carbs in the diet means that unless supplements are taken, fiber intake is low. Fiber is very important to our systems. High fiber intake can prevent some health conditions, including heart disease and some forms of cancer. Use some type of sugar-free fiber supplement to prevent any health problems and help you maintain regular bowel movements. The diet also reduces the volume of stool due to enhanced absorption and digestion of food; thus, fewer waste products are generated.

Fat regain

Dieting, in general, has very low long term success rates. There are some effects of getting out of a ketogenic diet like the regain of fat lost through calorific restriction alone. This is true for any diet based on calorific restriction. It is expected for weight to be regained after carb reintroduction. For people who use the weighing scale to measure their success, they may completely shun carbs as they think it is the main reason for the weight regain. You should understand that most of the initial weight gain is water and glycogen.

Immune system

There is a large variety in the immunity system response to ketogenic diets on different people. There has been some repost on reduction on some ailments such allergies and increased minor sickness susceptibility.

Optic neuropathy

This is optic nerve dysfunction. It has appeared in a few cases, but it is still existence. It was linked to the people not getting adequate amounts of calcium or vitamins supplements for about a year. All the cases were corrected by supplementation of adequate vitamin B, especially thiamine.

CHAPTER 3.
SOME TIPS FOR BEGINNER TO ACHIEVE KETO SUCCESS

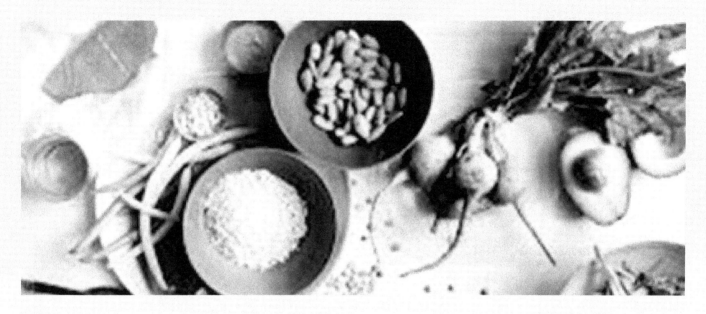

Nobody told you that life was going to be this way! But don't worry. There's still plenty of time to make amendments and take care of your health. Here are a couple of tips that will allow you to lead a healthier life in your fifties:

Start Building on Immunity

Every day, our body is exposed to free radicals and toxins from the environment. The added stress of work and family problems doesn't make it any easier for us. To combat this, it's essential that you start consuming healthy veggies that contain plenty of antioxidants and build a healthier immune system.

This helps ward off unwanted illnesses and diseases, allowing you to maintain good health.

Adding more healthy veggies to your Keto diet will help you obtain a variety of minerals, vitamins and antioxidants.

Consider Quitting Smoking

It's never too late to try to quit smoking even if you are in your fifties. Once a smoker begins to quit, the body quickly starts to heal the previous damages caused by smoking.

Once you start quitting, you'll notice how you'll be able to breathe easier, while acquiring a better sense of smell and taste. Over the period of time, eliminating the habit of smoking can greatly reduce the risks of high blood pressure, strokes and heart attack. Please note how these diseases are much more common among folks who are in the fifties and above when compared to younger folks.

Not to mention, quitting smoking will help you stay more active and enjoy better health with your friends and family.

Stay Social

We've already mentioned this before but it's worth pondering on again and again. Aging can be a daunting process and trying to get through it all on your own isn't particularly helpful. We urge you to stay in touch with friends and family or become a part of a local community club or network. Some older folks find it comforting to get an emotional support animal.

Being surrounded by people you love will give you a sense of belonging and will improve your mood. It'll also keep your mind and memory sharp as you engage in different conversations.

Health Screenings You Should Get After Your Fifties

Your fifties are considered the prime years of your life. Don't let the joy of these years be robbed away from you because of poor health. Getting simple tests done can go a long way in identifying any potential health problems that you may have. Here is a list of health screenings should get done:

Check Your Blood Pressure

Your blood pressure is a reliable indicator of your heart health. In simple words, blood pressure is a measure of how fast blood travels through the artery walls. Very high or even very low blood pressure can be a sign of an underlying problem. Once you hit your 40s, you should have your blood pressure checked more often.

EKG

The EKG reveals your heart health and activity. Short for electrocardiogram, the EKG helps identify problems in the heart. The process works by highlighting any rhythm problems that may be in the heart such as poor heart muscles, improper blood flow or any other form of abnormality. Getting an EKG is also a predictive measure for understanding the chances of a heart attack. Since people starting their fifties are at greater risk of getting a heart attack, you should get yourself checked more often.

Mammogram

Mammograms help rule out the risks of breast cancer. Women who enter their fifties should ideally get a mammogram after every ten years. However, if you have a family history, it is advisable that you get one much earlier to rule out the possibilities of cancer.

Blood Sugar Levels

If you're somebody who used to grab a fast food meal every once in a while before you switched to Keto, then you should definitely check your blood sugar levels more carefully. Blood sugar levels indicate whether or not you have diabetes. And you know how the saying goes, prevention is better than cure. It's best to clear these possibilities out of the way sooner than later.

Check for Osteoporosis

Unfortunately, as you grow older you also become susceptible to a number of bone diseases. Osteoporosis is a bone-related condition in which bones begin to lose mass, becoming frail and weak. Owing to this, seniors become more prone to fractures. This can make even the smallest of falls detrimental to your health.

Annual Physical Exam

Your insurance must be providing coverage for your annual physical exam. So, there's no reason you should not take advantage of it. This checkup helps identify the state of your health. You'll probably be surprised by how much doctors can tell from a single blood test.

Prostrate Screening Exam

Once men hit their fifties, they should be screened for prostate cancer (similar to how women should get a mammogram and pap smear). Getting a screening done becomes especially important if cancer runs in your family.

Eye Exam

As you start to age, you'll notice how your eyesight will start to deteriorate. It's quite likely that vision is not as sharp as it used to be. Ideally, you should have gotten your first eye exam during your 40s but it isn't too late. Get one as soon as possible to prevent symptoms from escalating.

Be Wary of Any Weird Moles

While skin cancer can become a problem at any age, older adults should pay closer attention to any moles or unusual skin tags in their bodies. While most cancers can be easily treated, melanoma can be particularly quite dangerous. If you have noticed any recent moles in your body that have changed in color, size or shape, make sure to visit the dermatologist.

Check Your Cholesterol Levels

Now, we've talked about this plenty of times but it's worth mentioning again. High cholesterol levels can be dangerous to your health and can be an indicator for a number of diseases, things become more complicated for conditions that don't show particular symptoms. Just to be on the safe side, your total cholesterol levels should be below 200 mg per deciliter. Your doctor will take a simple blood test and will give you a couple of guidelines with the results. In case there is something to worry about, you should make serious dietary and lifestyle changes in your life.

CHAPTER 4.
WHAT DOES THE KETOGENIC DIET MEAN TO WOMEN AFTER 50?

Why Keto for Women?

The health benefits of the Keto diet are not different for men or women, but the speed at which they are reached does differ. As mentioned, women's bodies are a lot different when it comes to the ways that they are able to burn fats and lose weight. For example, by design women have at least 10% more body fat than men. No matter how fit you are, this is just an aspect of being a woman that you must consider. Don't be hard on yourself if you notice that it seems like men can lose weight easier — that's because they can! What women have in additional body fat; men typically have the same in muscle mass. This is why men tend to see faster external results, because that added muscle mass means that their metabolism rates are higher. That increased metabolism means that fat and energy get burned faster. When you are on Keto, though, the internal change is happening right away.

Your metabolism is unique, but it is also going to be slower than a man's by nature. Since muscle is able to burn more calories than fat, the weight just seems to fall off of men, giving them the ability to reach the opportunity for muscle growth quickly. This should not be something that holds you back from starting your Keto journey. As long as you are keeping these realistic bodily factors in mind, you won't be left wondering why it is taking you a little bit longer to start losing weight. This point will come for you, but it will take a little bit more of a process that you must be committed to following through with.

Another unique condition that a woman can experience but a man cannot be PCOS or Polycystic Ovary Syndrome; a hormonal imbalance that causes the development of cysts. These cysts can cause pain, interfere with normal reproductive function, and, in extreme and dangerous cases, burst. PCOS is actually very common among women, affecting up to 10% of the entire female population. Surprisingly, most women are not even aware that they have the condition. Around 70% of women have PCOS that is undiagnosed. This condition can cause a significant hormonal imbalance, therefore affecting your metabolism. It can also inevitably lead to weight gain, making it even harder to see results while following diet plans. In order to stay on top of your health, you must make sure that you are going to the gynecologist regularly.

Menopause is another reality that must be faced by women, especially as we age. Most women begin the process of menopause in their mid-40s. Men do not go through menopause, so they are spared from yet another condition that causes slower metabolism and weight gain. When you start menopause, it is easy to gain weight and lose muscle. Most women, once menopause begins, lose muscle at a much faster rate, and conversely gain weight, despite dieting and exercise regimens. Keto can, therefore, be the right diet plan for you. Regardless of what your body is doing naturally, via processes like menopause, your internal systems are still going to be making the switch from running on carbs to deriving energy from fats.

Because a Keto diet reduces the amount of sugar you are consuming, it naturally lowers the amount of insulin in your bloodstream. This can actually have amazing effects on any existing PCOS and fertility issues, as well as menopausal symptoms and conditions like pre-diabetes and Type 2 diabetes. Once your body adjusts to a Keto diet, you are overcoming the things that are naturally in place that can be preventing you from losing weight and getting healthy. Even if you placed your body on a strict diet, if it isn't getting rid of sugars properly, you likely aren't going to see the same results that you will when you try Keto. This is a big reason why Keto can be so beneficial for women.

As we've deliberated, carbs and sugar can have a huge impact on your hormonal balance. You might not even realize that your hormones are not in balance until you experience a lifestyle that limits carbs and eliminates sugars. Keto is going to reset this balance for you, keeping your hormones at healthy levels. As a result of this, you will probably find yourself in a better general mood, and with much more energy to get through your days.

Why Keto for 50+?

As we age, we naturally look for ways to hold onto our youth and energy. It's not uncommon to think about things that promote anti-aging. Products and lifestyle changes are advertised everywhere, and they are designed to catch your attention, as you grapple with the reality of what it means to be a 50+ year-old woman in our society. Even if you aren't eating for the purposes of anti-aging yet, you have likely thought about it in terms of the way you treat your skin and hair, for example. The great thing about the Keto diet is that it supports maximum health, from the inside out; working hard to make sure that you are in the best shape that you can be in.

For instance, indigestion becomes common as you age. This happens because the body is not able to break down certain foods as well as it used to. With all of the additives and fillers, we all become used to putting our bodies through discomfort in an attempt to digest regular meals. You are probably not even aware that you are doing this to your body, but upon trying a Keto diet, you will realize how your digestion will begin to change. You will no longer feel bloated or uncomfortable after you eat. If you notice this as a common feeling, you are likely not eating food that is nutritious enough to satisfy your needs and is only resulting in excess calories.

Keto fills you up in all of the ways that you need, allowing your body to truly digest and metabolize all of the nutrients. When you eat your meals, you should not feel the need to overeat in order to overcompensate for not having enough nutrients. Anything that takes stress off of any system in your body is going to become a form of anti-aging. You will quickly find this benefit once you start your Keto journey, as it is one of the first-reported changes that most participants notice. In addition to a healthier digestive system, you will also experience more regular bathroom usage, with little to none of the problems often associated with age.

While weight loss is one of the more common desires for most 50+ women who start a diet plan, the way that the weight is lost matters. If you have ever shed a lot of weight before, you have probably experienced the adverse effects of sagging or drooping skin that you were left to deal with. Keto actually rejuvenates the elasticity in your skin. This means that you will be able to lose weight and your skin will be able to catch up. Instead of having to do copious amounts of exercise to firm up your skin, it should already be becoming firmer each day that you are on the Keto diet. This is something that a lot of participants are pleasantly surprised to find out.

Women also commonly report a natural reduction in wrinkles, and healthier skin and hair growth, in general. Many women who start the diet report that they actually notice reverse effects in their aging process. While the skin becomes healthier and more supple, it also becomes firmer. Even if you aren't presently losing weight, you will still be able to appreciate the effects that Keto brings to your skin and face. Because your internal systems are becoming healthier by the day, this tends to show on the outside in a short amount of time. You will also begin to feel healthier. While it is possible to read about the experiences of others, there is nothing like feeling this for yourself when you begin Keto.

Everyone, especially women over 50, has day-to-day tasks that are draining and require certain amounts of energy to complete. Aging can, unfortunately, take away from your energy reserve, even if you get enough sleep at night. It limits the way that you have to live your life, and this can become a very frustrating realization. Most diet plans bring about a sluggish feeling that you are simply supposed to get used to, for example. But Keto does the exact opposite. When you change your eating habits to fit the Keto guidelines, you are going to be hit with a boost of energy. Since your body is truly getting everything that it needs nutritionally, it will repay you with a sustained energy supply.

Another common complaint for women over 50 is that, seemingly overnight, your blood sugar levels are going to be more sensitive than usual. While it is important that everyone keeps an eye on these levels, it is especially important for those who are in their 50s and beyond. High blood sugar can be an indication that diabetes is on the way, but Keto can become a preventative measure, that we've already talked about. Additionally, naturally regulating elevated blood sugar levels, also reduces systemic inflammation, which is also common for women over 50. By balancing the immune system, of which inflammation is a part of, common aches and pains are reduced. Inflammation can also affect vital organs and is a precursor to cancer. Keto will support your path to an anti-inflammatory lifestyle.

Sugar is never great for us, but it turns out that sugar can become especially dangerous as we age. What is known as a "sugar sag" can occur when you get older because the excess sugar molecules will attach themselves to skin and protein in your body. This doesn't even necessarily happen because you are eating too much sugar. Average levels of sugar intake can also lead to this sagging as the sugar weakens the strength of your proteins that are supposed to hold you together. With sagging comes even more wrinkles and arterial stiffening.

If you have any anti-aging concerns, the Keto diet will likely be able to address your worries. It is a diet that works extremely hard while allowing you a fairly simple and direct guideline to follow in return. While your motivation is necessary in order to form a successful relationship with Keto, you won't need to worry about doing anything "wrong" or accidentally breaking from your diet. As long as you know how to give up your sugary foods and drinks while making sure that you are consuming the correct amount of carbs, you will be able to find your own success while on the diet.

As a woman over 50, you'll find that you will feel better, healthier and younger, by implementing the simple steps that will tune your body into processing excess fats for energy. You'll build muscle, lose fat, and look and feel younger. As we've touched on, a Keto diet helps balance your hormones, reversing and/or eliminating many common menopausal signs and symptoms.

CHAPTER 5.
WHAT KETO DOES TO AN OVER 50 WOMAN'S BODY

Women who are looking for a quick and effective way to shed excess weight, get high blood sugar levels under control, reduce overall inflammations, and improve physical and mental energy will do their best by following a ketogenic diet plan. But there are special considerations women must take into account when they are beginning the keto diet.

All women know it is much more difficult for women to lose weight than it is for men to lose weight. A woman will live on a starvation level diet and exercise like a triathlete and only lose five pounds. A man will stop putting dressing on his salad and will lose twenty pounds. It just is not fair. But we have the fact that we are women to blame. Women naturally have more standing between them and weight loss than men do.

The mere fact that we are women is the largest single contributor to the reason we find it difficult to lose weight. Since our bodies always think they need to be prepared for the possibility of pregnancy women will naturally have more body fat and less mass in our muscles than men will. Muscle cells burn more calories than fat cells do. So, because we are women, we will always lose weight more slowly than men will.

Being in menopause will also cause women to add more pounds to their bodies, especially in the lower half of the body. After menopause a woman's metabolism naturally slows down. Your hormones levels will decrease. These two factors alone will cause weight gain in the post-menopausal woman.

Women are a direct product of their hormones. Men also have hormones but not the ones like we have that regulate every function in our bodies. And the hormones in women will fluctuate around their everyday habits like lack of sleep, poor eating habits, and menstrual cycles. These hormones cause women to crave sweets around the time their periods occur. These cravings will wreck any diet plan. Staying true to the keto plan is challenging at this time because of the intense craving for sweets and carbs. Also having your period will often make you feel and look bloated because of the water your body holds onto during this time. And having cramps make you more likely to reach for a bag of cookies than a plate of steak and salad.

Because we are women, we may experience challenges on the keto diet that men will not face because they are men. One of these challenges is having weight loss plateau or even experiencing weight gain. This can happen because of the influence of hormones on weight loss in women. If this happens you will want to increase your consumption of good fats like ghee, butter, eggs, coconut oil, beef, avocados, and olive oil. Any food that is cooked or prepared using oil must be prepared in olive oil or avocado oil.

You can also use MCT oil. MCT stands for medium chain triglycerides. This is a form of fatty acid that is saturated and has many health benefits. MCT can help with many body functions from weight loss to improved brain function. MCTs are mostly missing from the typical American diet because we have been told that saturated fats are harmful to the body, and as a group they are. But certain saturated fats, like MCTs, are actually beneficial to the body, especially when they come from good foods like beef or coconut oil. They are easier to digest than most other saturated fats and may help improve heart and brain function and prevent obesity.

Many women on a keto diet will struggle with imbalances in their hormones. On the keto diet you do not rely on lowered calories to lose weight but on foods effect on your hormones. So, when women begin the keto diet any issues, they are already having with their hormones will be brought to attention and may cause the woman to give up before she really begins. Always remember that the keto diet is responsible for cleansing the system first so that the body can easily respond to the wonderful affects a keto diet has to offer.

Do not try to work toward the lean body that many men sport. It is best for overall function that women stay at twenty-two to twenty six percent body fat. Our hormones will function best in this range and we can't possibly function without our hormones. Women who are very lean, like gymnasts and extreme athletes, will find their hormones no longer function or function at a less than optimal rate. And remember that ideal weight may not be the right weight for you. Many women find that they perform their best when they are at their happy weight. If you find yourself fighting with yourself to lose the last few pounds you think you need to lose in order to have the perfect body then it may not be worth it. The struggle will affect your hormone function. Carefully observing the keto diet will allow time for your hormones to stabilize and regulate themselves back to their pre-obesity normal function.

Like any other diet plan the keto diet will work better if you are active. Regular exercise will allow the body to strengthen and tone muscles and will help to work off excess fat reserves. But exercise requires energy to accomplish. If you restrict your carb intake too much you might not have the energy needed to be physically able to make it all the way through the day and still be able to maintain an exercise routine. You might need to add in more carbs to your diet through the practice of carb cycling.

As a woman you know that sometimes your emotions get the better of you. This is true with your body, as you well know, and can be a major reason why women find it extremely difficult at times to lose weight the way they want to lose weight. We have been led to believe that not only can we do it all but that we must do it all. This gives many women unnecessary levels of pressure and can cause them to engage in emotional eating. Some women might have lowered feelings of self-worth and may not feel they are entitled to the benefits of the keto diet, and turning to food relieves the feelings of inadequacy that we try to hide from the world.

When you engage in the same activity for a long period of time it becomes a habit. When you reach for the bag of potato chips or the tub of ice cream whenever you are angry, upset, or depressed, then your brain will eventually tell you to reach for food whenever you feel an emotion that you don't want to deal with. Food acts as a security blanket against the world outside. It may be necessary to address any extreme emotional issues you are having before you begin the keto diet, so that you are better assured of success.

The basic act of staying on the keto diet can be very challenging for some women. Many women see beginning a new diet to lose weight as a punishment for being overweight. It may be worthwhile for you to work at changing the set of your mind if you are feeling this way. You may need to remind yourself daily that the keto diet is not a punishment but a blessing for your body. Tell yourself that you are not denying yourself certain foods because you can't eat them, but because you do not like the way those foods make your body feel. Don't watch other people eating their high carb diet and pity yourself. Instead, feel sorry for the people who have trapped themselves in a high calorie diet and are not experiencing the benefits that you are experiencing.

And for the first thirty days cut out all sweeteners, even the non-sugar ones that are allowed on the keto diet. While they may make food taste better, they also remind your brain that it needs sweet foods when it really doesn't. Cutting them out for at least thirty days will break the cycle that your body has fallen into and will cut the cravings for sweets in your diet.

It is very possible for women to be successful on the keto diet if they are prepared to follow a few simple adjustments that will make the diet look differently than your male partner might be eating but that will make you successful in the long run.

During the first one or two weeks you will need to consume extra fat than a man might need to. Doing this will have three important effects on your body. First it will cause your mitochondria to intensify their acceptance of your new way of finding energy. Mitochondria are tiny organisms that are found in cells and are responsible for using the fuel that insulin brings to the cell for fuel for the cell. Increasing your fat intake will also help make sure you are getting enough calories in your daily diet. This is important because if your body thinks you are starving it will begin to conserve calories and you will stop losing weight.

The third benefit from eating more fat, and perhaps the most important, is the psychological boost you will get from seeing that you can eat more fat and still lose weight and feel good. It will also reset your mindset that you formerly might have held against fat. For so long we have been told that low fat is the only way to lose weight. But an absence of dietary fat will lead to overeating and binge eating out of a feeling of deprivation. When you begin the diet by allowing yourself to eat a lot, or too much in your mind, fat, then you swing the pendulum around to the other side of the fat scale where it properly belongs. You teach yourself that fat can be good for you. Increasing the extra intake of fats should not last beyond the second week of the diet. Your body will improve its abilities to create and burn ketones and body fat, and then you will begin using your own body fat for fuel and you can begin to lower your reliance on dietary fat a little bit so that you will begin to lose weight.

The keto diet is naturally lower in calories if you follow the recommended levels of food intake. It is not necessary to try to restrict your intake of calories even further. All you need to do is to eat only until you are full and not one bite more. Besides losing weight the aim of the keto diet is to retrain your body on how to work properly. You will need to learn to trust your body and the signals it sends out to be able to readjust to a proper way of eating.

CHAPTER 6.
HOW CAN KETOGENIC DIET CAN AID WITH THE SIGN AND SYMPTOMS OF AGEING AND MENOPAUSE

How the ketogenic diet can aid with the signs and symptoms of ageing and menopause

For ageing women, menopause will bring severe changes and challenges, but the ketogenic diet can help you switch gears effortlessly to continue enjoying a healthy and happy life. Menopause can upset hormonal levels in women, which consequently affects brainpower and cognitive abilities. Furthermore, due to less production of estrogens and progesterone, your sex drive declines, and you suffer from sleep issues and mood problems. Let's have a look at how a ketogenic diet will help solve these side effects.

Enhanced Cognitive Functions

Usually, hormone estrogen ensures continuous flow of glucose into your brain. But after menopause, the estrogen levels begin to drop dramatically, so does the amount of glucose reaching the bran. As a result, your functional brainpower will start to deteriorate. However, by following the keto diet for women over 50, the problem of glucose intake is circumvented. This results in enhanced cognitive functions and brain activity.

Hormonal Balance

Usually, women face major symptoms of menopause due to hormonal imbalances. The keto diet for women over 50 works by stabilizing these imbalances such as estrogen. This aids in experiencing fewer and bearable menopausal symptoms like hot flashes. The keto diet also balances blood sugar levels and insulin and helps in controlling insulin sensitivity.

Intensified Sex Drive

The keto diet surges the absorption of vitamin D, which is essential for enhancing sex drive. Vitamin D ensures stable levels of testosterone and other sex hormones that could become unstable due to low levels of testosterone.

Better Sleep

Glucose disturbs your blood sugar levels dramatically, which in turn leads to poor quality of sleep. Along with other menopausal symptoms, good sleep becomes a huge problem as you age. The keto diet for women over 50 not only balances blood glucose levels, but also stabilizes other hormones like cortisol, melatonin, and serotonin warranting an improved and better sleep.

Reduces inflammation

Menopause can upsurge the inflammation levels by letting potential harmful invaders in our system, which result in uncomfortable and painful symptoms. Keto diet for women over 50 uses the healthy anti-inflammatory fats to reduce inflammation and lower pain in your joints and bones.

Fuel your brain

Are you aware that your brain is composed of 60% fat or more? This infers that it needs a larger amount of fat to keep it functioning optimally. In other words, the ketones from the keto diet serve as the energy source that fuels your brain cells.

Nutrient deficiencies

Ageing women tend to have higher deficiencies in essential nutrients such as, iron deficiency which leads to brain fog and fatigue; Vitamin B12 deficiency, which lead to neurological conditions like dementia; Fats deficiency, that can lead to problems with cognition, skin, vision; and Vitamin D deficiency that not only causes cognitive impairment in older adults and increase the risk of heart disease but also contribute to the risk of developing cancer. On a keto diet, the high-quality proteins ensure adequate and excellent sources of these important nutrients.

Controlling Blood Sugar

Research has suggested a link between poor blood sugar levels and brain diseases such as Alzheimer's disease, Parkinson's disease, or Dementia. Some factors contributing to Alzheimer's disease may include:

- Enormous intake of carbohydrates, especially from fructose—which is drastically reduced in the ketogenic diet.
- Lack of nutritional fats and good cholesterol — which are copious and healthy in the keto diet

Keto diet helps control blood sugar and improve nutrition; which in turn not only improve insulin response and resistance but also protect against memory loss which is often a part of ageing.

CHAPTER 7.
FOODS ALLOWED IN KETO DIET

To make the most of your diet, there are prohibited foods, and others that are allowed, but in limited quantities. Here are the foods allowed in the ketogenic diet:

Food allowed in unlimited quantities

Lean or fatty meats

No matter which meat you choose, it contains no carbohydrates so that you can have fun! Pay attention to the quality of your meat, and the amount of fat. Alternate between fatty meats and lean meats!

Here are some examples of lean meats:

- Beef: sirloin steak, roast beef, 5% minced steak, roast, flank steak, tenderloin, Grisons meat, tripe, kidneys
- Horse: roti, steak
- Pork: tenderloin, bacon, kidneys
- Veal: cutlet, shank, tenderloin, sweetbread, liver
- Chicken and turkey: cutlet, skinless thigh, ham
- Rabbit

Here are some examples of fatty meats:

- Lamb: leg, ribs, brain
- Beef: minced steak 10, 15, 20%, ribs, rib steak, tongue, marrow

- Pork: ribs, brain, dry ham, black pudding, white pudding, bacon, terrine, rillettes, salami, sausage, sausages, and merguez
- Veal: roast, paupiette, marrow, brain, tongue, dumplings
- Chicken and turkey: thigh with skin
- Guinea fowl
- Capon
- Turkey
- Goose: foie gras

Lean or fatty fish

The fish does not contain carbohydrates so that you can consume unlimited! As with meat, there are lean fish and fatty fish, pay attention to the amount of fat you eat and remember to vary your intake of fish. Oily fish have the advantage of containing a lot of good cholesterol, so it is beneficial for protection against cardiovascular disease! It will be advisable to consume fatty fish more than lean fish, to be able to manage your protein intake: if you consume lean fish, you will have a significant protein intake and little lipids, whereas with fatty fish, you will have a balanced protein and fat intake!

Here are some examples of lean fish:

- Cod
- Colin
- Sea bream
- Whiting
- Sole
- Turbot
- Limor career
- Location
- Pike
- Ray

Here are some examples of oily fish:

- Swordfish
- Salmon

- Tuna
- Trout
- Monkfish
- Herring
- Mackerel
- Cod
- Sardine

Eggs

The eggs contain no carbohydrates, so you can consume as much as you want. It is often said that eggs are full of cholesterol and that you have to limit their intake, but the more cholesterol you eat, the less your body will produce by itself! In addition, it's not just poor-quality cholesterol so that you can consume 6 per week without risk! And if you want to eat more but you are afraid for your cholesterol and I have not convinced you, remove the yellow!

Vegetables and raw vegetables

Yes, you can eat vegetables. But you have to be careful which ones: you can eat leafy vegetables (salad, spinach, kale, red cabbage, Chinese cabbage...) and flower vegetables (cauliflower, broccoli, Romanesco cabbage...) as well as avocado, cucumbers, zucchini or leeks, which do not contain many carbohydrates.

The oils

It's oil, so it's only fat, so it's unlimited to eat, but choose your oil wisely! Prefer olive oil, rapeseed, nuts, sunflower or sesame for example!

Foods authorized in moderate quantities.

The cold cuts

As you know, there is bad cholesterol in cold meats, so you will need to moderate your intake: eat it occasionally!

Fresh cheeses and plain yogurts

Consume with moderation because they contain carbohydrates.

Nuts and oilseeds

They have low levels of carbohydrates, but are rich in saturated fatty acids, that's why they should moderate their consumption. Choose almonds, hazelnuts, Brazil nuts or pecans.

Coconut (in oil, cream or milk)

It contains saturated fatty acids, that's why we limit its consumption. Cream and coconut oil contain a lot of medium chain triglycerides (MCTs), which increase the level of ketones, essential to stay in ketosis.

Berries and red fruits

They contain carbohydrates, in reasonable quantities, but you should not abuse them to avoid ketosis (blueberries, blackberries, raspberries...).

CHAPTER 8.
KETO GROCERY LIST

I've had people complain about the difficulty of switching their grocery list to one that's Ketogenic-friendly. The fact is that food is expensive — and most of the food you have in your fridge are probably packed full with carbohydrates. This is why if you're committing to a Ketogenic Diet, you need to do a clean sweep. That's right — everything that's packed with carbohydrates should be identified and set aside to make sure you're not eating more than you should. You can donate them to a charity before going out and buying your new Keto-friendly shopping list.

Seafood

Seafood means fish like sardines, mackerel, and wild salmon. It's also a good idea to add some shrimp, tuna, mussels, and crab into your diet. This is going to be a tad expensive but definitely worth it in the long run. What's the common denominator in all these food items? The secret is omega-3 fatty acids which is credited for lots of health benefits. You want to add food rich in omega-3 fatty acids in your diet.

Low-carb Vegetables

Not all vegetables are good for you when it comes to the Ketogenic Diet. The vegetable choices should be limited to those with low carbohydrate counts. Pack up your cart with items like spinach, eggplant, arugula, broccoli, and cauliflower. You can also put in bell peppers, cabbage, celery, kale, Brussels sprouts, mushrooms, zucchini, and fennel.

So what's in them? Well, aside from the fact that they're low-carb, these vegetable also contain loads of fiber which makes digestion easier. Of course, there's also the presence of vitamins, minerals, antioxidants, and various other nutrients that you need for day to day life. Which ones should you avoid? Steer clear of the starch-packed vegetables like carrots, turnips, and beets. As a rule, you go for the vegetables that are green and leafy.

Fruits Low in Sugar

During an episode of sugar-craving, it's usually a good idea to pick low-sugar fruit items. Believe it or not, there are lots of those in the market! Just make sure to stock up on any of these: avocado, blackberries, raspberries, strawberries, blueberries, lime, lemon, and coconut. Also note that tomatoes are fruits too so feel free to make side dishes or dips with loads of tomatoes! Keep in mind that these fruits should be eaten fresh and not out of a can. If you do eat them fresh off the can however, take a good look at the nutritional information at the back of the packaging. Avocadoes are particularly popular for those practicing the Ketogenic Diet because they contains LOTS of the good kind of fat.

Meat and Eggs

While some diets will tell you to skip the meat, the Ketogenic Diet actually encourages its consumption. Meat is packed with protein that will feed your muscles and give you a consistent source of energy through the day. It's a slow but sure burn when you eat protein as opposed to carbohydrates which are burned faster and therefore stored faster if you don't use them immediately.

But what kind of meat should you be eating? There's chicken, beef, pork, venison, turkey, and lamb. Keep in mind that quality plays a huge role here — you should be eating grass-fed organic beef or organic poultry if you want to make the most out of this food variety. The organic option lets you limit the possibility of ingesting toxins in your body due to the production process of these products. Plus, the preservation process also means there are added salt or sugar in the meat, which can throw off the whole diet.

Nuts and Seeds

Nuts and seeds you should definitely add in your cart include: chia seeds, Brazil nuts, macadamia nuts, flaxseed, walnuts, hemp seeds, pecans, sesame seeds, almonds, hazelnut, and pumpkin seeds. They also contain lots of protein and very little sugar so they're great if you have the munchies. They're the ideal snack because they're quick, easy, and will keep you full. They're high in calories though, which is why lots of people steer clear of them. As I mentioned earlier though — the Ketogenic Diet has nothing to do with calories and everything to do with the nutrient you're eating. So don't pay too much attention on the calorie count and just remember that they're a good source of fats and protein.

Dairy Products

OK — some people in their 50s already have a hard time processing dairy products, but for those who don't — you can happily add many of these to your diet. Make sure to consume sufficient amounts of cheese, plain Greek yogurt, cream butter, and cottage cheese. These dairy products are packed with calcium, protein, and the healthy kind of fat.

Oils

Nope, we're not talking about essentials oils but rather, MCT oil, coconut oil, avocado oil, nut oils, and even extra-virgin olive oil. You can start using those for your frying needs to create healthier food options. The beauty of these oils is that they add flavor to the food, making sure you don't get bored quickly with the recipes. Try picking up different types of Keto-friendly oils to add some variety to your cooking.

Coffee and Tea

The good news is that you don't have to skip coffee if you're going on a Ketogenic Diet. The bad news is that you can't go to Starbucks anymore and order their blended coffee choices. Instead, beverages would be limited to unsweetened tea or unsweetened coffee in order to keep the sugar consumption low. Opt for organic coffee and tea products to make the most out of these powerful antioxidants.

Dark Chocolate

Yes – chocolate is still on the menu, but it is limited to just dark chocolate. Technically, this means eating chocolate that is 70 percent cacao, which would make the taste a bit bitter.

Sugar Substitutes

Later in the recipes part of this book, you might be surprised at some of the ingredients required in the list. This is because while sweeteners are an important part of food preparation, you can't just use any kind of sugar in your recipe. Remember: the typical sugar is pure carbohydrate. Even if you're not eating carbohydrates, if you're dumping lots of sugar in your food – you're not really following the Ketogenic Diet principles.

So what do you do? You find sugar substitutes. The good news is that there are LOTS of those in the market. You can get rid of the old sugar and use any of these as a good substitute.

Stevia. This is perhaps the most familiar one in this list. It's a natural sweetener derived from plants and contains very few calories. Unlike your typical sugar, stevia may actually help lower the sugar levels instead of causing it to spike. Note though that it's sweeter than actual sugar so when cooking with stevia, you'll need to lower the amount used. Typically, the ratio is 200 grams of sugar per 1 teaspoon of powdered stevia.

Sucralose. It contains zero calories and zero carbohydrates. It's actually an artificial sweetener and does not metabolize – hence the complete lack of carbohydrates. Splenda is actually a sweetener derived from sucralose. Note though that you don't want to use this as a baking substitute for sugar. Its best use is for coffee, yogurt, and oatmeal sweetening. Note though that like stevia, it's also very sweet – in fact, it's actually 600 times sweeter than the typical sugar. Use sparingly.

Erythritol. It's a naturally occurring compound that interacts with the tongue's sweet taste receptors. Hence, it mimics the taste of sugar without actually being sugar. It does contain calories, but only about 5% of the calories you'll find in the typical sugar. Note though that it doesn't dissolve very well so anything prepared with this sweetener will have a gritty feeling. This can be problematic if you're using the product for baking. As for sweetness, the typical ratio is 1 1/3 cup for 1 cup of sugar.

Xylitol. Like erythritol, xylitol is a type of sugar alcohol that's commonly used in sugar-free gum. While it still contains calories, the calories are just 3 per gram. It's a sweetener that's good for diabetic patients because it doesn't raise the sugar levels or insulin in the body. The great thing about this is that you don't have to do any computations when using it for baking, cooking, or fixing a drink. The ratio of it with sugar is 1 to 1 so you can quickly make the substitution in the recipe.

What about Condiments?

Condiments are still on the table, but they won't be as tasty as you're used to. Your options include mustard, olive oil mayonnaise, oil-based salad dressings, and unsweetened ketchup. Of all these condiments, ketchup is the one with the most sugar, so make a point of looking for one with reduced sugar content. Or maybe avoid ketchup altogether and stick to mustard?

What about Snacks?

The good news is that there are packed snacks for those who don't have the time to make it themselves. Sugarless nut butters, dried seaweeds, nuts, and sugar-free jerky are all available in stores. The nuts and seeds discussed in a previous paragraph all make for excellent snack options.

What about Labels?

Let's not fool ourselves into thinking that we can cook food every single day. The fact is that there will be days when there will be purchases for the sake of convenience. There are also instances when you'll have problems finding the right ingredients for a given recipe. Hence, you'll need to find substitutes for certain ingredients without losing the "Keto friendly" vibe of the product.

So what should be done? Well, you need to learn how to read labels. Food doesn't have to be specially made to be keto-friendly, you just have to make sure that it doesn't contain any of the unfriendly nutrients or that the carbohydrate content is low enough.

CHAPTER 9. BREAKFAST

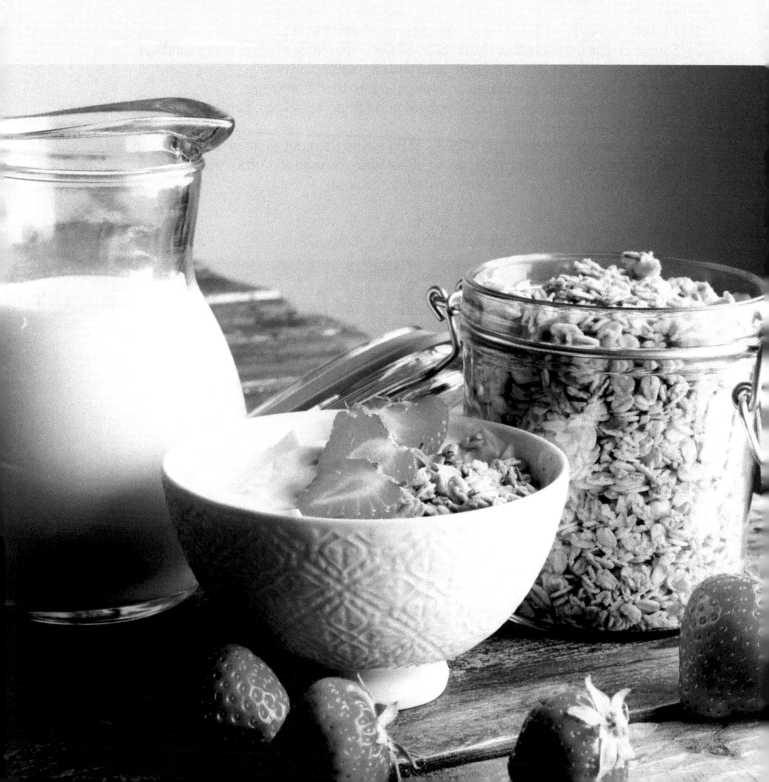

1. CHICKEN CORDON BLEU WITH CAULIFLOWER

PREPARATION: 10' **COOKING:** 45' **SERVES:** 4

INGREDIENTS

- 4 boneless chicken breast halves (about 12 ounces)
- 4 slices deli ham
- 4 slices Swiss cheese
- 1 large egg, whisked well
- 2 ounces pork rinds
- ¼ cup almond flour
- ¼ cup grated parmesan cheese
- ½ teaspoon garlic powder
- Salt and pepper
- 2 cups cauliflower florets

DIRECTIONS

1. Preheat the oven to 350 ° F and add a foil on a baking sheet.
2. Sandwich the breast half of the chicken between parchment parts and pound flat.
3. Spread the bits out and cover with ham and cheese sliced over.
4. Roll the chicken over the fillings and then dip into the beaten egg.
5. In a food processor, mix the pork rinds, almond flour, parmesan, garlic powder, salt and pepper,
6. And pulse into fine crumbs.
7. Roll the rolls of chicken in the mixture of pork rind then put them on the baking sheet.
8. Throw the cauliflower into the baking sheet with the melted butter and fold.
9. Bake for 45 minutes until the chicken is fully cooked.

NUTRITIONAL FACTS: Calories: 420 Fats: 2 3Protein: 7 Carbohydrates: 0

2. SESAME-CRUSTED TUNA WITH GREEN BEANS

PREPARATION: 15' **COOKING:** 5' **SERVES:** 4

INGREDIENTS

- ¼ cup white sesame seeds
- ¼ cup black sesame seeds
- 4 (6-ounce) ahi tuna steaks
- Salt and pepper
- 1 tablespoon olive oil
- 1 tablespoon coconut oil
- 2 cups green beans

DIRECTIONS

1. In a shallow dish, mix the two kinds of sesame seeds.
2. Season the tuna with pepper and salt.
3. Dredge the tuna in a mixture of sesame seeds.
4. Heat up to high heat the olive oil in a skillet, then add the tuna.
5. Cook for 1 to 2 minutes until it turns seared, then sear on the other side.
6. Remove the tuna from the skillet, and let the tuna rest while using the coconut oil to heat the skillet.
7. Fry the green beans in the oil for 5 minutes then use sliced tuna to eat.

NUTRITIONAL FACTS: Calories: 420 Fats: 23 Protein: 7 Carbohydrates: 0

3. ROSEMARY ROASTED PORK WITH CAULIFLOWER

PREPARATION: 10' **COOKING:** 20' **SERVES:** 4

INGREDIENTS
- 1 ½ pounds boneless pork tenderloin
- 1 tablespoon coconut oil
- 1 tablespoon fresh chopped rosemary
- Salt and pepper
- 1 tablespoon olive oil
- 2 cups cauliflower florets

DIRECTIONS
1. Rub the coconut oil into the pork, then season with the rosemary, salt, and pepper.
2. Heat up the olive oil over medium to high heat in a large skillet.
3. Add the pork on each side and cook until browned for 2 to 3 minutes.
4. Sprinkle the cauliflower over the pork in the skillet.
5. Reduce heat to low, then cover the skillet and cook until the pork is cooked through for 8 to 10 minutes.
6. Slice the pork with cauliflower and eat.

NUTRITIONAL FACTS: Calories: 320 Fats: 37 Protein: 3 Carbohydrates: 1

4. GRILLED SALMON AND ZUCCHINI WITH MANGO SAUCE

PREPARATION: 5' **COOKING:** 10' **SERVES:** 4

INGREDIENTS
- 4 (6-ounce) boneless salmon fillets
- 1 tablespoon olive oil
- Salt and pepper
- 1 large zucchini, sliced in coins
- 2 tablespoons fresh lemon juice
- ½ cup chopped mango
- ¼ cup fresh chopped cilantro
- 1 teaspoon lemon zest
- ½ cup canned coconut milk

DIRECTIONS
1. Preheat a grill pan to heat, and sprinkle with cooking spray liberally.
2. Brush with olive oil to the salmon and season with salt and pepper.
3. Apply lemon juice to the zucchini, and season with salt and pepper.
4. Put the zucchini and salmon fillets on the grill pan.
5. Cook for 5 minutes then turn all over and cook for another 5 minutes.
6. Combine the remaining ingredients in a blender and combine to create a sauce.
7. Serve the side-drizzled salmon filets with mango sauce and zucchini.

NUTRITIONAL FACTS: Calories: 350 Fats: 23 Protein: 7 Carbohydrates: 6

5. BEEF AND BROCCOLI STIR-FRY

PREPARATION: 20' **COOKING:** 15' **SERVES:** 4

INGREDIENTS

- ¼ cup soy sauce
- 1 tablespoon sesame oil
- 1 teaspoon garlic chili paste
- 1-pound beef sirloin
- 2 tablespoons almond flour
- 2 tablespoons coconut oil
- 2 cups chopped broccoli florets
- 1 tablespoon grated ginger
- 3 cloves garlic, minced

DIRECTIONS

1. In a small bowl, whisk the soy sauce, sesame oil, and chili paste together.
2. In a plastic freezer bag, slice the beef and mix with the almond flour.
3. Pour in the sauce and toss to coat for 20 minutes, then let rest.
4. Heat up the oil over medium to high heat in a large skillet.
5. In the pan, add the beef and sauce and cook until the beef is browned.
6. Move the beef to the skillet sides, then add the broccoli, ginger, and garlic.
7. Sauté until tender-crisp broccoli, then throw it all together and serve hot.

NUTRITIONAL FACTS: Calories: 350 Fats: 19 Protein: 37 Carbohydrates: 6

6. PARMESAN-CRUSTED HALIBUT WITH ASPARAGUS

PREPARATION: 10' **COOKING:** 15' **SERVES:** 4

INGREDIENTS

- 2 tablespoons olive oil
- ¼ cup butter, softened
- Salt and pepper
- ¼ cup grated Parmesan
- 1-pound asparagus, trimmed
- 2 tablespoons almond flour
- 4 (6-ounce) boneless halibut fillets
- 1 teaspoon garlic powder

DIRECTIONS

1. Preheat the oven to 400 F and line a foil-based baking sheet.
2. Throw the asparagus in olive oil and scatter over the baking sheet.
3. In a blender, add the butter, Parmesan cheese, almond flour, garlic powder, salt and pepper, and mix until smooth.
4. Place the fillets with the asparagus on the baking sheet, and spoon the Parmesan over the eggs.
5. Bake for 10 to 12 minutes, then broil until browned for 2 to 3 minutes.

NUTRITIONAL FACTS: Calories: 415 Fats: 26 Protein: 42 Carbohydrates: 3

7. HEARTY BEEF AND BACON CASSEROLE

PREPARATION: 25' **COOKING:** 30' **SERVES:** 8

INGREDIENTS

- 8 slices uncooked bacon
- 1 medium head cauliflower, chopped
- ¼ cup canned coconut milk
- Salt and pepper
- 2 pounds ground beef (80% lean)
- 8 ounces mushrooms, sliced
- 1 large yellow onion, chopped
- 2 cloves garlic, minced

DIRECTIONS

1. Preheat to 375 F on the oven.
2. Cook the bacon in a skillet until it crispness, then drain and chop on paper towels.
3. Bring to boil a pot of salted water, then add the cauliflower.
4. Boil until tender for 6 to 8 minutes then drain and add the coconut milk to a food processor.
5. Mix until smooth, then sprinkle with salt and pepper.
6. Cook the beef until browned in a pan, then wash the fat away.
7. Remove the mushrooms, onion, and garlic, then move to a baking platter.
8. Place on top of the cauliflower mixture and bake for 30 minutes.
9. Broil for 5 minutes on high heat, then sprinkle with bacon to serve.

NUTRITIONAL FACTS: Calories: 410 Fats: 25 Protein: 37 Carbohydrates: 6

8. SESAME WINGS WITH CAULIFLOWER

PREPARATION: 30' **COOKING:** 5' **SERVES:** 4

INGREDIENTS

- 2 ½ tablespoons soy sauce
- 2 tablespoons sesame oil
- 1 ½ teaspoons balsamic vinegar
- 1 teaspoon minced garlic
- 1 teaspoon grated ginger
- Salt
- 1-pound chicken wing, the wings itself
- 2 cups cauliflower florets

DIRECTIONS

1. In a freezer bag, mix the soy sauce, sesame oil, balsamic vinegar, garlic, ginger, and salt, then add the chicken wings.
2. Coat flip, then chill for 2 to 3 hours.
3. Preheat the oven to 400 F and line a foil-based baking sheet.
4. Spread the wings along with the cauliflower onto the baking sheet.
5. Bake for 35 minutes, then sprinkle on to serve with sesame seeds.

NUTRITIONAL FACTS: Calories: 400 Fats: 15 Protein: 5 Carbohydrates: 3

9. FRIED COCONUT SHRIMP WITH ASPARAGUS

PREPARATION: 15' **COOKING:** 10' **SERVES:** 6

INGREDIENTS

- 1 ½ cups shredded unsweetened coconut
- 2 large eggs
- Salt and pepper
- 1 ½ pounds large shrimp, peeled and deveined
- ½ cup canned coconut milk
- 1-pound asparagus, cut into 2-inch pieces

DIRECTIONS

1. Pour the coconut onto a shallow platter.
2. Beat the eggs in a bowl with a little salt and pepper.
3. Dip the shrimp into the egg first, then dredge with coconut.
4. Heat up coconut oil over medium-high heat in a large skillet.
5. Add the shrimp and fry over each side for 1 to 2 minutes until browned.
6. Remove the paper towels from the shrimp and heat the skillet again.
7. Remove the asparagus and sauté to tender-crisp with salt and pepper, then serve with the shrimp.

NUTRITIONAL FACTS: Calories: 535 Fats: 38 Protein: 16 Carbohydrates: 3

10. CREAMY QUESO DIP

PREPARATION: 15' **COOKING:** 5' **SERVES:** 8

INGREDIENTS

- 4 ounces chorizo, crumbled
- 1 clove garlic, minced
- ¼ cup heavy cream
- 6 ounces shredded white cheddar cheese
- 2 ounces shredded pepper jack cheese
- ¼ teaspoon xanthan gum
- Pinch salt
- 1 jalapeno, seeded and minced
- 1 small tomato, diced

DIRECTIONS

1. Cook the chorizo in a skillet until browned evenly, then scatter in a dish.
2. At medium-low heat, pressure the skillet and add the garlic–cook for 30 seconds.
3. Stir in the heavy cream, then add the cheese a little at a time, stirring frequently until it melts.
4. Sprinkle with salt and xanthan gum, then mix well, and cook until thickened.
5. Add the tomato and jalapeno, then serve, dipping with vegetables.

NUTRITIONAL FACTS: Calories: 195 Fats: 16 Protein: 12

11. COCONUT CHICKEN CURRY WITH CAULIFLOWER RICE

PREPARATION: 15' **COOKING:** 30' **SERVES:** 6

INGREDIENTS

- 1 tablespoon olive oil
- 1 medium yellow onion, chopped
- 1 ½ pounds boneless chicken thighs, chopped
- Salt and pepper
- 1 (14-ounce) can coconut milk
- 1 tablespoon curry powder
- 1 ¼ teaspoon ground turmeric
- 3 cups riced cauliflower

DIRECTIONS

1. Heat the oil over medium heat, in a large skillet.
2. Add the onions, and cook for about 5 minutes, until translucent.
3. Stir in the chicken and season with salt and pepper-cook for 6 to 8 minutes, stirring frequently until all sides are browned.
4. Pour the coconut milk into the pan, then whisk in the curry and turmeric powder.
5. Simmer until hot and bubbling, for 15 to 20 minutes.
6. Meanwhile, steam the cauliflower rice until tender with a few tablespoons of water.
7. Serve the cauliflower rice over the curry.

NUTRITIONAL FACTS: Calories: 430 Fats: 29 Protein: 9 Carbohydrates: 3

12. PUMPKIN SPICED ALMONDS

PREPARATION: 5' **COOKING:** 25' **SERVES:** 4

INGREDIENTS

- 1 tablespoon olive oil
- 1 ¼ teaspoon pumpkin pie spice
- Pinch salt
- 1 cup whole almonds, raw

DIRECTIONS

1. Preheat the oven to 300 ° F, and line a parchment baking sheet.
2. In a mixing bowl, whisk together the olive oil, pumpkin pie spice, and salt.
3. Toss in the almonds until coated evenly, then scatter onto the baking sheet.
4. Bake and place in an airtight container for 25 minutes then cool down completely.

NUTRITIONAL FACTS: Calories: 170 Fats: 15 Protein: 5 Carbohydrates: 3

13. TZATZIKI DIP WITH CAULIFLOWER

PREPARATION: 10' **COOKING:** 0' **SERVES:** 6

INGREDIENTS

- ½ (8-ounce) package cream cheese, softened
- 1 cup sour cream
- 1 tablespoon ranch seasoning
- 1 English cucumber, diced
- 2 tablespoons chopped chives
- 2 cups cauliflower florets

DIRECTIONS

1. Use an electric mixer to pound the cream cheese until smooth.
2. Stir in the sour cream and ranch seasoning, beat until smooth.
3. Fold in the cucumbers and chives, then chill with cauliflower florets for dipping before serving.

NUTRITIONAL FACTS: Calories: 125 Fats: 10 Protein: 5 Carbohydrates: 3

14. CLASSIC GUACAMOLE DIP

PREPARATION: 15' **COOKING:** 0' **SERVES:** 4

INGREDIENTS

- 2 mediums avocado, pitted
- 1 small yellow onion, diced
- 1 small tomato, diced
- ¼ cup fresh chopped cilantro
- 1 tablespoon fresh lime juice
- 1 jalapeno, seeded and minced
- 1 clove garlic, minced
- Salt
- Sliced veggies to serve

DIRECTIONS

1. Mash avocado flesh into a bowl.
2. Stir the onion, tomato, cilantro, lime juice, garlic, and jalapeno in a bowl
3. Season lightly with salt and spoon into a bowl – serve with sliced veggies.

NUTRITIONAL FACTS: Calories: 225 Fats: 20 Protein: 12 Carbohydrates: 3

15. EASY SKILLET PANCAKES

PREPARATION: 5'   **COOKING:** 5'   **SERVES:** 8

INGREDIENTS

- 8 ounces cream cheese
- 8 eggs
- 2 tablespoons coconut flour
- 2 teaspoons baking powder
- 1 teaspoon ground cinnamon
- ½ teaspoon vanilla extract
- 1 teaspoon liquid stevia or sweetener of choice (optional)
- 2 tablespoons butter

DIRECTIONS

1. In a blender, combine the cream cheese, eggs, coconut flour, baking powder, cinnamon, vanilla, and stevia (if using). Blend until smooth.
2. In a large skillet over medium heat, melt the butter.
3. Use half the mixture to pour four evenly sized pancakes and cook for about a minute, until you see bubbles on top. Flip the pancakes and cook for another minute. Remove from the pan and add more butter or oil to the skillet if needed. Repeat with the remaining batter.
4. Top with butter and eat right away, or freeze the pancakes in a freezer-safe resealable bag with sheets of parchment in between, for up to 1 month.

NUTRITIONAL FACTS: Calories: 179 Total Fat: 15g Protein: 8g Total Carbs: 3g Fiber: 1g Net Carbs: 2g

16. KETO EVERYTHING BAGELS

PREPARATION: 10'   **COOKING:** 15'   **SERVES:** 8

INGREDIENTS

- 2 cups shredded mozzarella cheese
- 2 tablespoons labneh cheese (or cream cheese)
- 1½ cups almond flour
- 1 egg
- 2 teaspoons baking powder
- ¼ teaspoon sea salt
- 1 tablespoon

DIRECTIONS

1. Preheat the oven to 400°F.
2. In a microwave-safe bowl, combine the mozzarella and labneh cheeses. Microwave for 30 seconds, stir, then microwave for another 30 seconds. Stir well. If not melted completely, microwave for another 10 to 20 seconds.
3. Add the almond flour, egg, baking powder, and salt to the bowl and mix well. Form into a dough using a spatula or your hands.
4. Cut the dough into 8 roughly equal pieces and form into balls.
5. Roll each dough ball into a cylinder, then pinch the ends together to seal.
6. Place the dough rings in a nonstick donut pan or arrange them on a parchment paper–lined baking sheet.
7. Sprinkle with the seasoning and bake for 12 to 15 minutes or until golden brown.
8. Store in plastic bags in the freezer and defrost overnight in the refrigerator. Reheat in the oven or toaster for a quick grab-and-go breakfast.

NUTRITIONAL FACTS: Calories: 241 Total Fat: 19g Protein: 12g Total Carbs: 5.5g Fiber: 2.5g Net Carbs: 3g

17. TURMERIC CHICKEN AND KALE SALAD WITH FOOD, LEMON AND HONEY

PREPARATION: 20'   COOKING: 15'   SERVES: 4

INGREDIENTS

For the chicken:
- 1 teaspoon of clarified butter or 1 tablespoon of coconut oil
- ½ medium brown onion, diced
- 250-300 g / 9 ounces minced chicken meat or diced chicken legs
- 1 large garlic clove, diced
- 1 teaspoon of turmeric powder
- 1 teaspoon of lime zest
- ½ lime juice
- ½ teaspoon of salt + pepper

For the salad:
- 6 stalks of broccoli or 2 cups of broccoli flowers
- 2 tablespoons of pumpkin seeds (seeds)
- 3 large cabbage leaves, stems removed and chopped
- ½ sliced avocado
- Handful of fresh coriander leaves, chopped
- Handful of fresh parsley leaves, chopped

For the dressing:
- 3 tablespoons of lime juice
- 1 small garlic clove, diced or grated
- 3 tablespoons of virgin olive oil (I used 1 tablespoon of avocado oil and 2 tablespoons of EVO)
- 1 teaspoon of raw honey
- ½ teaspoon whole or Dijon mustard
- ½ teaspoon of sea salt with pepper

DIRECTIONS

1. Heat the coconut oil in a pan. Add the onion and sauté over medium heat for 4-5 minutes, until golden brown. Add the minced chicken and garlic and stir 2-3 minutes over medium-high heat, separating.
2. Add your turmeric, lime zest, lime juice, salt and pepper, and cook, stirring consistently, for another 3-4 minutes. Set the ground beef aside.
3. While your chicken is cooking, put a small saucepan of water to the boil. Add your broccoli and cook for 2 minutes. Rinse with cold water and cut into 3-4 pieces each.
4. Add the pumpkin seeds to the chicken pan and toast over medium heat for 2 minutes, frequently stirring to avoid burning. Season with a little salt. Set aside. Raw pumpkin seeds are also good to use.
5. Put the chopped cabbage in a salad bowl and pour it over the dressing. Using your hands, mix, and massage the cabbage with the dressing. This will soften the cabbage, a bit like citrus juice with fish or beef Carpaccio: it "cooks" it a little.
6. Finally, mix the cooked chicken, broccoli, fresh herbs, pumpkin seeds, and avocado slices.

NUTRITIONAL FACTS: 232 calories Fat 11 Fiber 9 Carbs 8 Protein 14

18. OVERNIGHT "NOATS"

| PREPARATION: 5' + OVERNIGHT CHILLING | COOKING: 10' | SERVES: 1 |

INGREDIENTS

- 2 tablespoons hulled hemp seeds
- 1 tablespoon chia seeds
- ½ scoop (about 8 grams) collagen powder
- ½ cup unsweetened nut or seed milk (hemp, almond, coconut, and cashew)

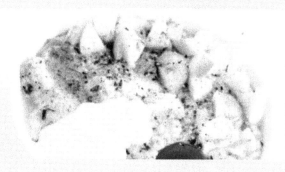

DIRECTIONS

1. In a small mason jar or glass container, combine the hemp seeds, chia seeds, collagen, and milk.
2. Secure tightly with a lid, shake well, and refrigerate overnight.

NUTRITIONAL FACTS: Calories: 263 Total Fat: 19g Protein: 16g Total Carbs: 7g Fiber: 5g Net Carbs: 2g

19. QUICK KETO BLENDER MUFFINS

| PREPARATION: 5' | COOKING: 25' | SERVES: 12 |

INGREDIENTS

- Butter, ghee, or coconut oil for greasing the pan
- 6 eggs
- 8 ounces cream cheese, at room temperature
- 2 scoops flavored collagen powder
- 1 teaspoon ground cinnamon
- 1 teaspoon baking powder
- Few drops or dash sweetener (optional)

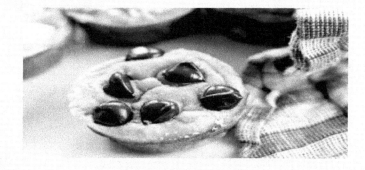

DIRECTIONS

1. Preheat the oven to 350°F. Grease a 12-cup muffin pan very well with butter, ghee, or coconut oil. Alternatively, you can use silicone cups or paper muffin liners.
2. In a blender, combine the eggs, cream cheese, collagen powder, cinnamon, baking powder, and sweetener (if using). Blend until well combined and pour the mixture into the muffin cups, dividing equally.
3. Bake for 22 to 25 minutes until the muffins are golden brown on top and firm.
4. Let cool then store in a glass container or plastic bag in the refrigerator for up to 2 weeks or in the freezer for up to 3 months.
5. To Servings refrigerated muffins, heat in the microwave for 30 seconds. To Servings from frozen, thaw in the refrigerator overnight and then microwave for 30 seconds, or microwave straight from the freezer for 45 to 60 seconds or until heated through.

NUTRITIONAL FACTS: Calories: 120 Total Fat: 10g Protein: 6g Total Carbs: 1.5g Fiber: 0g Net Carbs: 1.5g

20. BACON APPETIZERS

PREPARATION: 15'   COOKING: 2H   SERVES: 6

INGREDIENTS
- 1 pack Keto crackers
- ¾ cup Parmesan cheese, grated
- 1 lb. bacon, sliced thinly

DIRECTIONS
1. Preheat your oven to 250 degrees F.
2. Arrange the crackers on a baking sheet.
3. Sprinkle cheese on top of each cracker.
4. Wrap each cracker with the bacon.
5. Bake in the oven for 2 hours.

NUTRITIONAL FACTS: Calories 440 Total Fat 33.4g Saturated Fat 11g Cholesterol 86mg Sodium 1813mg Total Carbohydrate 3.7g Dietary Fiber 0.1g Total Sugars 0.1g Protein 29.4g Potassium 432mg

21. BUCKWHEAT SPAGHETTI WITH CHICKEN CABBAGE AND SAVORY FOOD RECIPES IN MASS SAUCE

PREPARATION: 15'   COOKING: 15'   SERVES: 2

INGREDIENTS

For the noodles:
- 2-3 handfuls of cabbage leaves (removed from the stem and cut)
- Buckwheat noodles 150g / 5oz (100% buckwheat, without wheat)
- 3-4 shiitake mushrooms, sliced
- 1 teaspoon of coconut oil or butter
- 1 brown onion, finely chopped
- 1 medium chicken breast, sliced or diced
- 1 long red pepper, thinly sliced (seeds in or out depending on how hot you like it)
- 2 large garlic cloves, diced
- 2-3 tablespoons of Tamari sauce (gluten-free soy sauce)

For the miso dressing:
- 1 tablespoon and a half of fresh organic miso
- 1 tablespoon of Tamari sauce
- 1 tablespoon of extra virgin olive oil
- 1 tablespoon of lemon or lime juice
- 1 teaspoon of sesame oil (optional)

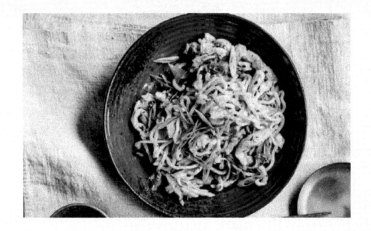

DIRECTIONS

1. Boil a medium saucepan of water. Add the black cabbage and cook 1 minute, until it is wilted. Remove and reserve, but reserve the water and return to boiling. Add your soba noodles and cook according to the directions on the package (usually about 5 minutes). Rinse with cold water and reserve.
2. In the meantime, fry the shiitake mushrooms in a little butter or coconut oil (about a teaspoon) for 2-3 minutes, until its color is lightly browned on each side. Sprinkle with sea salt and reserve.
3. In that same pan, heat more coconut oil or lard over medium-high heat. Fry the onion and chili for 2-3 minutes, and then add the chicken pieces. Cook 5 minutes on medium heat, stirring a few times, then add the garlic, tamari sauce, and a little water. Cook for another 2-3 minutes, stirring continuously until your chicken is cooked.
4. Finally, add the cabbage and soba noodles and stir the chicken to warm it.
5. Stir the miso sauce and sprinkle the noodles at the end of the cooking, in this way you will keep alive all the beneficial probiotics in the miso.

NUTRITIONAL FACTS: 305 calories Fat 11 Fiber 7 Carbs 9 Protein 12

22. FROZEN KETO COFFEE

PREPARATION: 5'   **COOKING:** 20'   **SERVES:** 1

INGREDIENTS

- 12 ounces coffee, chilled
- 1 scoop MCT powder (or 1 tablespoon MCT oil)
- 1 tablespoon heavy (whipping) cream
- Pinch ground cinnamon
- Dash sweetener (optional)
- ½ cup ice

DIRECTIONS

1. In a blender, combine the coffee, MCT powder, cream, cinnamon, sweetener (if using), and ice. Blend until smooth.

NUTRITIONAL FACTS: Calories: 127; Total Fat: 13g; Protein: 1g; Total Carbs: 1.5g; Fiber: 1g; Net Carbs: 0.5g

23. ASIAN KING JUMPED JAMP

PREPARATION: 15' **COOKING:** 10' **SERVES:** 4

INGREDIENTS

- 150 g / 5 oz. of raw shelled prawns, not chopped
- Two teaspoons of tamari (you can use soy sauce if you don't avoid gluten)
- Two teaspoons of extra virgin olive oil
- 75 g / 2.6 oz. soba (buckwheat pasta)
- 1 garlic clove, finely chopped
- 1 bird's eye chili, finely chopped
- 1 teaspoon finely chopped fresh ginger.
- 20 g / 0.7 oz. of sliced red onions
- 40 g / 1.4 oz. of celery, cut and sliced
- 75 g / 2.6 oz. of chopped green beans
- 50 g / 1.7 oz. of chopped cabbage
- 100 ml / ½ cup of chicken broth
- 5 g celery or celery leaves

DIRECTIONS

1. Heat a pan over high heat, and then cook the prawns in 1 teaspoon of tamari and 1 teaspoon of oil for 2-3 minutes. Transfer the prawns to a plate. Clean the pan with kitchen paper as it will be reused.
2. Cook your noodles in boiling water for 5-8 minutes or as indicated on the package. Drain and set aside.
3. Meanwhile, fry the garlic, chili and ginger, red onion, celery, beans, and cabbage in the remaining oil over medium-high heat for 2-3 minutes. Add your broth and allow it to boil, and then simmer for a minute or two, until the vegetables are cooked but crunchy.
4. Add shrimp, noodles and celery/celery leaves to the pan, bring to a boil again, then remove from the heat and serve.

NUTRITIONAL FACTS: Calories 223 Protein 34 Fat 2 Carbs 6

24. BUCKWHEAT PASTA SALAD

PREPARATION: 10' **COOKING:** 30' **SERVES:** 4

INGREDIENTS

- 50 g / 1.7 oz. buckwheat pasta
- Large handful of rockets
- A small handful of basil leaves
- Eight cherry tomatoes halved
- 1/2 avocado, diced
- Ten olives
- 1 tablespoon. extra olive virgin oil
- 20 g / 0.70 oz. pine nuts

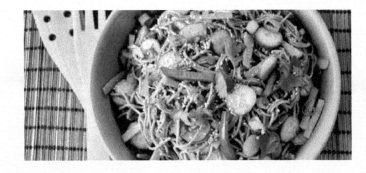

DIRECTIONS

1. Combine all the ingredients except your pine nuts. Arrange your combination on a plate, and then scatter the pine nuts over the top.

NUTRITIONAL FACTS: 125 calories Fat 6 Fiber 5 Carbs 10 Protein 11

25. GREEK SALAD SKEWERS

PREPARATION: 35' **COOKING:** 0' **SERVES:** 2

INGREDIENTS

- Two wooden skewers, soaked in water for 30 minutes before use
- Eight large black olives
- Eight cherry tomatoes
- 1 yellow pepper, cut into eight squares.
- ½ red onions, you can cut in half and separated into eight pieces
- 100 g / 3.5 oz. (about 10cm) cucumber, cut into four slices and halved
- 100 g / 3.5 oz. feta, cut into eight cubes

For the dressing:
- 1 tablespoon. extra olive virgin oil
- Juice of ½ lemons
- 1 teaspoon. of your balsamic vinegar
- ½ clove garlic, ensure it peeled and crushed
- Basil leaves chopped (or ½ teaspoon. dried mixed herbs to replace basil and oregano)
- Oregano leaves,
- Salt and grounded black pepper

DIRECTIONS

1. Blend each skewer with the salad ingredients in the order
2. Put all your dressing ingredients into a bowl and mix thoroughly. Pour over the skewers.

NUTRITIONAL FACTS: Calories 99 Protein 34 Fat 4 Carbs 5

26. ANTIPASTI SKEWERS

PREPARATION: 10' **COOKING:** 0' **SERVES:** 6

INGREDIENTS

- 6 small mozzarella balls
- 1 tablespoon olive oil
- Salt to taste
- 1/8 teaspoon dried oregano
- 2 roasted yellow peppers, sliced into strips and rolled
- 6 cherry tomatoes
- 6 green olives, pitted
- 6 Kalamata olives, pitted
- 2 artichoke hearts, sliced into wedges
- 6 slices salami, rolled
- 6 leaves fresh basil

DIRECTIONS

1. Toss the mozzarella balls in olive oil.
2. Season with salt and oregano.
3. Thread the mozzarella balls and the rest of the ingredients into skewers.
4. Serve in a platter.

NUTRITIONAL FACTS: Calories 180 Total Fat 11.8g Saturated Fat 4.5g Cholesterol 26mg Sodium 482mg Total Carbohydrate 11.7g Dietary Fiber 4.8g Total Sugars 4.1g Protein 9.2g Potassium 538mg

27. KALE, EDAMAME AND TOFU CURRY

PREPARATION: 20' **COOKING:** 40' **SERVES:** 3

INGREDIENTS

- 1 tablespoon rapeseed oil
- 1 large onion, chopped
- Four cloves garlic, peeled and grated
- 1 large thumb (7cm) fresh ginger, peeled and grated
- 1 red chili, deseeded and thinly sliced
- 1/2 teaspoon ground turmeric
- 1/4 teaspoon cayenne pepper
- 1 teaspoon paprika
- 1/2 teaspoon ground cumin
- 1 teaspoon salt
- 250 g / 9 oz. dried red lentils
- 1-liter boiling water
- 50 g / 1.7 oz. frozen soya beans
- 200 g / 7 oz. firm tofu, chopped into cubes
- Two tomatoes, roughly chopped
- Juice of 1 lime
- 200 g / 7 oz. kale leaves stalk removed and torn

DIRECTIONS

1. Put the oil in a pan over low heat. Add your onion and cook for 5 minutes before adding the garlic, ginger, and chili and cooking for a further 2 minutes. Add your turmeric, cayenne, paprika, cumin, and salt and Stir through before adding the red lentils and stirring again.
2. Pour in the boiling water and allow it to simmer for 10 minutes, reduce the heat and cook for about 20-30 minutes until the curry has a thick '•porridge' consistency.
3. Add your tomatoes, tofu and soya beans and cook for a further 5 minutes. Add your kale leaves and lime juice and cook until the kale is just tender.

NUTRITIONAL FACTS: Calories 133 Carbohydrate 54 Protein 43

28. CHOCOLATE CUPCAKES WITH MATCHA ICING

PREPARATION: 35' **COOKING:** 0' **SERVES:** 4

INGREDIENTS

- 150g / 5 oz. self-rising flour
- 200 g / 7 oz. caster sugar
- 60 g / 2.1 oz. cocoa
- ½ teaspoon. salt
- ½ teaspoon. fine espresso coffee, decaf if preferred
- 120 ml / ½ cup milk
- ½ teaspoon. vanilla extract
- 50 ml / ¼ cup vegetable oil
- 1 egg
- 120 ml / ½ cup of water

For the icing:
- 50 g / 1.7 oz. butter,
- 50 g / 1.7 oz. icing sugar
- 1 tablespoon matcha green tea powder
- ½ teaspoon vanilla bean paste
- 50 g / 1.7 oz. soft cream cheese

DIRECTIONS

1. Heat the oven and Line a cupcake tin with paper
2. Put the flour, sugar, cocoa, salt, and coffee powder in a large bowl and mix well.
3. Add milk, vanilla extract, vegetable oil, and egg to dry ingredients and use an electric mixer to beat until well combined. Gently pour the boiling water slowly and beat on low speed until completely combined. Use the high speed to beat for another minute to add air to the dough. The dough is much more liquid than a normal cake mix. Have faith; It will taste fantastic!
4. Arrange the dough evenly between the cake boxes. Each cake box must not be more than ¾ full. Bake for 15-18 minutes, until the dough resumes when hit. Remove from oven and allow cooling completely before icing.
5. To make the icing, beat your butter and icing sugar until they turn pale and smooth. Add the matcha powder and vanilla and mix again. Add the cream cheese and beat until it is smooth. Pipe or spread on the cakes.

NUTRITIONAL FACTS: calories435 Fat 5 Fiber 3 Carbs 7 Protein 9

29. SESAME CHICKEN SALAD

PREPARATION: 20'   **COOKING:** 0'   **SERVES:** 4

INGREDIENTS

- 1 tablespoon of sesame seeds
- 1 cucumber, peeled, halved lengthwise, without a teaspoon, and sliced.
- 100 g / 3.5 oz. cabbage, chopped
- 60 g pak choi, finely chopped
- ½ red onion, thinly sliced
- Large parsley (20 g / 0.7 oz.), chopped.
- 150 g / 5 oz. cooked chicken, minced

For the dressing:

- 1 tablespoon of extra virgin olive oil
- 1 teaspoon of sesame oil
- 1 lime juice
- 1 teaspoon of light honey
- 2 teaspoons soy sauce

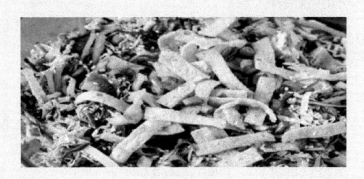

DIRECTIONS

1. Roast your sesame seeds in a dry pan for 2 minutes until they become slightly golden and fragrant.
2. Transfer to a plate to cool.
3. In a small bowl, mix olive oil, sesame oil, lime juice, honey, and soy sauce to prepare the dressing.
4. Place the cucumber, black cabbage, pak choi, red onion, and parsley in a large bowl and mix gently.
5. Pour over the dressing and mix again.
6. Distribute the salad between two dishes and complete with the shredded chicken. Sprinkle with sesame seeds just before serving.

NUTRITIONAL FACTS: Calories 345 Fat 5 Fiber 2 Carbs 10 Protein 4

30. JALAPENO POPPERS

PREPARATION: 30' COOKING: 60' SERVES: 10

INGREDIENTS
- 5 fresh jalapenos, sliced and seeded
- 4 oz. package cream cheese
- ¼ lb. bacon, sliced in half

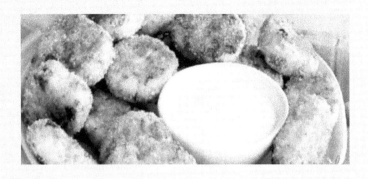

DIRECTIONS
1. Preheat your oven to 275 degrees F.
2. Place a wire rack over your baking sheet.
3. Stuff each jalapeno with cream cheese and wrap in bacon.
4. Secure with a toothpick.
5. Place on the baking sheet.
6. Bake for 1 hour and 15 minutes.

NUTRITIONAL FACTS: Calories 103 Total Fat 8.7g Saturated Fat 4.1g Cholesterol 25mg Sodium 296mg Total Carbohydrate 0.9g Dietary Fiber 0.2g Total Sugars 0.3g Protein 5.2g Potassium 93mg

31. BLT PARTY BITES

PREPARATION: 35' COOKING: 0' SERVES: 8

INGREDIENTS
- 4 oz. bacon, chopped
- 3 tablespoons panko breadcrumbs
- 1 tablespoon Parmesan cheese, grated
- 1 teaspoon mayonnaise
- 1 teaspoon lemon juice
- Salt to taste
- ½ heart Romaine lettuce, shredded
- 6 cocktail tomatoes

DIRECTIONS
1. Put the bacon in a pan over medium heat.
2. Fry until crispy.
3. Transfer bacon to a plate lined with paper towel.
4. Add breadcrumbs and cook until crunchy.
5. Transfer breadcrumbs to another plate also lined with paper towel.
6. Sprinkle Parmesan cheese on top of the breadcrumbs.
7. Mix the mayonnaise, salt and lemon juice.
8. Toss the Romaine in the mayo mixture.
9. Slice each tomato on the bottom to create a flat surface so it can stand by itself.
10. Slice the top off as well.
11. Scoop out the insides of the tomatoes.
12. Stuff each tomato with the bacon, Parmesan, breadcrumbs and top with the lettuce.

NUTRITIONAL FACTS: Calories 107 Total Fat 6.5g Saturated Fat 2.1g Cholesterol 16mg Sodium 360mg Total Carbohydrate 5.4g Dietary Fiber 1.5g Total Sugars 3.3g Protein 6.5g Potassium 372mg

32. STRAWBERRIES AND CREAM SMOOTHIE

PREPARATION: 5' COOKING: 15' SERVES: 1

INGREDIENTS
- 5 medium strawberries, hulled
- 3 tablespoons heavy (whipping) cream
- 3 ice cubes
- Your favorite vanilla-flavored sweetener

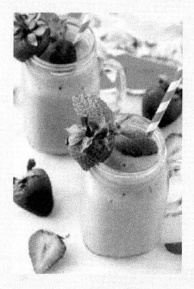

DIRECTIONS
1. In a blender, combine all the ingredients and blend until smooth. Enjoy right away!

NUTRITIONAL FACTS: Calories: 176 Total Fat: 16g Protein: 2g Total Carbs: 6g Fiber: 1g Net Carbs: 5g

33. CAULI FLITTERS

PREPARATION: 10' COOKING: 15' SERVES: 2

INGREDIENTS
- 2 eggs
- 1 head of cauliflower
- 1 tbsp. yeast
- sea salt, black pepper
- 1-2 tbsp. ghee
- 1 tbsp. turmeric
- 2/3 cup almond flour

DIRECTIONS
1. Place the cauliflower into a large pot and start to boil it for 8 mins. Add the florets into a food processor and pulse them.
2. Add the eggs, almond flour, yeast, turmeric, salt and pepper to a mixing bowl. Stir well. Form into patties.
3. Heat your ghee to medium in a skillet. Form your fritters and cook until golden on each side (3-4 mins).
4. Serve it while hot.

NUTRITIONAL FACTS: Calories: 238 kcal Fat: 23 g Carbs: 5 g Protein: 6 g

34. BACON WRAPPED CHICKEN BREAST

PREPARATION: 10' COOKING: 45' SERVES: 4

INGREDIENTS

- 4 boneless, skinless chicken breast
- 8 oz. sharp cheddar cheese
- 8 slices bacon
- 4 oz. sliced jalapeno peppers
- 1 tsp garlic powder
- Salt and pepper to taste

DIRECTIONS

1. Preheat the oven at around 3500F. Ensure to season both sides of chicken breast well with salt, garlic powder, and pepper. Place the chicken breast on a non-stick baking sheet (foil-covered). Cover the chicken with cheese and add jalapeno slices. Cut the bacon slices in half and then place the four halves over each piece of chicken. Bake for around 30 to 45 minutes at most. If the chicken is set but the bacon still feels undercooked, you may want to put it under the broiler for a few minutes. Once done, serve hot with a side of low carb garlic parmesan roasted asparagus.

NUTRITIONAL FACTS: Calories: 640 Fat: 48g Carbohydrates: 6g Fiber: 3g Net carbs: 3g Protein: 47g

35. NO-BAKE KETO POWER BARS

PREPARATION: 10' OVERNIGHT TO CHILL COOKING: 20' SERVES: 12 BARS

INGREDIENTS

- ½ cup pili nuts
- ½ cup whole hazelnuts
- ½ cup walnut halves
- ¼ cup hulled sunflower seeds
- ¼ cup unsweetened coconut flakes or chips
- ¼ cup hulled hemp seeds
- 2 tablespoons unsweetened cacao nibs
- 2 scoops collagen powder (I use 1 scoop Perfect Keto vanilla collagen and 1 scoop Perfect Keto unflavored collagen powder)
- ½ teaspoon ground cinnamon
- ½ teaspoon sea salt
- ¼ cup coconut oil, melted
- 1 teaspoon vanilla extract
- Stevia or monk fruit to sweeten (optional if you are using unflavored collagen powder)

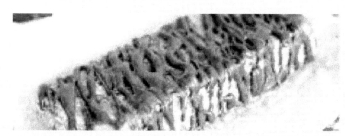

DIRECTIONS

1. Line a 9-inch square baking pan with parchment paper.
2. In a food processor or blender, combine the pili nuts, hazelnuts, walnuts, sunflower seeds, coconut, hemp seeds, cacao nibs, collagen powder, cinnamon, and salt and pulse a few times.
3. Add the coconut oil, vanilla extract, and sweetener (if using). Pulse again until the ingredients are combined. Do not over pulse or it will turn to mush. You want the nuts and seeds to still have some texture.
4. Pour the mixture into the prepared pan and press it into an even layer. Cover with another piece of parchment (or fold over extra from the first piece) and place a heavy pan or dish on top to help press the bars together.
5. Refrigerate overnight and then cut into 12 bars. Store the bars in individual storage bags in the refrigerator for a quick grab-and-go breakfast.

NUTRITIONAL FACTS: Calories: 242 Total Fat: 22g Protein: 6.5g Total Carbs: 4.5g Fiber: 2.5g Net Carbs: 2g

KETO WOMEN over 50   **54**

36. AVOCADO TOAST

PREPARATION: 20'   **COOKING:** 40'   **SERVES:** 2

INGREDIENTS

- ½ cup grass-fed butter
- 2 tbsp coconut oil
- 7 large eggs
- 1 tsp baking powder
- 2 cups almond flour
- ½ tsp xanthan gum
- ½ tsp kosher salt
- 1 medium avocado

DIRECTIONS

1. Preheat over at 3500F. Beat eggs for around two minutes with a mixer at high speed. Then, add coconut oil and butter (both melted) to the eggs and continue beating. Ensure that oil and butter are not too warm to cook the eggs. Add remaining bread ingredients and mix well. Now, the batter should become thick. Pour batter in a non-stick loaf pan lined with parchment paper. Let it bake for 45 minutes or until the fork comes clean through the middle.
2. For topping, toast two slices of your keto bread to your liking. Slice the whole avocado thinly, without the skin or pit. Use these to make one long strip of overlapping slices. Roll these into a spiral and that is it! Enjoy your keto bread with avocado topping.

NUTRITIONAL FACTS: Calories: 350 Fat: 32g Carbohydrates: 7g Fiber: 4g Net carbs: 3g Protein: 10g

37. ALMOND FLOUR PANCAKES

PREPARATION: 5'   **COOKING:** 5'   **SERVES:** 4

INGREDIENTS

- ½ cup almond flour
- ½ cup cream cheese
- 4 medium eggs
- ½ tsp cinnamon
- ½ tsp granulated sweetener
- 1 tsp grass-fed butter
- 1 tbsp sugar-free syrup

DIRECTIONS

1. Add all the ingredients into a blender and let them blend in well. Once done, set the batter aside.
2. On a non-stick pan at medium heat, fry pancakes with melted butter. Once the center starts to bubble, turn over. Once done with the pancake, move on to the rest, using the batter.
3. Finally, serve your pancakes warm, along with some low carb fruit or with an exquisite side of sugar-free syrup to enjoy a healthy and tasty breakfast.

NUTRITIONAL FACTS: Calories: 234 Fat: 20g Carbohydrates: 4g Fiber: 1.5gNet carbs: 2.5g Protein: 11g

38. CHICKEN AVOCADO EGG BACON SALAD

PREPARATION: 10'   COOKING: 10'   SERVES: 4

INGREDIENTS

- 12 oz. cooked chicken breast
- 6 slices crumbled bacon
- 3 boiled eggs cut into cubes
- 1 cup cherry tomatoes cut into halves
- 1/2 small sliced red onion
- 1 large avocado(s)
- 1/2 stick finely chopped celery

Salad Dressing
- 1/2 cup olive oil mayonnaise
- 2 tbsp. sour cream
- 1 tsp Dijon mustard
- 4 tbsp. extra virgin olive oil
- 2 cloves minced garlic
- 2 tsp lemon juice
- 4 cups lettuce
- Salt and pepper to taste

DIRECTIONS

1. Combine all the ingredients together and mix them well for the salad dressing. Then, combine chicken, tomatoes, bacon, eggs, red onions, and celery together. Add about ¾ of the salad dressing and mix them well. Add the avocado and toss together gently. Check the taste and, if needed, add the remainder of the salad dressing as well. Finally, add salt and pepper to taste and then serve it over lettuce.

NUTRITIONAL FACTS: Calories: 387 Fat: 27g Carbohydrates: 2.5g Fiber: 1g Net carbs: 1.5g Protein: 24g

39. KETO FLU COMBAT SMOOTHIE

PREPARATION: 5'   COOKING: 15'   SERVES: 1

INGREDIENTS

- ½ cup unsweetened nut or seed milk (hemp, almond, coconut, and cashew)
- 1 cup spinach
- ½ medium avocado (about 75 grams), pitted and peeled
- 1 scoop MCT powder (or 1 tablespoon MCT oil)
- ½ tablespoon unsweetened cacao powder
- ¼ teaspoon of sea salt
- Dash sweetener (optional)
- ½ cup ice

DIRECTIONS

1. In a blender, combine the milk, spinach, avocado, MCT powder, cacao powder, salt, sweetener (if using), and ice and blend until smooth.

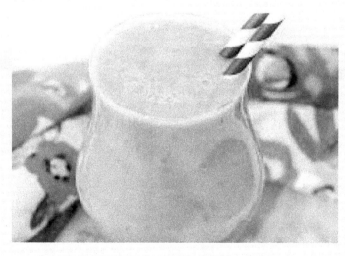

NUTRITIONAL FACTS: Calories: 249 Total Fat: 21g Protein: 5g Total Carbs: 10g Fiber: 8g Net Carbs: 2g

KETO WOMEN over 50 56

40. BACON HASH

PREPARATION: 5' COOKING: 10' SERVES: 2

INGREDIENTS

- Small green pepper (1)
- Jalapenos (2)
- Small onion (1)
- Eggs (4)
- Bacon slices (6)

DIRECTIONS

1. Chop the bacon into chunks using a food processor. Set aside for now. Slice the onions and peppers into thin strips. Dice the jalapenos as small as possible.
2. Heat a skillet and fry the veggies. Once browned, combine the fixings and cook until crispy. Place on a serving dish with the eggs.

NUTRITIONAL FACTS: Carbohydrates: 9 grams Protein: 23 grams Fats: 24 grams Calories: 366

41. EGG SALAD

PREPARATION: 15' COOKING: 10' SERVES: 4

INGREDIENTS

- 6 eggs
- 2 tbsp mayonnaise
- 1 tsp Dijon mustard
- 1 tsp lemon juice
- Salt and pepper to taste

DIRECTIONS

1. In a medium saucepan, place the solid eggs gently.
2. Add some cold water so that the eggs are covered around an inch. Boil them for around 10 minutes.
3. Once done, remove them from the heat and let them cool. Peel the eggs while running them under cold water. Now add these in a food processor and pulse until they are chopped.
4. Add and stir mayonnaise, lemon juice, mustard, and salt and pepper. Ensure to taste and then adjust as necessary.
5. Finally, serve them with a bit of lettuce leaves and, if needed, bacon for wrapping.

NUTRITIONAL FACTS: Calories: 222 Fat: 19g Net carbs: 1g Protein: 13g

42. BAGELS WITH CHEESE

PREPARATION: 10'   COOKING: 15'   SERVES: 6

INGREDIENTS
- Mozzarella cheese (2.5 cups)
- Baking powder (1 tsp.)
- Cream cheese (3 oz.)
- Almond flour (1.5 cups)
- Eggs (2)

DIRECTIONS
1. Shred the mozzarella and combine with the flour, baking powder, and cream cheese in a mixing container. Pop into the microwave for about one minute. Mix well.
2. Let the mixture cool and add the eggs. Break apart into six sections and shape into round bagels. Note: You can also sprinkle with a seasoning of your choice or pinch of salt if desired.
3. Bake them for approximately 12 to 15 minutes. Serve or cool and store.

NUTRITIONAL FACTS: Carbohydrates: 8 grams Protein: 19 grams Fats: 31 grams Calories: 374

43. CAPICOLA EGG CUPS

PREPARATION: 5'   COOKING: 15'   SERVES: 4

INGREDIENTS
- 8 eggs
- 1 cup cheddar cheese
- 4 oz. capicola or bacon (slices)
- salt, pepper, basil

DIRECTIONS
1. Preheat the oven to 400°F. You will need 8 wells of a standard-size muffin pan.
2. Place the slices in the 8 wells, forming a cup shape. Sprinkle into each cup some of the cheese, according to your liking.
3. Crack an egg into each cup, season them with salt and pepper.
4. Bake for 10-15 mins. Serve hot, top it with basil.

NUTRITIONAL FACTS: Carbs: 1 g Fat: 11 g Protein: 16 g Calories: 171 kcal

KETO WOMEN over 50   58

44. SCRAMBLED EGGS

PREPARATION: 2'   COOKING: 8'   SERVES: 4

INGREDIENTS
- 4 oz. butter
- 8 eggs
- salt and pepper for taste

DIRECTIONS
1. Crack the eggs in a bowl, and whisk them together, while seasoning it.
2. Melt the butter in a skillet over medium heat, but don't turn it into brown.
3. Pour the eggs into the skillet and cook it for 1-2 mins, until they look and feel fluffy and creamy.
4. Tip: If you want to shake things up, you can pair this one up with bacon, salmon, or maybe avocado as well.

NUTRITIONAL FACTS: Carbs: 1 g Fat: 31 g Protein: 11 g Calories: 327 kcal

45. FRITTATA WITH SPINACH

PREPARATION: 5'   COOKING: 30'   SERVES: 4

INGREDIENTS
- 8 eggs
- 8 ozs. fresh spinach
- 5 ozs. diced bacon
- 5 ozs. shredded cheese
- 1 cup heavy whipping cream
- 2 tbsps. butter
- salt and pepper

DIRECTIONS
1. Preheat the oven to 350 °F
2. Fry the bacon until crispy, add the spinach and cook until wilted. Set them aside.
3. Whisk the cream and eggs together, and pour it into the baking dish.
4. Add the cheese, spinach, and bacon on the top, and place in the oven. Bake for 25-30 minutes, until golden brown on top.

NUTRITIONAL FACTS: Carbs: 4 g Fat: 59 g Protein: 27 g Calories: 661 kcal

46. CHEESE OMELET

PREPARATION: 5' COOKING: 10' SERVES: 2

INGREDIENTS
- 6 eggs
- 3 ozs. ghee
- 7 ozs. shredded cheddar cheese
- salt and pepper

DIRECTIONS
1. Whisk the eggs until smooth. Compound half of the cheese and season it with salt and pepper.
2. Melt the butter in a pan. Pour in the mixture and let it sit for a few minutes (3-4)
3. When the mixture is looking good, add the other half of the cheese. Serve immediately.

NUTRITIONAL FACTS: Carbs: 4 g Fat: 80 g Protein: 40 g Calories: 897 kcal

CHAPTER 10.
LUNCH

47. BUTTERED COD

PREPARATION: 5' **COOKING:** 5' **SERVES:** 4

INGREDIENTS

- 1 ½ lb. cod fillets, sliced
- 6 tablespoons butter, sliced
- ¼ teaspoon garlic powder
- ¾ teaspoon ground paprika
- Salt and pepper to taste
- Lemon slices
- Chopped parsley

DIRECTIONS

1. Mix the garlic powder, paprika, salt and pepper in a bowl.
2. Season cod pieces with seasoning mixture.
3. Add 2 tablespoons butter in a pan over medium heat.
4. Let half of the butter melt.
5. Add the cod and cook for 2 minutes per side.
6. Top with the remaining slices of butter.
7. Cook for 3 to 4 minutes.
8. Garnish with parsley and lemon slices before serving.

NUTRITIONAL FACTS: Calories 295 Total Fat 19g Saturated Fat 11g Cholesterol 128mg Sodium 236mg Total Carbohydrate 1.5g Dietary Fiber 0.7g Total Sugars 0.3g Protein 30.7g Potassium 102mg

48. SALMON WITH RED CURRY SAUCE

PREPARATION: 10' **COOKING:** 22' **SERVES:** 4

INGREDIENTS

- 4 salmon fillets
- 2 tablespoons olive oil
- Salt and pepper to taste
- 1 ½ tablespoons red curry paste
- 1 tablespoon fresh ginger, chopped
- 14 oz. coconut cream
- 1 ½ tablespoons fish sauce

DIRECTIONS

1. Preheat your oven to 350 degrees F.
2. Cover baking sheet with foil.
3. Brush both sides of salmon fillets with olive oil and season with salt and pepper.
4. Place the salmon fillets on the baking sheet.
5. Bake salmon in the oven for 20 minutes.
6. In a pan over medium heat, mix the curry paste, ginger, coconut cream and fish sauce.
7. Sprinkle with salt and pepper.
8. Simmer for 2 minutes.
9. Pour the sauce over the salmon before serving.

NUTRITIONAL FACTS: Calories 553 Total Fat 43.4g Saturated Fat 24.1g Cholesterol 78mg Sodium 908mg Total Carbohydrate 7.9g Dietary Fiber 2.4g Total Sugars 3.6g Protein 37.3g Potassium 982mg

49. SALMON TERIYAKI

PREPARATION: 15' **COOKING:** 25' **SERVES:** 6

INGREDIENTS

- 3 tablespoons sesame oil
- 2 teaspoons fish sauce
- 3 tablespoons coconut amino
- 2 teaspoons ginger, grated
- 4 cloves garlic, crushed
- 2 tablespoons xylitol
- 1 tablespoon green lime juice
- 2 teaspoons green lime zest
- Cayenne pepper to taste
- 6 salmon fillets
- 1 teaspoon arrowroot starch
- ¼ cup water
- Sesame seeds

DIRECTIONS

1. Preheat your oven to 400 degrees F.
2. Combine the sesame oil, fish sauce, coconut amino, ginger, garlic, xylitol, green lime juice, zest and cayenne pepper in a mixing bowl.
3. Create 6 packets using foil.
4. Add half of the marinade in the packets.
5. Add the salmon inside.
6. Place in the baking sheet and cook for about 20 to 25 minutes.
7. Add the remaining sauce in a pan over medium heat.
8. Dissolve arrowroot in water, and add to the sauce.
9. Simmer until the sauce has thickened.
10. Place the salmon on a serving platter and pour the sauce on top.
11. Sprinkle sesame seeds on top before serving.

NUTRITIONAL FACTS: Calories 312 Total Fat 17.9g Saturated Fat 2.6g Cholesterol 78mg Sodium 242mg Total Carbohydrate 3.5g Dietary Fiber 0.1g Total Sugars 0.1g Protein 34.8g Potassium 706mg

50. PESTO SHRIMP WITH ZUCCHINI NOODLES

PREPARATION: 10' **COOKING:** 15' **SERVES:** 3

INGREDIENTS

- Pesto sauce
- 3 cups basil leaves
- ¾ cup pine nuts
- 2 cloves garlic
- ½ lemon, juiced
- 1 teaspoon lemon zest
- Salt to taste
- ¼ cup olive oil
- Shrimp and Zoodles
- 3 zucchinis
- Salt to taste
- 1 lb. shrimp
- 2 tablespoons avocado oil

DIRECTIONS

1. Put all the pesto ingredients in a blender.
2. Blend until smooth.
3. Spiralize the zucchini into noodle form.
4. Season with salt.
5. Drain water from the zucchini noodles.
6. Season the shrimp with salt and pepper.
7. Add half of the oil in a pan over medium heat.
8. Once the oil is hot, add the shrimp and cook for 1 to 2 minutes.
9. Add the remaining oil to the pan.
10. Add the zucchini noodles and cook for 3 minutes.
11. Add the pesto and toss to coat the noodles evenly with the sauce.
12. Season with salt.

NUTRITIONAL FACTS: Calories 304 Total Fat 22.2g Saturated Fat 2.6g Cholesterol 159mg Sodium 223mg Total Carbohydrate 8g Dietary Fiber 2.3g Total Sugars 2.5g Protein 21.3g Potassium 547mg

51. CRAB CAKES

PREPARATION: 1H 20' COOKING: 20' SERVES: 8

INGREDIENTS

- 2 tablespoons butter
- 2 cloves garlic, minced
- ½ cup bell pepper, chopped
- 1 rib celery, chopped
- 1 shallot, chopped
- Salt and pepper to taste
- 2 tablespoons mayonnaise
- 1 egg, beaten
- 1 teaspoon mustard
- 1 tablespoon Worcestershire sauce
- 1 teaspoon hot sauce
- ½ cup Parmesan cheese, grated
- ½ cup pork rinds, crushed
- 1 lb. crabmeat
- 2 tablespoons olive oil

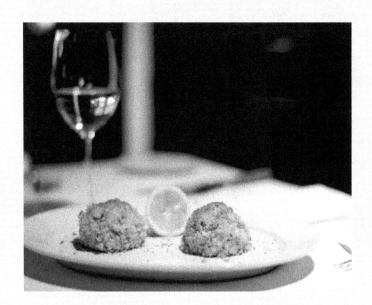

DIRECTIONS

1. Add the butter to the pan over medium heat.
2. Add the garlic, bell pepper, celery, shallot, salt and pepper.
3. Cook for 10 minutes.
4. In a bowl, mix the mayo, egg, Worcestershire, mustard and hot sauce.
5. Add the sautéed vegetables to this mixture.
6. Mix well.
7. Add the cheese and pork rind.
8. Fold in the crabmeat.
9. Line the baking sheet with foil.
10. Create patties from the mixture.
11. Place the patties on the baking sheet.
12. Cover the baking sheet with foil.
13. Refrigerate for 1 hour.
14. Fry in olive oil in a pan over medium heat.
15. Cook until crispy and golden brown.

NUTRITIONAL FACTS: Calories 150 Total Fat 9.2g Saturated Fat 3.2g Cholesterol 43mg Sodium 601mg Total Carbohydrate 10.8g Dietary Fiber 0.5g Total Sugars 4.6g Protein 6.4g Potassium 80mg

52. TUNA SALAD

PREPARATION: 5' COOKING: 0' SERVES: 2

INGREDIENTS

- 1 cup tuna flakes
- 3 tablespoons mayonnaise
- 1 teaspoon onion flakes
- Salt and pepper to taste
- 3 cups Romaine lettuce

DIRECTIONS

1. Mix the tuna flakes, mayonnaise, onion flakes, salt and pepper in a bowl.
2. Serve with lettuce.

NUTRITIONAL FACTS: Calories 130 Total Fat 7.8g Saturated Fat 1.1g Cholesterol 13mg Sodium 206mg Total Carbohydrate 8.5g Dietary Fiber 0.6g Total Sugars 2.6g Protein 8.2g Potassium 132mg

53. KETO FROSTY

PREPARATION: 45' **COOKING:** 0' **SERVES:** 4

INGREDIENTS

- 1 ½ cups heavy whipping cream
- 2 tablespoons cocoa powder (unsweetened)
- 3 tablespoons Swerve
- 1 teaspoon pure vanilla extract
- Salt to taste

DIRECTIONS

1. In a bowl, combine all the ingredients.
2. Use a hand mixer and beat until you see stiff peaks forming.
3. Place the mixture in a Ziploc bag.
4. Freeze for 35 minutes.
5. Serve in bowls or dishes.

NUTRITIONAL FACTS: Calories 164 Total Fat 17g Saturated Fat 10.6g Cholesterol 62mg Sodium 56mg Total Carbohydrate 2.9g Dietary Fiber 0.8g Total Sugars 0.2g Protein 1.4g Potassium 103mg

54. KETO SHAKE

PREPARATION: 15' **COOKING:** 0' **SERVES:** 1

INGREDIENTS

- ¾ cup almond milk
- ½ cup ice
- 2 tablespoons almond butter
- 2 tablespoons cocoa powder (unsweetened)
- 2 tablespoons Swerve
- 1 tablespoon chia seeds
- 2 tablespoons hemp seeds
- ½ tablespoon vanilla extract
- Salt to taste

DIRECTIONS

1. Blend all the ingredients in a food processor.
2. Chill in the refrigerator before serving.

NUTRITIONAL FACTS: Calories 104 Total Fat 9.5g Saturated Fat 5.1g Cholesterol 0mg Sodium 24mg Total Carbohydrate 3.6g Dietary Fiber 1.4g Total Sugars 1.1g Protein 2.9g Potassium 159mg

55. KETO FAT BOMBS

PREPARATION: 30' **COOKING:** 0' **SERVES:** 10

INGREDIENTS

- 8 tablespoons butter
- ¼ cup Swerve
- ½ teaspoon vanilla extract
- Salt to taste
- 2 cups almond flour
- 2/3 cup chocolate chips

DIRECTIONS

1. In a bowl, beat the butter until fluffy.
2. Stir in the sugar, salt and vanilla.
3. Mix well.
4. Add the almond flour.
5. Fold in the chocolate chips.
6. Cover the bowl with cling wrap and refrigerate for 20 minutes.
7. Create balls from the dough.

NUTRITIONAL FACTS: Calories 176 Total Fat 15.2g Saturated Fat 8.4g Cholesterol 27mg Sodium 92mg Total Carbohydrate 12.9g Dietary Fiber 1g Total Sugars 10.8g Protein 2.2g Potassium 45mg

56. AVOCADO ICE POPS

PREPARATION: 20' **COOKING:** 0' **SERVES:** 10

INGREDIENTS

- 3 avocados
- ¼ cup lime juice
- 3 tablespoons Swerve
- ¾ cup coconut milk
- 1 tablespoon coconut oil
- 1 cup keto friendly chocolate

DIRECTIONS

1. Add all the ingredients except the oil and chocolate in a blender.
2. Blend until smooth.
3. Pour the mixture into the popsicle mold.
4. Freeze overnight.
5. In a bowl, mix oil and chocolate chips.
6. Melt in the microwave. And then let cool.
7. Dunk the avocado popsicles into the chocolate before serving.

NUTRITIONAL FACTS: Calories 176 Total Fat 17.4g Saturated Fat 7.5g Cholesterol 0mg Sodium 6mg Total Carbohydrate 10.8g Dietary Fiber 4.5g Total Sugars 5.4g Protein 1.6g Potassium 341mg

57. CARROT BALLS

PREPARATION: 1H 10' **COOKING:** 0' **SERVES:** 8

INGREDIENTS

- 8 oz. block cream cheese
- ¾ cup coconut flour
- ½ teaspoon pure vanilla extract
- 1 teaspoon stevia
- ¼ teaspoon ground nutmeg
- 1 teaspoon cinnamon
- 1 cup carrots, grated
- 1/2 cup pecans, chopped
- 1 cup coconut, shredded

DIRECTIONS

1. Use a hand mixer to beat the cream cheese, coconut flour, vanilla, stevia, nutmeg and cinnamon.
2. Fold in the carrots and pecans.
3. Form into balls.
4. Refrigerate for 1 hour.
5. Roll into shredded coconut before serving.

NUTRITIONAL FACTS: Calories 390 Total Fat 35g Saturated Fat 17g Cholesterol 60mg Sodium 202mg Total Carbohydrate 17.2g Dietary Fiber 7.8g Total Sugars 6g Protein 7.8g Potassium 154mg

58. COCONUT CRACK BARS

PREPARATION: 2' **COOKING:** 3' **SERVES:** 20

INGREDIENTS

- 3 cups coconut flakes (unsweetened)
- 1 cup coconut oil
- ¼ cup maple syrup

DIRECTIONS

1. Line a baking sheet with parchment paper.
2. Put coconut in a bowl.
3. Add the oil and syrup.
4. Mix well.
5. Pour the mixture into the pan.
6. Refrigerate until firm.
7. Slice into bars before serving.

NUTRITIONAL FACTS: Calories 147 Total Fat 14.9g Saturated Fat 13g Cholesterol 0mg Sodium 3mg Total Carbohydrate 4.5g Dietary Fiber 1.1g Total Sugars 3.1g Protein 0.4g Potassium 51mg

59. STRAWBERRY ICE CREAM

PREPARATION: 1H 20' **COOKING:** 0' **SERVES:** 4

INGREDIENTS

- 17 oz. coconut milk
- 16 oz. frozen strawberries
- ¾ cup Swerve
- ½ cup fresh strawberries

DIRECTIONS

1. Put all the ingredients except fresh strawberries in a blender.
2. Pulse until smooth.
3. Put the mixture in an ice cream maker.
4. Use ice cream maker according to directions.
5. Add the fresh strawberries a few minutes before the ice cream is done.
6. Freeze for 1 hour before serving.

NUTRITIONAL FACTS: Calories 320 Total Fat 28.8g Saturated Fat 25.5g Cholesterol 0mg Sodium 18mg Total Carbohydrate 25.3g Dietary Fiber 5.3g Total Sugars 19.1g Protein 2.9g Potassium 344mg

60. KEY LIME PUDDING

PREPARATION: 20' **COOKING:** 1H 15' **SERVES:** 2

INGREDIENTS

- 1 cup hot water
- 2/4 cup erythrytol syrup
- 6 drops stevia
- 1 teaspoon almond extract
- 1 teaspoon vanilla extract
- ¼ teaspoon Xanthan gum powder
- 2 ripe avocados, sliced
- 1 ½ oz. lime juice
- 3 tablespoons coconut oil
- Salt to taste

DIRECTIONS

1. Add water, erythritol, stevia, almond extract and vanilla extract to a pot.
2. Bring to a boil.
3. Simmer until the syrup has been reduced and has thickened.
4. Turn the heat off.
5. Add the gum powder.
6. Mix until thickened.
7. Add the avocado into a food processor.
8. Add the rest of the ingredients.
9. Pulse until smooth.
10. Place the mixture in ramekins.
11. Refrigerate for 1 hour.
12. Pour the syrup over the pudding before serving.

NUTRITIONAL FACTS: Calories 299 Total Fat 29.8g Saturated Fat 12.9g Cholesterol 0mg Sodium 47mg Total Carbohydrate 9.7g Dietary Fiber 6.8g Total Sugars 0.8g Protein 2g Potassium 502mg

61. CHICKEN, BACON AND AVOCADO CLOUD SANDWICHES

PREPARATION: 10' **COOKING:** 25' **SERVES:** 6

INGREDIENTS

For cloud bread
- 3 large eggs
- 4 oz. cream cheese
- ½ tablespoon. ground psyllium husk powder
- ½ teaspoon baking powder
- A pinch of salt
- To assemble sandwich
- 6 slices of bacon, cooked and chopped
- 6 slices pepper Jack cheese
- ½ avocado, sliced
- 1 cup cooked chicken breasts, shredded
- 3 tablespoons. mayonnaise

DIRECTIONS

1. Preheat your oven to 300 degrees.
2. Prepare a baking sheet by lining it with parchment paper.
3. Separate the egg whites and egg yolks, and place into separate bowls.
4. Whisk the egg whites until very stiff. Set aside.
5. Combined egg yolks and cream cheese.
6. Add the psyllium husk powder and baking powder to the egg yolk mixture. Gently fold in.
7. Add the egg whites into the egg mixture and gently fold in.
8. Dollop the mixture onto the prepared baking sheet to create 12 cloud bread. Use a spatula to gently spread the circles around to form ½-inch thick pieces.
9. Bake for 25 minutes or until the tops are golden brown.
10. Allow the cloud bread to cool completely before serving. Can be refrigerated for up to 3 days of frozen for up to 3 months. If food prepping, place a layer of parchment paper between each bread slice to avoid having them getting stuck together. Simply toast in the oven for 5 minutes when it is time to serve.
11. To assemble sandwiches, place mayonnaise on one side of one cloud bread. Layer with the remaining sandwich ingredients and top with another slice of cloud bread.

NUTRITIONAL FACTS: Calories: 333 kcal Carbs: 5g Fat: 26g Protein: 19.9g

62. ROASTED LEMON CHICKEN SANDWICH

PREPARATION: 15' COOKING: 1H 30' SERVES: 12

INGREDIENTS

- 1 kg whole chicken
- 5 tablespoons. butter
- 1 lemon, cut into wedges
- 1 tablespoon. garlic powder
- Salt and pepper to taste
- 2 tablespoons. mayonnaise
- Keto-friendly bread

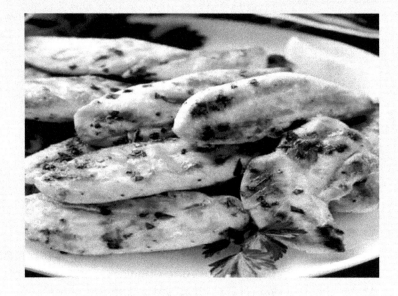

DIRECTIONS

1. Preheat the oven to 350 degrees F.
2. Grease a deep baking dish with butter.
3. Ensure that the chicken is patted dry and that the gizzards have been removed.
4. Combine the butter, garlic powder, salt and pepper.
5. Rub the entire chicken with it, including in the cavity.
6. Place the lemon and onion inside the chicken and place the chicken in the prepared baking dish.
7. Bake for about 1½ hours, depending on the size of the chicken.
8. Baste the chicken often with the drippings. If the drippings begin to dry, add water. The chicken is done when a thermometer, insert it into the thickest part of the thigh reads 165 degrees F or when the clear juices run when the thickest part of the thigh is pierced.
9. Allow the chicken to cool before slicing.
10. To assemble sandwich, shred some of the breast meat and mix with the mayonnaise. Place the mixture between the two bread slices.
11. To save the chicken, refrigerated for up to 5 days or freeze for up to 1 month.

NUTRITIONAL FACTS: Calories: 214 kcal Carbs: 1.6 gFat: 11.8 gProtein: 24.4 g.

63. KETO-FRIENDLY SKILLET PEPPERONI PIZZA

PREPARATION: 10' **COOKING:** 6' **SERVES:** 4

INGREDIENTS

For Crust
- ½ cup almond flour
- ½ teaspoon baking powder
- 8 large egg whites, whisked into stiff peaks
- Salt and pepper to taste

Toppings
- 3 tablespoons. Unsweetened tomato sauce
- ½ cup shredded cheddar cheese
- ½ cup pepperoni

DIRECTIONS

1. Gently incorporate the almond flour into the egg whites. Ensure that no lumps remain.
2. Stir in the remaining crust ingredients.
3. Heat a nonstick skillet over medium heat. Spray with nonstick spray.
4. Pour the batter into the heated skillet to cover the bottom of the skillet.
5. Cover the skillet with a lid and cook the pizza crust to cook for about 4 minutes or until bubbles that appear on the top.
6. Flip the dough and add the toppings, starting with the tomato sauce and ending with the pepperoni
7. Cook the pizza for 2 more minutes.
8. Allow the pizza to cool slightly before serving.
9. Can be stored in the refrigerator for up to 5 days and frozen for up to 1 month.

NUTRITIONAL FACTS: Calories: 175 kcal Carbs: 1.9 g Fat: 12 g Protein: 14.3 g.

64. CHEESY CHICKEN CAULIFLOWER

PREPARATION: 5' **COOKING:** 10' **SERVES:** 4

INGREDIENTS

- 2 cups cauliflower florets, chopped
- ½ cup red bell pepper, chopped
- 1 cup roasted chicken, shredded (Lunch Recipes: Roasted Lemon Chicken Sandwich)
- ¼ cup shredded cheddar cheese
- 1 tablespoon. butter
- 1 tablespoon. sour cream
- Salt and pepper to taste

DIRECTIONS

1. Stir fry the cauliflower and peppers in the butter over medium heat until the veggies are tender.
2. Add the chicken and cook until the chicken is warmed through.
3. Add the remaining ingredients and stir until the cheese is melted.
4. Serve warm.

NUTRITIONAL FACTS: Calories: 144 kcal Carbs: 4 g Fat: 8.5 g Protein: 13.2 g.

65. CHICKEN SOUP

PREPARATION: 10' **COOKING:** 25' **SERVES:** 6

INGREDIENTS

- 4 cups roasted chicken, shredded (Lunch Recipes: Roasted Lemon Chicken Sandwich)
- 2 tablespoons. butter
- 2 celery stalks, chopped
- 1 cup mushrooms, sliced
- 4 cups green cabbage, sliced into strips
- 2 garlic cloves, minced
- 6 cups chicken broth
- 1 carrot, sliced
- Salt and pepper to taste
- 1 tablespoon. garlic powder
- 1 tablespoon. onion powder

DIRECTIONS

1. Sauté the celery, mushrooms and garlic in the butter in a pot over medium heat for 4 minutes.
2. Add broth, carrots, garlic powder, onion powder, salt, and pepper.
3. Simmer for 10 minutes or until the vegetables are tender.
4. Add the chicken and cabbage and simmer for another 10 minutes or until the cabbage is tender.
5. Serve warm.
6. Can be refrigerated for up to 3 days or frozen for up to 1 month.

NUTRITIONAL FACTS: Calories: 279 kcal Carbs: 7.5 g Fat: 12.3 g Protein: 33.4 g.

66. CHICKEN AVOCADO SALAD

PREPARATION: 7' **COOKING:** 10' **SERVES:** 4

INGREDIENTS

- 1 cup roasted chicken, shredded (Lunch Recipes: Roasted Lemon Chicken Sandwich)
- 1 bacon strip, cooked and chopped
- 1/2 medium avocado, chopped
- ¼ cup cheddar cheese, grated
- 1 hard-boiled egg, chopped
- 1 cup romaine lettuce, chopped
- 1 tablespoon. olive oil
- 1 tablespoon. apple cider vinegar
- Salt and pepper to taste

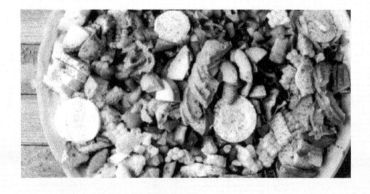

DIRECTIONS

1. Create the dressing by mixing apple cider vinegar, oil, salt and pepper.
2. Combine all the other ingredients in a mixing bowl.
3. Drizzle with the dressing and toss.
4. Can be refrigerated for up to 3 days.

NUTRITIONAL FACTS: Calories: 220 kcal Carbs: 2.8 g Fat: 16.7 gProtein: 14.8 g.

67. CHICKEN BROCCOLI DINNER

PREPARATION: 10' **COOKING:** 5' **SERVES:** 1

INGREDIENTS

- 1 roasted chicken leg (Lunch Recipes: Roasted Lemon Chicken Sandwich)
- ½ cup broccoli florets
- ½ tablespoon. unsalted butter, softened
- 2 garlic cloves, minced
- Salt and pepper to taste

DIRECTIONS

1. Boil the broccoli in lightly salted water for 5 minutes. Drain the water from the pot and keep the broccoli in the pot. Keep the lid on to keep the broccoli warm.
2. Mix all the butter, garlic, salt and pepper in a small bowl to create garlic butter.
3. Place the chicken, broccoli and garlic butter.

NUTRITIONAL FACTS: Calories: 257 kcal Carbs: 5.1 g Fat: 14 g Protein: 27.4 g.

68. EASY MEATBALLS

PREPARATION: 10' **COOKING:** 20' **SERVES:** 4

INGREDIENTS

- 1 lb. ground beef
- 1 egg, beaten
- Salt and pepper to taste
- 1 teaspoon garlic powder
- 1 teaspoon onion powder
- 2 tablespoons. butter
- ¼ cup mayonnaise
- ¼ cup pickled jalapeños
- 1 cup cheddar cheese, grated

DIRECTIONS

1. Combine the cheese, mayonnaise, pickled jalapenos, salt, pepper, garlic powder and onion powder in a large mixing bowl.
2. Add the beef and egg and combine using clean hands.
3. Form large meatballs. Makes about 12.
4. Fry the meatballs in the butter over medium heat for about 4 minutes on each side or until golden brown.
5. Serve warm with a keto-friendly side.
6. The meatball mixture can also be used to make a meatloaf. Just preheat your oven to 400 degrees F, press the mixture into a loaf pan and bake for about 30 minutes or until the top is golden brown.
7. Can be refrigerated for up to 5 days or frozen for up to 3 months.

NUTRITIONAL FACTS: Calories: 454 kcal Carbs: 5 g Fat: 28.2 g Protein: 43.2 g.

69. CHICKEN CASSEROLE

PREPARATION: 10' **COOKING:** 40' **SERVES:** 8

INGREDIENTS

- 1 lb. boneless chicken breasts, cut into 1" cubes
- 2 tablespoons. butter
- 4 tablespoons. green pesto
- 1 cup heavy whipping cream
- ¼ cup green bell peppers, diced
- 1 cup feta cheese, diced
- 1 garlic clove, minced
- Salt and pepper to taste

DIRECTIONS

1. Preheat your oven to 400 degrees F.
2. Season the chicken with salt and pepper then batch fry in the butter until golden brown.
3. Place the fried chicken pieces in a baking dish. Add the feta cheese, garlic and bell peppers.
4. Combine the pesto and heavy cream in a bowl. Pour on top of the chicken mixture and spread with a spatula.
5. Bake for 30 minutes or until the casserole is light brown around the edges.
6. Serve warm.
7. Can be refrigerated for up to 5 days and frozen for 2 weeks.

NUTRITIONAL FACTS: Calories: 294 kcal Carbs: 1.7 g Fat: 22.7 g Protein: 20.1 g.

70. LEMON BAKED SALMON

PREPARATION: 10' **COOKING:** 30' **SERVES:** 4

INGREDIENTS

- 1 lb. salmon
- 1 tablespoon. olive oil
- Salt and pepper to taste
- 1 tablespoon. butter
- 1 lemon, thinly sliced
- 1 tablespoon. lemon juice

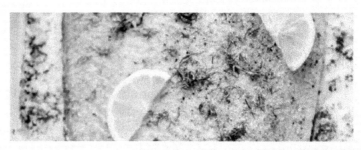

DIRECTIONS

1. Preheat your oven to 400 degrees F.
2. Grease a baking dish with the olive oil and place the salmon skin-side down.
3. Season the salmon with salt and pepper then top with the lemon slices.
4. Slice half the butter and place over the salmon.
5. Bake for 20minutes or until the salmon flakes easily.
6. Melt the remaining butter in a saucepan. When it starts to bubble, remove from heat and allow to cool before adding the lemon juice.
7. Drizzle the lemon butter over the salmon and Serve warm.

NUTRITIONAL FACTS: Calories: 211 kcal Carbs: 1.5 g Fat: 13.5 g Protein: 22.2 g.

71. ITALIAN SAUSAGE STACKS

PREPARATION: 10' COOKING: 25' SERVES: 3

INGREDIENTS

- 6 Italian sausage patties
- 4 tablespoon olive oil
- 2 ripe avocados, pitted
- 2 teaspoon fresh lime juice
- Salt and black pepper to taste
- 6 fresh eggs
- Red pepper flakes to garnish

DIRECTIONS

1. In a skillet, warm the oil over medium heat and fry the sausage patties about 8 minutes until lightly browned and firm. Remove the patties to a plate.
2. Spoon the avocado into a bowl, mash with the lime juice, and season with salt and black pepper. Spread the mash on the sausages.
3. Boil 3 cups of water in a wide pan over high heat, and reduce to simmer (don't boil).
4. Crack each egg into a small bowl and gently put the egg into the simmering water; poach for 2 to 3 minutes. Use a perforated spoon to remove from the water on a paper towel to dry. Repeat with the other 5 eggs. Top each stack with a poached egg, sprinkle with chili flakes, salt, black pepper, and chives. Serve with turnip wedges.

NUTRITIONAL FACTS: Kcal 378, Fat 23g, Net Carbs 5g, Protein 16g

72. BAKED SALMON

PREPARATION: 10' COOKING: 10' SERVES: 4

INGREDIENTS

- Cooking spray
- 3 cloves garlic, minced
- ¼ cup butter
- 1 teaspoon lemon zest
- 2 tablespoons lemon juice
- 4 salmon fillets
- Salt and pepper to taste
- 2 tablespoons parsley, chopped

DIRECTIONS

1. Preheat your oven to 425 degrees F.
2. Grease the pan with cooking spray.
3. In a bowl, mix the garlic, butter, and lemon zest and lemon juice.
4. Sprinkle salt and pepper on salmon fillets.
5. Drizzle with the lemon butter sauce.
6. Bake in the oven for 12 minutes.
7. Garnish with parsley before serving.

NUTRITIONAL FACTS: Calories 345 Total Fat 22.7g Saturated Fat 8.9g Cholesterol 109mg Sodium 163mg Total Carbohydrate 1.2g Dietary Fiber 0.2g Total Sugars 0.2g Protein 34.9g Potassium 718mg

73. TUNA PATTIES

PREPARATION: 10' COOKING: 10' SERVES: 8

INGREDIENTS
- 20 oz. canned tuna flakes
- ¼ cup almond flour
- 1 egg, beaten
- 2 tablespoons fresh dill, chopped
- 2 stalks green onion, chopped
- Salt and pepper to taste
- 1 tablespoon lemon zest
- ¼ cup mayonnaise
- 1 tablespoon lemon juice
- 2 tablespoons avocado oil

DIRECTIONS
1. Combine all the ingredients except avocado oil, lemon juice and avocado oil in a large bowl.
2. Form 8 patties from the mixture.
3. In a pan over medium heat, add the oil.
4. Once the oil starts to sizzle, cook the tuna patties for 3 to 4 minutes per side.
5. Drain each patty on a paper towel.
6. Spread mayo on top and drizzle with lemon juice before serving.

NUTRITIONAL FACTS: Calories 101 Total Fat 4.9g Saturated Fat 1.2g Cholesterol 47mg Sodium 243mg Total Carbohydrate 3.1g Dietary Fiber 0.5g Total Sugars 0.7g Protein 12.3g Potassium 60mg

74. CAULIFLOWER MASH

PREPARATION: 10' COOKING: 5' SERVES: 8

INGREDIENTS
- 4 cups cauliflower florets, chopped
- 1 cup grated parmesan cheese
- 6 tablespoons. butter
- ½ lemon, juice and zest
- Salt and pepper to taste

DIRECTIONS
1. Boil the cauliflower in lightly salted water over high heat for 5 minutes or until the florets are tender but still firm.
2. Strain the cauliflower in a colander and add the cauliflower to a food processor
3. Add the remaining ingredients and pulse the mixture to a smooth and creamy consistency
4. Serve with protein like salmon, chicken or meatballs.
5. Can be refrigerated for up to 3 days.

NUTRITIONAL FACTS: Calories: 101 kcal Carbs: 3.1 g Fat: 9.5 g Protein: 2.2 g.

75. ALMOND WAFFLES WITH CINNAMON CREAM

PREPARATION: 10' **COOKING:** 25' **SERVES:** 3

INGREDIENTS

For the Spread
- 8 oz. cream cheese, at room temperature
- 1 teaspoon cinnamon powder
- 3 tablespoon swerve brown sugar
- Cinnamon powder for garnishing

For the Waffles
- 5 tablespoon melted butter
- 1 ½ cups unsweetened almond milk
- 7 large eggs
- ¼ teaspoon liquid stevia
- ½ teaspoon baking powder
- 1 ½ cups almond flour

DIRECTIONS

1. Combine the cream cheese, cinnamon, and swerve with a hand mixer until smooth. Cover and chill until ready to use.
2. To make the waffles, whisk the butter, milk, and eggs in a medium bowl. Add the stevia and baking powder and mix. Stir in the almond flour and combine until no lumps exist. Let the batter sit for 5 minutes to thicken. Spritz a waffle iron with a non-stick cooking spray.
3. Ladle a ¼ cup of the batter into the waffle iron and cook according to the manufacturer's instructions until golden, about 10 minutes in total. Repeat with the remaining batter.
4. Slice the waffles into quarters; apply the cinnamon spread in between each of two waffles and snap. Sprinkle with cinnamon powder and serve.

NUTRITIONAL FACTS: Kcal 307, Fat 24g, Net Carbs 8g, Protein 12g

76. GRILLED MAHI WITH LEMON BUTTER SAUCE

PREPARATION: 20' **COOKING:** 10' **SERVES:** 6

INGREDIENTS

- 6 mahi fillets
- Salt and pepper to taste
- 2 tablespoons olive oil
- 6 tablespoons butter
- ¼ onion, minced
- ½ teaspoon garlic, minced
- ¼ cup chicken stock
- 1 tablespoon lemon juice

DIRECTIONS

1. Preheat your grill to medium heat.
2. Season fish fillets with salt and pepper.
3. Coat both sides with olive oil.
4. Grill for 3 to 4 minutes per side.
5. Place fish on a serving platter.
6. In a pan over medium heat, add the butter and let it melt.
7. Add the onion and sauté for 2 minutes.
8. Add the garlic and cook for 30 seconds.
9. Pour in the chicken stock.
10. Simmer until the stock has been reduced to half.
11. Add the lemon juice.
12. Pour the sauce over the grilled fish fillets.

NUTRITIONAL FACTS: Calories 234 Total Fat 17.2g Saturated Fat 8.3g Cholesterol 117mg Sodium 242mg Total Carbohydrate 0.6g Dietary Fiber 0.1g Total Sugars 0.3g Protein 19.1g Potassium 385mg

77. SHRIMP SCAMPI

PREPARATION: 15' **COOKING:** 10' **SERVES:** 6

INGREDIENTS

- 2 tablespoons olive oil
- 2 tablespoons butter
- 1 tablespoon garlic, minced
- ½ cup dry white wine
- ¼ teaspoon red pepper flakes
- Salt and pepper to taste
- 2 lb. large shrimp, peeled and deveined
- ¼ cup fresh parsley, chopped
- 1 teaspoon lemon zest
- 2 tablespoons lemon juice
- 3 cups spaghetti squash, cooked

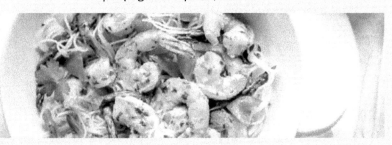

DIRECTIONS

1. In a pan over medium heat, add the oil and butter.
2. Cook the garlic for 2 minutes.
3. Pour in the wine.
4. Add the red pepper flakes, salt and pepper.
5. Cook for 2 minutes.
6. Add the shrimp.
7. Cook for 2 to 3 minutes.
8. Remove from the stove.
9. Add the parsley, lemon zest and lemon juice.
10. Serve on top of spaghetti squash.

NUTRITIONAL FACTS: Calories 232 Total Fat 8.9g Saturated Fat 3.2g Cholesterol 226mg Sodium 229mg Total Carbohydrate 7.6g Dietary Fiber 0.2g Total Sugars 0.3g Protein 28.9g Potassium 104mg

78. DARK CHOCOLATE SMOOTHIE

PREPARATION: 10' **COOKING:** 25' **SERVES:** 3

INGREDIENTS

- 8 pecans
- ¾ cup coconut milk
- ¼ cup water
- 1 ½ cups watercress
- 2 teaspoon vegan protein powder
- 1 tablespoon chia seeds
- 1 tablespoon unsweetened cocoa powder
- 4 fresh dates, pitted

DIRECTIONS

1. In a blender, add all ingredients and process until creamy and uniform. Place into two glasses and chill before serving.

NUTRITIONAL FACTS: Kcal 335; Fat: 31.7g Net Carbs: 12.7g, Protein: 7g

79. FIVE GREENS SMOOTHIE

PREPARATION: 10'   **COOKING:** 25'   **SERVES:** 3

INGREDIENTS

- 6 kale leaves, chopped
- 3 stalks celery, chopped
- 1 ripe avocado, skinned, pitted, sliced
- 1 cup ice cubes
- 2 cups spinach, chopped
- 1 large cucumber, peeled and chopped
- Chia seeds to garnish

DIRECTIONS

1. In a blender, add the kale, celery, avocado, and ice cubes, and blend for 45 seconds. Add the spinach and cucumber, and process for another 45 seconds until smooth.
2. Pour the smoothie into glasses, garnish with chia seeds and serve the drink immediately.

NUTRITIONAL FACTS: Kcal 124, Fat 7.8g, Net Carbs 2.9g, Protein 3.2g

80. SMOKED SALMON ROLLS WITH DILL CREAM CHEESE

PREPARATION: 10'   **COOKING:** 25'   **SERVES:** 3

INGREDIENTS

- 3 tablespoon cream cheese, softened
- 1 small lemon, zested and juiced
- 3 teaspoon chopped fresh dill
- Salt and black pepper to taste
- 3 (7-inch) low carb tortillas
- 6 slices smoked salmon

DIRECTIONS

1. In a bowl, mix the cream cheese, lemon juice, zest, dill, salt, and black pepper.
2. Lay each tortilla on a plastic wrap (just wide enough to cover the tortilla), spread with cream cheese mixture, and top each (one) with two salmon slices. Roll up the tortillas and secure both ends by twisting.
3. Refrigerate for 2 hours, remove plastic, cut off both ends of each wrap, and cut wraps into wheels.

NUTRITIONAL FACTS: Kcal 250, Fat 16g, Net Carbs 7g, Protein 18g

81. PAN-SEARED HALIBUT WITH CITRUS BUTTER SAUCE

PREPARATION: 10' **COOKING:** 15' **SERVES:** 3

INGREDIENTS

- 4 (5-ounce) halibut fillets, each about 1 inch thick
- Sea salt
- Freshly ground black pepper
- ¼ cup butter
- 2 teaspoons minced garlic
- 1 shallot, minced
- 3 tablespoons dry white wine
- 1 tablespoon freshly squeezed lemon juice
- 1 tablespoon freshly squeezed orange juice
- 2 teaspoons chopped fresh parsley
- 2 tablespoons olive oil

DIRECTIONS

1. Pat the fish dry with paper towels and then lightly season the fillets with salt and pepper. Set aside on a paper towel–lined plate.
2. Place a small saucepan over medium heat and melt the butter.
3. Sauté the garlic and shallot until tender, about 3 minutes.
4. Whisk in the white wine, lemon juice, and orange juice and bring the sauce to a simmer, cooking until it thickens slightly, about 2 minutes.
5. Remove the sauce from the heat and stir in the parsley; set aside.
6. Place a large skillet over medium-high heat and add the olive oil.
7. Panfry the fish until lightly browned and just cooked through, turning them over once, about 10 minutes in total.
8. Serve the fish immediately with a spoonful of sauce for each.

NUTRITIONAL FACTS: Calories: 319 Fat: 26g Protein: 22g Carbohydrates: 2g Fiber: 0g

82. LEMON BUTTER CHICKEN

PREPARATION: 10' **COOKING:** 40' **SERVES:** 4

INGREDIENTS

- 4 bone-in, skin-on chicken thighs
- Sea salt
- Freshly ground black pepper
- 2 tablespoons butter, divided
- 2 teaspoons minced garlic
- ½ cup Herbed Chicken Stock
- ½ cup heavy (whipping) cream
- Juice of ½ lemon

DIRECTIONS

1. Preheat the oven to 400°F.
2. Lightly season the chicken thighs with salt and pepper.
3. Place a large ovenproof skillet over medium-high heat and add 1 tablespoon of butter.
4. Brown the chicken thighs until golden on both sides, about 6 minutes in total. Remove the thighs to a plate and set aside.
5. Add the remaining 1 tablespoon of butter and sauté the garlic until translucent, about 2 minutes.
6. Whisk in the chicken stock, heavy cream, and lemon juice.
7. Bring the sauce to a boil and then return the chicken to the skillet.
8. Place the skillet in the oven, covered, and braise until the chicken is cooked through, about 30 minutes.

NUTRITIONAL FACTS: Calories: 294 Fat: 26g Protein: 12g Carbohydrates: 4g Fiber: 1g

83. SIMPLE FISH CURRY

PREPARATION: 10' **COOKING:** 25' **SERVES:** 4

INGREDIENTS

- 2 tablespoons coconut oil
- 1½ tablespoons grated fresh ginger
- 2 teaspoons minced garlic
- 1 tablespoon curry powder
- ½ teaspoon ground cumin
- 2 cups coconut milk
- 16 ounces firm white fish, cut into 1-inch chunks
- 1 cup shredded kale
- 2 tablespoons chopped cilantro

DIRECTIONS

1. Place a large saucepan over medium heat and melt the coconut oil.
2. Sauté the ginger and garlic until lightly browned, about 2 minutes.
3. Stir in the curry powder and cumin and sauté until very fragrant, about 2 minutes.
4. Stir in the coconut milk and bring the liquid to a boil.
5. Reduce the heat to low and simmer for about 5 minutes to infuse the milk with the spices.
6. Add the fish and cook until the fish is cooked through, about 10 minutes.
7. Stir in the kale and cilantro and simmer until wilted, about 2 minutes.
8. Serve.

NUTRITIONAL FACTS: Calories: 416 Fat: 31g Protein: 26g Carbohydrates: 5g Fiber: 1g]

84. ROASTED SALMON WITH AVOCADO SALSA

PREPARATION: 15' **COOKING:** 12' **SERVES:** 4

INGREDIENTS

For the Salsa
- 1 avocado, peeled, pitted, and diced
- 1 scallion, white and green parts, chopped
- ½ cup halved cherry tomatoes
- Juice of 1 lemon
- Zest of 1 lemon

For the Fish
- 1 teaspoon ground cumin
- ½ teaspoon ground coriander
- ½ teaspoon onion powder
- ¼ teaspoon sea salt
- Pinch freshly ground black pepper
- Pinch cayenne pepper
- 4 (4-ounce) boneless, skinless salmon fillets
- 2 tablespoons olive oil

DIRECTIONS

To Make the Salsa

1. In a small bowl, stir together the avocado, scallion, tomatoes, lemon juice, and lemon zest until mixed.
2. Set aside.

To Make the Fish

3. Preheat the oven to 400°F. Line a baking sheet with aluminum foil and set aside.
4. In a small bowl, stir together the cumin, coriander, onion powder, salt, black pepper, and cayenne until well mixed.
5. Rub the salmon fillets with the spice mix and place them on the baking sheet.
6. Drizzle the fillets with the olive oil and roast the fish until it is just cooked through, about 15 minutes.
7. Serve the salmon topped with the avocado salsa.

NUTRITIONAL FACTS: Calories: 320 Fat: 26g Protein: 22g Carbohydrates: 4g Fiber: 3g

85. SOLE ASIAGO

PREPARATION: 10' **COOKING:** 8' **SERVES:** 4

INGREDIENTS
- 4 (4-ounce) sole fillets
- ¾ cup ground almonds
- ¼ cup Asiago cheese
- 2 eggs, beaten
- 2½ tablespoons melted coconut oil

DIRECTIONS
1. Preheat the oven to 350°F. Line a baking sheet with parchment paper and set aside.
2. Pat the fish dry with paper towels.
3. Stir together the ground almonds and cheese in a small bowl.
4. Place the bowl with the beaten eggs in it next to the almond mixture.
5. Dredge a sole fillet in the beaten egg and then press the fish into the almond mixture so it is completely coated. Place on the baking sheet and repeat until all the fillets are breaded.
6. Brush both sides of each piece of fish with the coconut oil.
7. Bake the sole until it is cooked through, about 8 minutes in total.
8. Serve immediately.

NUTRITIONAL FACTS: Calories: 406 Fat: 31g Protein: 29g Carbohydrates: 6 g Fiber: 3g

86. BAKED COCONUT HADDOCK

PREPARATION: 10' **COOKING:** 12' **SERVES:** 4

INGREDIENTS
- 4 (5-ounce) boneless haddock fillets
- Sea salt
- Freshly ground black pepper
- 1 cup shredded unsweetened coconut
- ¼ cup ground hazelnuts
- 2 tablespoons coconut oil, melted

DIRECTIONS
1. Preheat the oven to 400°F. Line a baking sheet with parchment paper and set aside.
2. Pat the fillets very dry with paper towels and lightly season them with salt and pepper.
3. Stir together the shredded coconut and hazelnuts in a small bowl.
4. Dredge the fish fillets in the coconut mixture so that both sides of each piece are thickly coated.
5. Place the fish on the baking sheet and lightly brush both sides of each piece with the coconut oil.
6. Bake the haddock until the topping is golden and the fish flakes easily with a fork, about 12 minutes total.
7. Serve.

PREP TIP the breading of the fish can be done ahead, up to 1 day, if you just want to pop the fish in the oven when you get home. Place the breaded fish on the baking sheet and cover it with plastic wrap in the refrigerator until you wish to bake it.

NUTRITIONAL FACTS: Calories: 299 Fat: 24g Protein: 20g Carbohydrates: 4g Fiber: 3g

87. CHEESY GARLIC SALMON

PREPARATION: 15'   **COOKING:** 12'   **SERVES:** 4

INGREDIENTS

- ½ cup Asiago cheese
- 2 tablespoons freshly squeezed lemon juice
- 2 tablespoons butter, at room temperature
- 2 teaspoons minced garlic
- 1 teaspoon chopped fresh basil
- 1 teaspoon chopped fresh oregano
- 4 (5-ounce) salmon fillets
- 1 tablespoon olive oil

DIRECTIONS

1. Preheat the oven to 350°F. Line a baking sheet with parchment paper and set aside.
2. In a small bowl, stir together the Asiago cheese, lemon juice, butter, garlic, basil, and oregano.
3. Pat the salmon dry with paper towels and place the fillets on the baking sheet skin-side down. Divide the topping evenly between the fillets and spread it across the fish using a knife or the back of a spoon.
4. Drizzle the fish with the olive oil and bake until the topping is golden and the fish is just cooked through, about 12 minutes.
5. Serve.

NUTRITIONAL FACTS: Calories: 357 Fat: 28g Protein: 24g Carbohydrates: 2g Fiber: 0g

88. CHICKEN BACON BURGERS

PREPARATION: 10'   **COOKING:** 25'   **SERVES:** 4

INGREDIENTS

- 1-pound ground chicken
- 8 bacon slices, chopped
- ¼ cup ground almonds
- 1 teaspoon chopped fresh basil
- ¼ teaspoon sea salt
- Pinch freshly ground black pepper
- 2 tablespoons coconut oil
- 4 large lettuce leaves
- 1 avocado, peeled, pitted, and sliced

DIRECTIONS

1. Preheat the oven to 350°F. Line a baking sheet with parchment paper and set aside.
2. In a medium bowl, combine the chicken, bacon, ground almonds, basil, salt, and pepper until well mixed.
3. Form the mixture into 6 equal patties.
4. Place a large skillet over medium-high heat and add the coconut oil.
5. Pan sear the chicken patties until brown on both sides, about 6 minutes in total.
6. Place the browned patties on the baking sheet and bake until completely cooked through, about 15 minutes.
7. Serve on the lettuce leaves, topped with the avocado slices.

NUTRITIONAL FACTS: Calories: 374 Fat: 33g Protein: 18g Carbohydrates: 3g Fiber: 2g

89. HERB BUTTER SCALLOPS

PREPARATION: 10' **COOKING:** 10' **SERVES:** 3

INGREDIENTS

- 1 pound sea scallops, cleaned
- Freshly ground black pepper
- 8 tablespoons butter, divided
- 2 teaspoons minced garlic
- Juice of 1 lemon
- 2 teaspoons chopped fresh basil
- 1 teaspoon chopped fresh thyme

DIRECTIONS

1. Pat the scallops dry with paper towels and season them lightly with pepper.
2. Place a large skillet over medium heat and add 2 tablespoons of butter.
3. Arrange the scallops in the skillet, evenly spaced but not too close together, and sear each side until they are golden brown, about 2½ minutes per side.
4. Remove the scallops to a plate and set aside.
5. Add the remaining 6 tablespoons of butter to the skillet and sauté the garlic until translucent, about 3 minutes.
6. Stir in the lemon juice, basil, and thyme and return the scallops to the skillet, turning to coat them in the sauce.
7. Serve immediately.

NUTRITIONAL FACTS: Calories: 306 Fat: 24g Protein: 19g Carbohydrates: 4g Fiber: 0g

90. PAPRIKA CHICKEN

PREPARATION: 10' **COOKING:** 25' **SERVES:** 4

INGREDIENTS

- 4 (4-ounce) chicken breasts, skin-on
- Sea salt
- Freshly ground black pepper
- 1 tablespoon olive oil
- ½ cup chopped sweet onion
- ½ cup heavy (whipping) cream
- 2 teaspoons smoked paprika
- ½ cup sour cream
- 2 tablespoons chopped fresh parsley

DIRECTIONS

1. Lightly season the chicken with salt and pepper.
2. Place a large skillet over medium-high heat and add the olive oil.
3. Sear the chicken on both sides until almost cooked through, about 15 minutes in total. Remove the chicken to a plate.
4. Add the onion to the skillet and sauté until tender, about 4 minutes.
5. Stir in the cream and paprika and bring the liquid to a simmer.
6. Return the chicken and any accumulated juices to the skillet and simmer the chicken for 5 minutes until completely cooked.
7. Stir in the sour cream and remove the skillet from the heat.
8. Serve topped with the parsley.

NUTRITIONAL FACTS: Calories: 389 Fat: 30g Protein: 25g Carbohydrates: 4g Fiber: 0g

91. TROUT AND CHILI NUTS

PREPARATION: 10' **COOKING:** 0' **SERVES:** 3

INGREDIENTS
- 1.5kg of rainbow trout
- 300gr shelled walnuts
- 1 bunch of parsley
- 9 cloves of garlic
- 7 tablespoons of olive oil
- 2 fresh hot peppers
- The juice of 2 lemons
- Halls

DIRECTIONS
1. Clean and dry the trout then place them in a baking tray.
2. Chop the walnuts, parsley and chili peppers then mash the garlic cloves.
3. Mix the ingredients by adding olive oil, lemon juice and a pinch of salt.
4. Stuff the trout with some of the sauce and use the rest to cover the fish.
5. Bake at 180° for 30/40 minutes.
6. Serve the trout hot or cold.

NUTRITIONAL FACTS: Calories 226 Fat 5 Fiber 2 Carbs 7 Protein 8

92. NUT GRANOLA & SMOOTHIE BOWL

PREPARATION: 10' **COOKING:** 40' **SERVES:** 3

INGREDIENTS
- 6 cups Greek yogurt
- 4 tablespoon almond butter
- A handful toasted walnuts
- 3 tablespoon unsweetened cocoa powder
- 4 teaspoon swerve brown sugar
- 2 cups nut granola for topping

DIRECTIONS
1. Combine the Greek yogurt, almond butter, walnuts, cocoa powder, and swerve brown sugar in a smoothie maker; puree in high-speed until smooth and well mixed.
2. Share the smoothie into four breakfast bowls, top with a half cup of granola each, and serve.

NUTRITIONAL FACTS: Kcal 361, Fat 31.2g, Net Carbs 2g, Protein 13g

93. BACON AND EGG QUESADILLAS

PREPARATION: 10' **COOKING:** 30' **SERVES:** 3

INGREDIENTS

- 8 low carb tortilla shells
- 6 eggs
- 1 cup water
- 3 tablespoon butter
- 1 ½ cups grated cheddar cheese
- 1 ½ cups grated Swiss cheese
- 5 bacon slices
- 1 medium onion, thinly sliced
- 1 tablespoon chopped parsley

DIRECTIONS

1. Bring the eggs to a boil in water over medium heat for 10 minutes. Transfer the eggs to an ice water bath, peel the shells, and chop them; set aside.
2. Meanwhile, as the eggs cook, fry the bacon in a skillet over medium heat for 4 minutes until crispy. Remove and chop. Plate and set aside too.
3. Fetch out 2/3 of the bacon fat and sauté the onions in the remaining grease over medium heat for 2 minutes; set aside. Melt 1 tablespoon of butter in a skillet over medium heat.
4. Lay one tortilla in a skillet; sprinkle with some Swiss cheese. Add some chopped eggs and bacon over the cheese, top with onion, and sprinkle with some cheddar cheese. Cover with another tortilla shell. Cook for 45 seconds, then carefully flip the quesadilla, and cook the other side too for 45 seconds. Remove to a plate and repeat the cooking process using the remaining tortilla shells.
5. Garnish with parsley and serve warm.

NUTRITIONAL FACTS: Kcal 449, Fat 48.7g, Net Carbs 6.8g, Protein 29.1g

94. BACON AND CHEESE FRITTATA

PREPARATION: 10' **COOKING:** 20' **SERVES:** 3

INGREDIENTS

- 10 slices bacon
- 10 fresh eggs
- 3 tablespoon butter, melted
- ½ cup almond milk
- Salt and black pepper to taste
- 1 ½ cups cheddar cheese, shredded
- ¼ cup chopped green onions

DIRECTIONS

1. Preheat the oven to 400°F and grease a baking dish with cooking spray. Cook the bacon in a skillet over medium heat for 6 minutes. Once crispy, remove from the skillet to paper towels and discard grease. Chop into small pieces. Whisk the eggs, butter, milk, salt, and black pepper. Mix in the bacon and pour the mixture into the baking dish.
2. Sprinkle with cheddar cheese and green onions, and bake in the oven for 10 minutes or until the eggs are thoroughly cooked. Remove and cool the frittata for 3 minutes, slice into wedges, and serve warm with a dollop of Greek yogurt.
3.

NUTRITIONAL FACTS: Kcal 325, Fat 28g, Net Carbs 2g, Protein 15g

95. SPICY EGG MUFFINS WITH BACON & CHEESE

PREPARATION: 10' **COOKING:** 20' **SERVES:** 3

INGREDIENTS

- 12 eggs
- ¼ cup coconut milk
- Salt and black pepper to taste
- 1 cup grated cheddar cheese
- 12 slices bacon
- 4 jalapeño peppers, seeded and minced

DIRECTIONS

1. Preheat oven to 370°F.
2. Crack the eggs into a bowl and whisk with coconut milk until combined. Season with salt and pepper, and evenly stir in the cheddar cheese.
3. Line each hole of a muffin tin with a slice of bacon and fill each with the egg mixture two-thirds way up. Top with the jalapeno peppers and bake in the oven for 18 to 20 minutes or until puffed and golden. Remove, allow cooling for a few minutes, and serve with arugula salad.

NUTRITIONAL FACTS: Kcal 302, Fat 23.7g, Net Carbs 3.2g, Protein 20g

96. HAM & EGG BROCCOLI BAKE

PREPARATION: 10' **COOKING:** 25' **SERVES:** 3

INGREDIENTS

- 2 heads broccoli, cut into small florets
- 2 red bell peppers, seeded and chopped
- ¼ cup chopped ham
- 2 teaspoon ghee
- 1 teaspoon dried oregano + extra to garnish
- Salt and black pepper to taste
- 8 fresh eggs

DIRECTIONS

1. Preheat oven to 425°F.
2. Melt the ghee in a frying pan over medium heat; brown the ham, stirring frequently, about 3 minutes.
3. Arrange the broccoli, bell peppers, and ham on a foil-lined baking sheet in a single layer, toss to combine; season with salt, oregano, and black pepper. Bake for 10 minutes until the vegetables have softened.
4. Remove, create eight indentations with a spoon, and crack an egg into each. Return to the oven and continue to bake for an additional 5 to 7 minutes until the egg whites are firm.
5. Season with salt, black pepper, and extra oregano, share the bake into four plates and serve with strawberry lemonade (optional).

NUTRITIONAL FACTS: Kcal 344, Fat 28g, Net Carbs 4.2g, Protein 11g

97. HOT BUFFALO WINGS

PREPARATION: 10' COOKING: 47' SERVES: 3

INGREDIENTS

- Hot sauce ¼ cup
- Coconut oil 4 tablespoons, plus more for rubbing on the wings
- Chicken wings 12 (fresh or frozen)
- Garlic 1 clove, minced
- Salt ¼ teaspoon
- Paprika ¼ teaspoon
- Cayenne pepper ¼ teaspoon
- Ground black pepper 1 dash

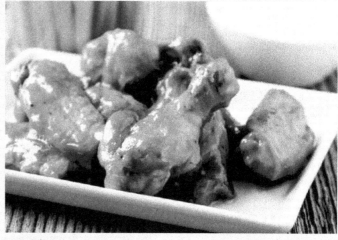

DIRECTIONS

1. Preheat your oven to 400 degrees F (200 degrees C).
2. Evenly spread chicken wings on a wire rack placed on a baking dish (it will save wings to become soggy on the bottom).
3. Rub each chicken wing with olive oil and season with salt and pepper, then bake for 45 minutes, or until crispy.
4. Meanwhile, in a saucepan combine coconut oil and garlic and cook over medium heat for 1 minute, or until fragrant.
5. Remove from heat and stir in hot sauce, salt, paprika, cayenne pepper and black pepper.
6. Remove wings from the oven and transfer to a large bowl.
7. Pour hot sauce mixture over wings and toss until each wing is coated with the sauce.
8. Serve immediately.

NUTRITIONAL FACTS: Calories: 391 Carbohydrates: 1 g Fats: 33 g Protein: 31 g

98. TURKEY MEATBALLS

PREPARATION: 30' COOKING: 0' SERVES: 4

INGREDIENTS

- 255g turkey sausage
- 2 tablespoons of extra virgin olive oil
- One can of 425g chickpeas, rinsed and drained…
- 1/2 medium onion, chopped, 2/3 cup
- 2 cloves of garlic, finely chopped
- 1 teaspoon of cumin
- 1/2 cup flour
- 1/2 teaspoon instant yeast for desserts
- Salt and ground black pepper
- 1 cup of Greek yogurt
- 2 tablespoons of lime juice
- 2 radicchio hearts, chopped
- Hot sauce

DIRECTIONS

1. Preheat the oven to 200°C.
2. In a processor, blend the chickpeas, onion, garlic, cumin, 1 teaspoon salt and 1/2 teaspoon pepper until all the ingredients are finely chopped. Add the flour, baking powder and blend to make everything mix well. Transfer to a medium bowl and add the sausage, stirring together with your hands. Cover and refrigerate for 30 minutes.
3. Once cold, take the mixture in spoonful, forming 1-inch balls with wet hands. Heat the olive oil in a pan over medium heat. In two groups, put the falafel in the pan and cook until slightly brown, about a minute and a half per side. Transfer to a baking tray and bake in the oven until well cooked, for about 10 minutes.
4. Mix together the yogurt, lime juice, 1/2 teaspoon salt and 1/4 teaspoon pepper. Divide the lettuce into 4 plates, season with some yogurt sauce.

NUTRITIONAL FACTS: Calories 189 Fat 5 Protein 77 Sugar 3

99. CHICKEN IN SWEET AND SOUR SAUCE WITH CORN SALAD

PREPARATION: 10'   **COOKING:** 15'   **SERVES:** 4

INGREDIENTS

- 2 cups plus 2 tablespoons of unflavored low-fat yoghurt
- 2 cups of frozen mango chunks
- 3 tablespoons of honey
- ¼ cup plus 1 tablespoon apple cider vinegar
- ¼ cup sultana
- 2 tablespoons of olive oil, plus an amount to be brushed
- ¼ teaspoon of cayenne pepper
- 5 dried tomatoes (not in oil)
- 2 small cloves of garlic, finely chopped
- 4 cobs, peeled
- 8 peeled and boned chicken legs, peeled (about 700g)
- Halls
- 6 cups of mixed salad
- 2 medium carrots, finely sliced

DIRECTIONS

1. For the smoothie: in a blender, mix 2 cups of yogurt, 2 cups of ice, 1 cup of mango and all the honey until the mixture becomes completely smooth. Divide into 4 glasses and refrigerate until ready to use. Rinse the blender.
2. Preheat the grill to medium-high heat. Mix the remaining cup of mango, ¼ cup water, ¼ cup vinegar, sultanas, olive oil, cayenne pepper, tomatoes and garlic in a microwave bowl. Cover with a piece of clear film and cook in the microwave until the tomatoes become soft, for about 3 minutes. Leave to cool slightly and pass in a blender. Transfer to a small bowl. Leave 2 tablespoons aside to garnish, turn the chicken into the remaining mixture.
3. Put the corn on the grill, cover and bake, turning it over if necessary, until it is burnt, about 10 minutes. Remove and keep warm.
4. Brush the grill over medium heat and brush the grills with a little oil. Turn the chicken legs into half the remaining sauce and ½ teaspoon of salt. Put on the grill and cook until the cooking marks appear and the internal temperature reaches 75°C on an instantaneous thermometer, 8 to 10 minutes per side. Bart and sprinkle a few times with the remaining sauce while cooking.
5. While the chicken is cooking, beat the remaining 2 tablespoons of yogurt, the 2 tablespoons of sauce set aside, the remaining spoonful of vinegar, 1 tablespoon of water and ¼ teaspoon of salt in a large bowl. Mix the mixed salad with the carrots. Divide chicken, corn and salad into 4 serving dishes. Garnish the salad with the dressing set aside. Serve each plate with a mango smoothie.

NUTRITIONAL FACTS: Calories 346 Protein 56 Fat 45

100. CHINESE CHICKEN SALAD

PREPARATION: 15'   COOKING: 30'   SERVES: 4

INGREDIENTS

For the chicken salad:
- 4 divided chicken breasts with skin and bones
- Olive oil of excellent quality
- Salt and freshly ground black pepper
- 500 g asparagus, with the ends removed and cut into three parts diagonally
- 1 red pepper, peeled
- Chinese condiment, recipe to follow
- 2 spring onions (both the white and the green part), sliced diagonally
- 1 tablespoon of white sesame seeds, toasted

For Chinese dressing:
- 120 ml vegetable oil
- 60 ml of apple cider vinegar of excellent quality
- 60 ml soy sauce
- 1 ½ tablespoon of black sesame
- ½ tablespoon of honey
- 1 clove of garlic, minced
- ½ teaspoon of fresh peeled and grated ginger
- ½ tablespoon sesame seeds, toasted
- 60 g peanut butter
- 2 teaspoons of salt
- ½ teaspoons freshly ground black pepper

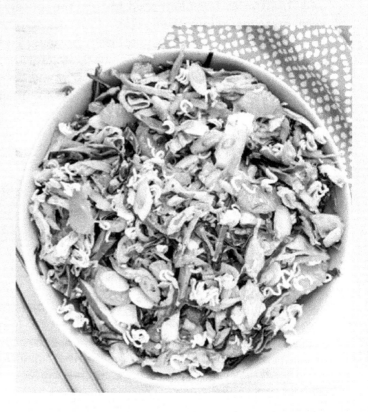

DIRECTIONS

For the chicken salad:
1. Heat the oven to 180°C (or 200°C for gas oven). Put the chicken breast on a baking tray and rub the skin with a little olive oil. Season freely with salt and pepper.
2. Brown for 35 to 40 minutes, until the chicken is freshly cooked. Let it cool down as long as it takes to handle it. Remove the meat from the bones, remove the skin and chop the chicken into medium-sized pieces.
3. Blanch the asparagus in a pot of salted water for 3-5 minutes until tender. Soak them in water with ice to stop cooking. Drain them. Cut the peppers into strips the same size as the asparagus. In a large bowl, mix the chopped chicken, asparagus and peppers.
4. Spread the Chinese dressing on chicken and vegetables. Add the spring onions and sesame seeds, and season to taste. Serve cold or at room temperature.

For Chinese dressing:
5. Mix all ingredients and set aside until use.

NUTRITIONAL FACTS: Calories 222 Protein 28 Fat 10 Sugar 6

101. CHICKEN SALAD

PREPARATION: 15' **COOKING:** 25' **SERVES:** 4

INGREDIENTS

For the Buffalo chicken salad:
- 2 chicken breasts (225 g) peeled, boned, cut in half
- 2 tablespoons of hot cayenne pepper sauce (or another type of hot sauce), plus an addition depending on taste
- 2 tablespoons of olive oil
- 2 romaine lettuce heart, cut into 2 cm strips
- 4 celery stalks, finely sliced
- 2 carrots, roughly grated
- 2 fresh onions, only the green part, sliced
- 125 ml of blue cheese dressing, recipe to follow

For the seasoning of blue cheese
- 2 tablespoons mayonnaise
- 70 ml of partially skimmed buttermilk
- 70 ml low-fat white yoghurt
- 1 tablespoon of wine vinegar
- ½ teaspoon of sugar
- 35 g of chopped blue cheese
- Salt and freshly ground black pepper

DIRECTIONS

For the Buffalo chicken salad:
1. Preheat the grid.
2. Place the chicken between 2 sheets of baking paper and beat it with a meat tenderizer so that it is about 2 cm thick, then cut the chicken sideways creating 1 cm strips.
3. In a large bowl, add the hot sauce and oil, add the chicken and turn it over until it is well soaked. Place the chicken on a baking tray and grill until well cooked, about 4-6 minutes, turning it once.
4. In a large bowl, add the lettuce, celery, grated carrots and fresh onions. Add the seasoning of blue cheese. Distribute the vegetables in 4 plates and arrange the chicken on each of the dishes. Serve with hot sauce on the side.

For the blue cheese dressing:
5. Cover a small bowl with absorbent paper folded in four. Spread the yoghurt on the paper and put it in the fridge for 20 minutes to drain and firm it.
6. In a medium bowl, beat the buttermilk and firm yogurt with mayonnaise until well blended. Add the vinegar and sugar and keep beating until well blended. Add the blue cheese and season with salt and pepper to taste.

NUTRITIONAL FACTS: 321 calories Fat 3 Fiber 5 Carbs 7 Protein 4

102. AVOCADO AND KALE EGGS

PREPARATION: 10' **COOKING:** 30' **SERVES:** 3

INGREDIENTS
- 1 teaspoon ghee
- 1 red onion, sliced
- 4 oz. chorizo, sliced into thin rounds
- 1 cup chopped kale
- 1 ripe avocado, pitted, peeled, chopped
- 4 eggs
- Salt and black pepper to season

DIRECTIONS
1. Preheat oven to 370°F.
2. Melt ghee in a cast iron pan over medium heat and sauté the onion for 2 minutes. Add the chorizo and cook for 2 minutes more, flipping once.
3. Introduce the kale in batches with a splash of water to wilt, season lightly with salt, stir and cook for 3 minutes. Mix in the avocado and turn the heat off.
4. Create four holes in the mixture, crack the eggs into each hole, sprinkle with salt and black pepper, and slide the pan into the preheated oven to bake for 6 minutes until the egg whites are set or firm and yolks still runny. Season to taste with salt and pepper, and serve right away with low carb toasts.

NUTRITIONAL FACTS: Kcal 274, Fat 23g, Net Carbs 4g, Protein 13g

103. TOFU MEAT AND SALAD

PREPARATION: 15'   **COOKING:** 20'   **SERVES:** 3

INGREDIENTS

- 1 tablespoon of garlic sauce and chili in a bottle
- 1 1/2 tablespoon sesame oil
- 3 tablespoons of low-sodium soy sauce
- 60 ml hoisin sauce
- 2 tablespoons rice vinegar
- 2 tablespoons of sherry or Chinese cooking wine
- 225 g of extra-solid tofu
- 2 teaspoons of rapeseed oil
- 2 tablespoons of finely chopped fresh ginger
- 4 spring onions, with the green part chopped and set aside, in thin slices
- 225 g of minced lean beef (90% or more lean)
- 25 g of diced Chinese water chestnuts
- 1 large head of cappuccino lettuce, with the leaves separated, but without the outer ones
- 1 red pepper, diced

DIRECTIONS

1. In a bowl, mix together the garlic and chili sauce, sesame oil, soy sauce, hoisin sauce, vinegar and sherry.
2. Cut the tofu into 1 cm thick slices and place them on a kitchen towel. Use the cloth to dab the tofu well to remove as much water as possible. Should take a couple of minutes and about three dish towels. Chop the dry tofu well and set aside.
3. Heat the oil in a wok or in a very large pan and medium flame. Add the ginger and the white part of the spring onions and cook until the spring onions become translucent and the ginger fragrant, for about 2-3 minutes. Add the beef and tofu and cook, stirring, until the meat becomes dull and freshly cooked, for about 4-5 minutes. Add the sauce set aside. Reduce the flame and simmer slowly, stirring, for another 3-4 minutes. Add the chestnuts and mix well to incorporate.
4. Fill each lettuce leaf with stuffing. Serve by decorating with the green part of the spring onions, red pepper and peanuts.

NUTRITIONAL FACTS: Calories 122 Fat 2 Protein 66

104 ASPARAGUS AND PISTACHIOS VINAIGRETTE

PREPARATION: 10'   **COOKING:** 5'   **SERVES:** 2

INGREDIENTS

- Two 455g bunches of large asparagus, without the tip
- 1 tablespoon of olive oil
- Salt and freshly ground black pepper
- 6 tablespoons of sliced pistachios blanched and boiled
- 1 1/2 tablespoon lemon juice
- 1/4 teaspoon of sugar
- 1 1/2 teaspoon lemon zest

DIRECTIONS

1. Preheat the oven to 220°C. Put the grill in the top third of the oven. Place the asparagus on a baking tray covered with baking paper. Sprinkle with olive oil and season with a little salt and pepper. Bake for 15 minutes, until soft.
2. Meanwhile, blend 5 tablespoons of almonds, lemon juice, sugar and 6 tablespoons of water for 1 minute until smooth. Taste and regulate salt. Pour the sauce on a plate and put the spinach on the sauce. Decorate with peel and the remaining spoon of pistachios

NUTRITIONAL FACTS: Calories 560 Fat 5 Fiber 2 Carbs 3 Protein 9

CHAPTER 11. DINNER

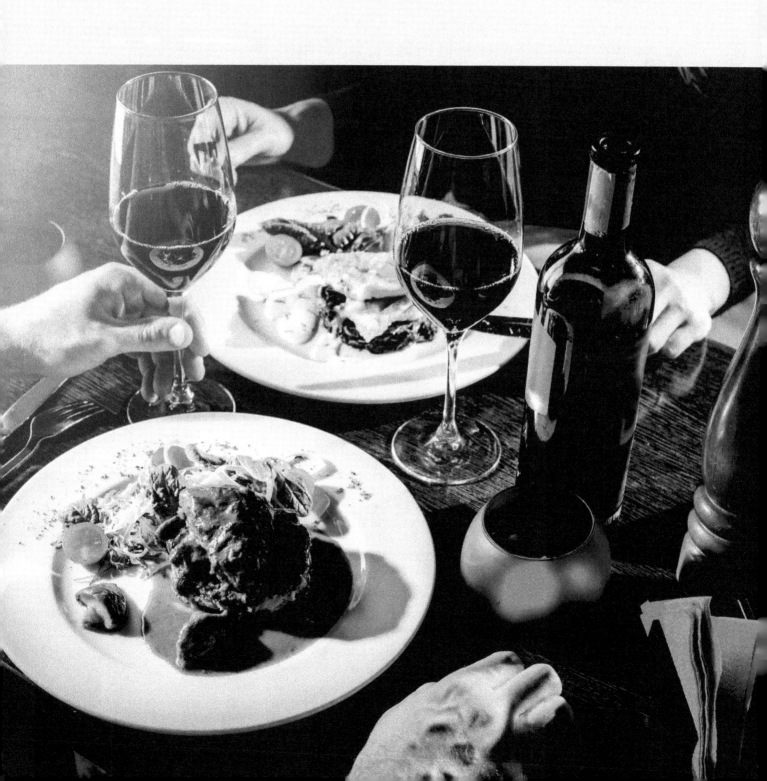

105. BEEF-STUFFED MUSHROOMS

PREPARATION: 20' **COOKING:** 25' **SERVES:** 4

INGREDIENTS

- 4 mushrooms, stemmed
- 3 tablespoons olive oil, divided
- 1 yellow onion, sliced thinly
- 1 red bell pepper, sliced into strips
- 1 green bell pepper, sliced into strips
- Salt and pepper to taste
- 8 oz. beef, sliced thinly
- 3 oz. provolone cheese, sliced
- Chopped parsley

DIRECTIONS

1. Preheat your oven to 350 degrees F.
2. Arrange the mushrooms on a baking pan.
3. Brush with oil.
4. Add the remaining oil to a pan over medium heat.
5. Cook onion and bell peppers for 5 minutes.
6. Season with salt and pepper.
7. Place onion mixture on a plate.
8. Cook the beef in the pan for 5 minutes.
9. Sprinkle with salt and pepper.
10. Add the onion mixture back to the pan.
11. Mix well.
12. Fill the mushrooms with the beef mixture and cheese.
13. Bake in the oven for 15 minutes.

NUTRITIONAL FACTS: Calories 333 Total Fat 20.3 g Saturated Fat 6.7 g Cholesterol 61 mg Sodium 378 mg Total Carbohydrate 8.2 g Dietary Fiber 3.7 g Protein 25.2 g   Total Sugars 7 g Potassium 789 mg

106. RIB ROAST

PREPARATION: 15' **COOKING:** 3H **SERVES:** 8

INGREDIENTS

- 1 rib roast
- Salt to taste
- 12 cloves garlic, chopped
- 2 teaspoons lemon zest
- 6 tablespoons fresh rosemary, chopped
- 5 sprigs thyme

DIRECTIONS

1. Preheat your oven to 325 degrees F.
2. Season all sides of rib roast with salt.
3. Place the rib roast in a baking pan.
4. Sprinkle with garlic, lemon zest and rosemary.
5. Add herb sprigs on top.
6. Roast for 3 hours.
7. Let rest for a few minutes and then slice and serve.

NUTRITIONAL FACTS: Calories 329 Total Fat 27 g Saturated Fat 9 g Cholesterol 59 mg Sodium 498 mg Total Carbohydrate 5.3 g Dietary Fiber 1.8 g Protein 18 g Total Sugars 2 gPotassium 493 mg

107. BEEF STIR FRY

PREPARATION: 15' **COOKING:** 10' **SERVES:** 4

INGREDIENTS

- 1 tablespoon soy sauce
- 1 tablespoon ginger, minced
- 1 teaspoon cornstarch
- 1 teaspoon dry sherry
- 12 oz. beef, sliced into strips
- 1 teaspoon toasted sesame oil
- 2 tablespoons oyster sauce
- 1 lb. baby bok choy, sliced
- 3 tablespoons chicken broth

DIRECTIONS

1. Mix soy sauce, ginger, cornstarch and dry sherry in a bowl.
2. Toss the beef in the mixture.
3. Pour oil into a pan over medium heat.
4. Cook the beef for 5 minutes, stirring.
5. Add oyster sauce, bok choy and chicken broth to the pan.
6. Cook for 1 minute.

NUTRITIONAL FACTS: Calories 247 Total Fat 15.8 g Saturated Fat 4 g Cholesterol 69 mg Sodium 569 mg Total Carbohydrate 6.3 g Dietary Fiber 1.1 g Protein 25 g

108. SWEET & SOUR PORK

PREPARATION: 15' **COOKING:** 15' **SERVES:** 4

INGREDIENTS

- 1 lb. pork chops
- Salt and pepper to taste
- ½ cup sesame seeds
- 2 tablespoons peanut oil
- 2 tablespoons soy sauce
- 3 tablespoons apricot jam
- Chopped scallions

DIRECTIONS

1. Season pork chops with salt and pepper.
2. Press sesame seeds on both sides of pork.
3. Pour oil into a pan over medium heat.
4. Cook pork for 3 to 5 minutes per side.
5. Transfer to a plate.
6. In a bowl, mix soy sauce and apricot jam.
7. Simmer for 3 minutes.
8. Pour sauce over the pork and garnish with scallions before serving.

NUTRITIONAL FACTS: Calories 414 Total Fat 27.5 g Saturated Fat 5.6 g Cholesterol 68 mg Sodium 607 mg Total Carbohydrate 12.9 g Dietary Fiber 1.8 g Protein 29 g   Total Sugars 9 g Potassium 332 mg

109. GRILLED PORK WITH SALSA

PREPARATION: 30' COOKING: 15' SERVES: 4

INGREDIENTS

- Salsa
- 1 onion, chopped
- 1 tomato, chopped
- 1 peach, chopped
- 1 apricot, chopped
- 1 tablespoon olive oil
- 1 tablespoon lime juice
- 2 tablespoons fresh cilantro, chopped
- Salt and pepper to taste
- Pork
- 1 lb. pork tenderloin, sliced
- 1 tablespoon olive oil
- Salt and pepper to taste
- ½ teaspoon ground cumin
- ¾ teaspoon chili powder

DIRECTIONS

1. Combine salsa ingredients in a bowl.
2. Cover and refrigerate.
3. Brush pork tenderloin with oil.
4. Season with salt, pepper, cumin and chili powder.
5. Grill pork for 5 to 7 minutes per side.
6. Slice pork and serve with salsa.

NUTRITIONAL FACTS: Calories 219 Total Fat 9.5 g Saturated Fat 1.8 g Cholesterol 74 mg Sodium 512 mg Total Carbohydrate 8.3 g Dietary Fiber 1.5 g Protein 24 g Total Sugars 6 gPotassium 600 mg

110. GARLIC PORK LOIN

PREPARATION: 15' COOKING: 1H SERVES: 6

INGREDIENTS

- 1 ½ lb. pork loin roast
- 4 cloves garlic, sliced into slivers
- Salt and pepper to taste

DIRECTIONS

1. Preheat your oven to 425 degrees F.
2. Make several slits all over the pork roast.
3. Insert garlic slivers.
4. Sprinkle with salt and pepper.
5. Roast in the oven for 1 hour.

NUTRITIONAL FACTS: Calories 235 Total Fat 13.3 g Saturated Fat 2.6 g Cholesterol 71 mg Sodium 450 mg Total Carbohydrate 1.7 g Dietary Fiber 0.3 g Protein 25.7 g Total Sugars 3 g Potassium 383 mg

111. CHICKEN PESTO

PREPARATION: 15' **COOKING:** 25' **SERVES:** 4

INGREDIENTS

- 1 lb. chicken cutlet
- Salt and pepper to taste
- 1 tablespoon olive oil
- ½ cup onion, chopped
- ½ cup heavy cream
- ½ cup dry white wine
- 1 tomato, chopped
- ¼ cup pesto
- 2 tablespoons basil, chopped

DIRECTIONS

1. Season chicken with salt and pepper.
2. Pour oil into a pan over medium heat.
3. Cook chicken for 3 to 4 minutes per side.
4. Place the chicken on a plate.
5. Add the onion to the pan.
6. Cook for 1 minute.
7. Stir in the rest of the ingredients.
8. Bring to a boil.
9. Simmer for 15 minutes.
10. Put the chicken back to the pan.
11. Cook for 2 more minutes and then serve.

NUTRITIONAL FACTS: Calories 371 Total Fat 23.7 g Saturated Fat 9.2 g Cholesterol 117 mg Sodium 361 mg Total Carbohydrate 5.7 g Dietary Fiber 1 g Protein 27.7 g Total Sugars 3 g Potassium 567 mg

112. GARLIC PARMESAN CHICKEN WINGS

PREPARATION: 20' **COOKING:** 20' **SERVES:** 8

INGREDIENTS

- Cooking spray
- ½ cup all-purpose flour
- Pepper to taste
- 2 tablespoons garlic powder
- 3 eggs, beaten
- 1 ¼ cups Parmesan cheese, grated
- 2 cups breadcrumbs
- 2 lb. chicken wings

DIRECTIONS

1. Preheat your oven to 450 degrees F.
2. Spray baking pan with oil.
3. In a bowl, mix the flour, pepper and garlic powder.
4. Add eggs to another bowl.
5. Mix the Parmesan cheese and breadcrumbs in another bowl.
6. Dip the chicken wings in the first, second and third bowls.
7. Spray chicken wings with oil.
8. Bake in the oven for 20 minutes.

NUTRITIONAL FACTS: Calories 221 Total Fat 11.6 g Saturated Fat 3.9 g Cholesterol 122 mg Sodium 242 mg Total Carbohydrate 8 g Dietary Fiber 0.4 g Protein 16 g Total Sugars 3 g Potassium 163 mg

113. CRISPY BAKED SHRIMP

PREPARATION: 15'   **COOKING:** 10'   **SERVES:** 4

INGREDIENTS

- ¼ cup whole-wheat breadcrumbs
- 3 tablespoons olive oil, divided
- 1 ½ lb. jumbo shrimp, peeled and deveined
- Salt and pepper to taste
- 2 tablespoons lemon juice
- 1 tablespoon garlic, chopped
- 2 tablespoons butter
- ¼ cup Parmesan cheese, grated
- 2 tablespoons chives, chopped

DIRECTIONS

1. Preheat your oven to 425 degrees F.
2. Add breadcrumbs to a pan over medium heat.
3. Cook until toasted.
4. Transfer to a plate.
5. Coat baking pan with 1 tablespoon oil.
6. Arrange shrimp in a single layer in a baking pan.
7. Season with salt and pepper.
8. Mix lemon juice, garlic and butter in a bowl.
9. Pour mixture on top of the shrimp.
10. Add Parmesan cheese and chives to the breadcrumbs.
11. Sprinkle breadcrumbs on top of the shrimp.
12. Bake for 10 minutes.

NUTRITIONAL FACTS: Calories 340 Total Fat 18.7 g Saturated Fat 6 g Cholesterol 293 mg Sodium 374 mg Total Carbohydrate 6 g Dietary Fiber 0.8 g Protein 36.9 g Total Sugars 2 g Potassium 483 mg

114. HERBED MEDITERRANEAN FISH FILLET

PREPARATION: 20'   **COOKING:** 1H   **SERVES:** 6

INGREDIENTS

- 3 lb. sea bass fillet
- Salt to taste
- 2 tablespoons tarragon, chopped
- ¼ cup dry white wine
- 3 tablespoons olive oil, divided
- 1 tablespoon butter
- 2 cloves garlic, minced
- 2 cups whole-wheat breadcrumbs
- 3 tablespoons parsley, chopped
- 3 tablespoons oregano, chopped
- 3 tablespoons fresh basil, chopped

DIRECTIONS

1. Preheat your oven to 350 degrees F.
2. Season fish with salt and tarragon.
3. Pour half of oil into a roasting pan.
4. Stir in wine.
5. Add the fish in the roasting pan.
6. Bake in the oven for 50 minutes.
7. Add remaining oil to a pan over medium heat.
8. Cook herbs, breadcrumbs and salt.
9. Spread breadcrumb mixture on top of fish and bake for 5 minutes.

NUTRITIONAL FACTS: Calories 288 Total Fat 12.7 g Saturated Fat 2.9 g Cholesterol 65 mg Sodium 499 mg Total Carbohydrate 10.4 g Dietary Fiber 1.8 g Protein 29.5 g Total Sugars 1 g Potassium 401 mg

115. MUSHROOM STUFFED WITH RICOTTA

PREPARATION: 10' **COOKING:** 10' **SERVES:** 4

INGREDIENTS
- 4 large mushrooms, stemmed
- 1 tablespoon olive oil
- Salt and pepper to taste
- ¼ cup basil, chopped
- 1 cup ricotta cheese
- ¼ cup Parmesan cheese, grated

DIRECTIONS
1. Preheat your grill.
2. Coat the mushrooms with oil.
3. Season with salt and pepper.
4. Grill for 5 minutes.
5. Stuff each mushroom with a mixture of basil, ricotta cheese and Parmesan cheese.
6. Grill for another 5 minutes.

NUTRITIONAL FACTS: Calories 259 Total Fat 17.3 g Saturated Fat 5.4 g Cholesterol 24 mg Sodium 509 mg Total Carbohydrate 14.9 g Dietary Fiber 2.6 g Protein 12.2 g Total Sugars 7 g Potassium 572 mg

116. THAI CHOPPED SALAD

PREPARATION: 15' **COOKING:** 0' **SERVES:** 4

INGREDIENTS
- 10 oz. kale and cabbage mix
- 14 oz. tofu, sliced into cubes and fried crispy
- ½ cup vinaigrette

DIRECTIONS
1. Arrange kale and cabbage in a serving platter.
2. Top with the tofu cubes.
3. Drizzle with the vinaigrette.

NUTRITIONAL FACTS: Calories 332 Total Fat 15 g Saturated Fat 1.5 g Cholesterol 0 mg Sodium 236 mg   Total Carbohydrate 26.3 g Dietary Fiber 7.6 g Protein 1.3 g Total Sugars 13 g Potassium 41 mg

117. LEMON & ROSEMARY SALMON

PREPARATION: 10' COOKING: 15' SERVES: 4

INGREDIENTS
- 4 salmon fillets
- Salt and pepper to taste
- 4 tablespoons butter
- 1 lemon, sliced
- 8 rosemary sprigs

DIRECTIONS
1. Season salmon with salt and pepper.
2. Place salmon on a foil sheet.
3. Top with butter, lemon slices and rosemary sprigs.
4. Fold the foil and seal.
5. Bake in the oven at 450 degrees F for 15 minutes.

NUTRITIONAL FACTS: Calories 365 Total Fat 22 g Saturated Fat 6 g Cholesterol 86 mg Sodium 445 mg Total Carbohydrate 5 g Dietary Fiber 1.9 g Protein 29.8 g Total Sugars 3 g Potassium 782 mg

118. CHICKEN KURMA

PREPARATION: 20' COOKING: 25' SERVES: 6

INGREDIENTS
- 1 tablespoon olive oil
- 1 onion, diced
- 3 cloves garlic, sliced thinly
- 1 ginger, minced
- 2 tomatoes, diced
- 1 serrano pepper, minced
- Salt and pepper to taste
- 1 teaspoon ground turmeric
- 1 tablespoon tomato paste
- 1 ½ lb. chicken, sliced
- 1 red bell pepper, chopped

DIRECTIONS
1. Pour oil into a pan over medium heat.
2. Cook onion for 3 minutes.
3. Add garlic, ginger, tomatoes, Serrano pepper, salt, pepper, and turmeric and tomato paste.
4. Bring to a boil.
5. Reduce heat and simmer for 10 minutes.
6. Add chicken and cook for 5 minutes.
7. Stir in red bell pepper.
8. Cook for 5 minutes.

NUTRITIONAL FACTS: Calories 175 Total Fat 15.2 g Saturated Fat 3 g Cholesterol 115 mg Sodium 400 mg Total Carbohydrate 7 g Dietary Fiber 1.8 g Protein 24 g Total Sugars 3 g Potassium 436 mg

119. PORK CHOPS WITH BACON & MUSHROOMS

PREPARATION: 10'   COOKING: 20'   SERVES: 4

INGREDIENTS

- 6 strips bacon, chopped
- 4 pork chops
- Salt and pepper to taste
- 2 cloves garlic, minced
- 8 oz. mushrooms, sliced
- 1 tablespoon olive oil
- 5 sprigs fresh thyme
- 2/3 cup chicken broth
- 1/2 cup heavy cream

DIRECTIONS

1. Cook bacon in a pan until crispy.
2. Transfer bacon on a plate.
3. Sprinkle salt and pepper on the pork chops.
4. Cook the pork chops in bacon fat for 4 minutes per side.
5. Transfer pork chops on a plate.
6. Add the garlic and mushrooms in the pan.
7. Add the olive oil
8. Cook for 5 minutes.
9. Pour in the broth and let the mixture boil.
10. Stir in the heavy cream and reduce the heat to low.
11. Put the bacon and pork chops back to the pan.
12. Cook for 3 more minutes before serving.

NUTRITIONAL FACTS: Calories 516 Total Fat 41.3g Saturated Fat 15.4g Cholesterol 121mg Sodium 851mg Total Carbohydrate 4.2g Dietary Fiber 1.1g Total Sugars 1.2g Protein 31.7g Potassium 679mg

120. PORK

PREPARATION: 10'   COOKING: 20'   SERVES: 4

INGREDIENTS

- A single pound of pork tenderloin
- A quarter cup of oil
- 3 medium shallots (chop them finely)

DIRECTIONS

1. Slice your pork into thick slices (go for about a half-inch thick).
2. Chop up your shallots before placing them on a plate.
3. Get a cast-iron skillet and warm up the oil
4. Press your pork into your shallots on both sides. Press firmly to make sure that they stick.
5. Place the slices of pork with shallots into the warm oil and then cook until it's done. The shallots may burn, but they will still be fine.
6. Make sure the pork is cooked through thoroughly.

NUTRITIONAL FACTS: Calories-519 Fat-36 grams Protein-46 grams Carbs-7 grams

121. GARLIC SHRIMP

PREPARATION: 10' COOKING: 30' SERVES: 4

INGREDIENTS

- 2 minced garlic cloves
- 2 whole garlic cloves
- The juice from half a lemon
- 2 tablespoons of oil (olive)
- 2 tablespoons of butter
- ¾ pounds of either small or medium shrimp (it needs to be both shelled and deveined)
- A quarter of a teaspoon of paprika
- A quarter of a teaspoon of pepper flakes (red ones)
- 2 tablespoons of parsley that is chopped.

DIRECTIONS

1. Sprinkle your shrimp with a teaspoon of salt (fine grain sea salt) and let it sit for ten minutes.
2. Get a skillet.
3. Heat the butter with olive oil over a heat that is medium-high.
4. Add the flakes and garlic.
5. Sauté for half a minute.
6. Add your shrimp and cook until they have turned pink. This will take approximately two minutes. Stir constantly.
7. Add paprika and juice from the lemon.
8. Cook for another sixty seconds.

NUTRITIONAL FACTS: Per serving Calories-260 Fat-18 grams Carbs-none Protein-24 protein

122. PORK CHOP

PREPARATION: 10' COOKING: 30' SERVES: 2

INGREDIENTS

- A dozen pork chop (boneless and thin cut)
- 2 cups of spinach (you should use baby spinach for this)
- 4 cloves of garlic
- A dozen slices provolone cheese

DIRECTIONS

1. Preheat your oven to a temperature of 350.
2. Press the garlic cloves using a garlic press. The cloves should go through the press and into a small bowl.
3. Spread the garlic that you have made onto one side of the pork chops.
4. Flip half a dozen chops while making sure the garlic side is down.
5. You should do this on a baking sheet that is rimmed.
6. Divide your spinach between the half dozen chops.
7. Fold cheese slices in half.
8. Put them on top of the spinach.
9. Put a second pork chop on top of the first set, but this time make sure that the garlic side is up.
10. Bake for 20 minutes.
11. Cover each chop with another piece of cheese.
12. Bake another 15 minutes.
13. Your meat meter should be at 160 degrees when you check with a thermometer.

NUTRITIONAL FACTS: Calories-436 Fat-25 grams Carbs-2 grams Protein-47 grams

123. CITRUS EGG SALAD

PREPARATION: 10' **COOKING:** 20' **SERVES:** 3

INGREDIENTS
- Half a dozen eggs (6)
- A single teaspoon of mustard (go with Dijon)
- 2 tablespoons of mayo
- A single teaspoon of lemon juice

DIRECTIONS
1. Place the eggs gently in a medium saucepan.
2. Add cold water until your eggs are covered by an inch.
3. Bring to a boil.
4. You should do this for ten minutes. Remove from your heat and cool. Peel your eggs under running water that is cold.
5. Put your eggs in a food processor. Pulse until they are chopped.
6. Stir in condiments and juice.

NUTRITIONAL FACTS: Calories-222 Fat-19 grams Protein-13 grams Carbs-1 gram

124. CHOWDER

PREPARATION: 10' **COOKING:** 30' **SERVES:** 4

INGREDIENTS
- A single tablespoon of butter
- 5 minced garlic cloves
- An entire head of cauliflower (cut it into florets that are small)
- Half of a teaspoon of oregano (use dried)
- Half a cup of carrots that have been diced
- Half a cup of onions that have been diced
- A cup and a half of broth (use vegetable)
- A quarter cup of cream cheese

DIRECTIONS
1. Get a soup pot.
2. Heat your butter.
3. Add garlic and onions.
4. Sauté for a few moments.
5. Add the rest of the ingredients to the pot.
6. Bring to a boil.
7. Slow the heat and put it on a simmer.
8. Cook for 15 minutes.
9. Shut off the flame.
10. Use a hand blender to blend the soup partly in the pot.
11. Switch the flame back on.
12. Add a cup of broth.
13. Add the cream cheese.
14. Simmer for 10 minutes and switch off the flame again.

NUTRITIONAL FACTS: Calories-143 Fat-8.4 grams Carbs-15.2 grams Protein-4.5 grams

125. BULGUR APPETIZER SALAD

PREPARATION: 30' **COOKING:** 0' **SERVES:** 4

INGREDIENTS

- 1 cup bulgur
- 2 cups hot water
- Black pepper to the taste
- 2 cups corn
- 1 cucumber, chopped
- 2 tablespoons lemon juice
- 2 tablespoons balsamic vinegar
- ¼ cup olive oil

DIRECTIONS

1. In a bowl, mix bulgur with the water, cover, leave aside for 30 minutes, fluff with a fork and transfer to a salad bowl.
2. Add corn, cucumber, oil with lemon juice, vinegar and pepper, toss, divide into small cups and serve.

NUTRITIONAL FACTS: Calories 130 Fat 2 Fiber 2 Carbs 7 Protein 6

126. COCOA BARS

PREPARATION: 2H **COOKING:** 0' **SERVES:** 12

INGREDIENTS

- 1 cup unsweetened cocoa chips
- 2 cups rolled oats
- 1 cup low-fat peanut butter
- ½ cup chia seeds
- ½ cup raisins
- ¼ cup coconut sugar
- ½ cup coconut milk

DIRECTIONS

1. Put 1 and ½ cups oats in your blender, pulse well, transfer this to a bowl, add the rest of the oats, cocoa chips, chia seeds, raisins, sugar and milk, stir really well, spread this into a square pan, press well, keep in the fridge for 2 hours, slice into 12 bars and serve.

NUTRITIONAL FACTS: Calories 198 Fat 5 Fiber 4 Carbs 10 Protein 89

127. CINNAMON APPLE CHIPS

PREPARATION: 10' **COOKING:** 2H **SERVES:** 4

INGREDIENTS
- Cooking spray
- 2 teaspoons cinnamon powder
- 2 apples, cored and thinly sliced

DIRECTIONS
1. Arrange apple slices on a lined baking sheet, spray them with cooking oil, sprinkle cinnamon, introduce in the oven and bake at 300 degrees F for 2 hours.
2. Divide into bowls and serve as a snack.

NUTRITIONAL FACTS: Calories 80 Fat 0 Fiber 3 Carbs 7 Protein 4

128. GREEK PARTY DIP

PREPARATION: 10' **COOKING:** 0' **SERVES:** 4

INGREDIENTS
- ½ cup coconut cream
- 1 cup fat-free Greek yogurt
- 2 teaspoons dill, dried
- 2 teaspoons thyme, dried
- 1 teaspoon sweet paprika
- 2 teaspoons no-salt-added sun-dried tomatoes, chopped
- 2 teaspoons parsley, chopped
- 2 teaspoons chives, chopped
- Black pepper to the taste

DIRECTIONS
1. In a bowl, mix cream with yogurt, dill with thyme, paprika, tomatoes, parsley, chives and pepper, stir well, divide into smaller bowls and serve as a dip.

NUTRITIONAL FACTS: Calories 100 Fat 1 Fiber 4 Carbs 8 Protein 3

129. SPICY PUMPKIN SEEDS BOWLS

PREPARATION: 10' **COOKING:** 20' **SERVES:** 6

INGREDIENTS

- ½ tablespoon chili powder
- ½ teaspoon cayenne pepper
- 2 cups pumpkin seeds
- 2 teaspoons lime juice

DIRECTIONS

1. Spread pumpkin seeds on a lined baking sheet, add lime juice, cayenne and chili powder, toss well, introduce in the oven, roast at 275 degrees F for 20 minutes, divide into small bowls and serve as a snack.

NUTRITIONAL FACTS: Calories 170 Fat 2 Fiber 7 Carbs 12 Protein 6

130. APPLE AND PECANS BOWLS

PREPARATION: 10' **COOKING:** 0' **SERVES:** 4

INGREDIENTS

- 4 big apples, cored, peeled and cubed
- 2 teaspoons lemon juice
- ¼ cup pecans, chopped

DIRECTIONS

1. In a bowl, mix apples with lemon juice and pecans, toss, divide into small bowls and serve as a snack.

NUTRITIONAL FACTS: Calories 120 Fat 4 Fiber 3 Carbs 12 Protein 3

131. SHRIMP MUFFINS

PREPARATION: 10' **COOKING:** 45' **SERVES:** 6

INGREDIENTS

- 1 spaghetti squash, peeled and halved
- 2 tablespoons avocado mayonnaise
- 1 cup low-fat mozzarella cheese, shredded
- 8 ounces' shrimp, peeled, cooked and chopped
- 1 and ½ cups almond flour
- 1 teaspoon parsley, dried
- 1 garlic clove, minced
- Black pepper to the taste
- Cooking spray

DIRECTIONS

1. Arrange the squash on a lined baking sheet, introduce in the oven at 375 degrees F, bake for 30 minutes, scrape flesh into a bowl, add pepper, parsley flakes, flour, shrimp, mayo and mozzarella and stir well, divide this mix into a muffin tray greased with cooking spray, bake in the oven at 375 degrees F for 15 minutes and serve them cold as a snack.

NUTRITIONAL FACTS: Calories 140 Fat 2 Fiber 4 Carbs 14 Protein 12

132. ZUCCHINI BOWLS

PREPARATION: 10' **COOKING:** 20' **SERVES:** 12

INGREDIENTS

- Cooking spray
- ½ cup dill, chopped
- 1 egg
- ½ cup whole wheat flour
- Black pepper to the taste
- 1 yellow onion, chopped
- 2 garlic cloves, minced
- 3 zucchinis, grated

DIRECTIONS

1. In a bowl, mix zucchinis with garlic, onion, flour, pepper, egg and dill, stir well, shape small bowls out of this mix, arrange them on a lined baking sheet, grease them with some cooking spray, bake at 400 degrees F for 20 minutes, flipping them halfway, divide them into bowls and serve as a snack.

NUTRITIONAL FACTS: Calories 120, Fat 1 Fiber 4 Carbs 12 Protein 6

133. CHEESY MUSHROOMS CAPS

PREPARATION: 10'   **COOKING:** 30'   **SERVES:** 20

INGREDIENTS

- 20 white mushroom caps
- 1 garlic clove, minced
- 3 tablespoons parsley, chopped
- 2 yellow onions, chopped
- Black pepper to the taste
- ½ cup low-fat parmesan, grated
- ¼ cup low-fat mozzarella, grated
- A drizzle of olive oil
- 2 tablespoons non-fat yogurt

DIRECTIONS

1. Heat up a pan with some oil over medium heat, add garlic and onion, stir, cook for 10 minutes and transfer to a bowl.
2. Add black pepper, garlic, parsley, mozzarella, parmesan and yogurt, stir well, stuff the mushroom caps with this mix, arrange them on a lined baking sheet, bake in the oven at 400 degrees F for 20 minutes and serve them as an appetizer.

NUTRITIONAL FACTS: Calories 120, Fat 1 Fiber 3 Carbs 11 Protein 7

134. MOZZARELLA CAULIFLOWER BARS

PREPARATION: 10'   **COOKING:** 40'   **SERVES:** 12

INGREDIENTS

- 1 big cauliflower head, riced
- ½ cup low-fat mozzarella cheese, shredded
- ¼ cup egg whites
- 1 teaspoon Italian seasoning
- Black pepper to the taste

DIRECTIONS

1. Spread the cauliflower rice on a lined baking sheet, cook in the oven at 375 degrees F for 20 minutes, transfer to a bowl, add black pepper, cheese, seasoning and egg whites, stir well, spread into a rectangle pan and press well on the bottom.
2. Introduce in the oven at 375 degrees F, bake for 20 minutes, cut into 12 bars and serve as a snack.

NUTRITIONAL FACTS: Calories 140 Fat 1 Fiber 3 Carbs 6 Protein 6

135. SHRIMP AND PINEAPPLE SALSA

PREPARATION: 10' COOKING: 40' SERVES: 4

INGREDIENTS
- 1-pound large shrimp, peeled and deveined
- 20 ounces canned pineapple chunks
- 1 tablespoon garlic powder
- 1 cup red bell peppers, chopped
- Black pepper to the taste

DIRECTIONS
1. Place shrimp in a baking dish, add pineapple, garlic, bell peppers and black pepper, toss a bit, introduce in the oven, bake at 375 degrees F for 40 minutes, divide into small bowls and serve cold.

NUTRITIONAL FACTS: Calories 170 Fat 5 Fiber 4 Carbs 15 Protein 11

136. STRAWBERRY BUCKWHEAT PANCAKES

PREPARATION: 20' COOKING: 5' SERVES: 4

INGREDIENTS
- 100g (3½oz) strawberries, chopped
- 100g (3½ oz.) buckwheat flour
- 1 egg
- 250mls (8fl oz.) milk
- 1 teaspoon olive oil
- 1 teaspoon olive oil for frying
- Freshly squeezed juice of 1 orange
- 175 calories per serving

DIRECTIONS
1. Pour the milk into a bowl and mix in the egg and a teaspoon of olive oil. Sift in the flour to the liquid mixture until smooth and creamy. Allow it to rest for 15 minutes. Heat a little oil in a pan and pour in a quarter of the mixture (or to the size you prefer.) Sprinkle in a quarter of the strawberries into the batter. Cook for around 2 minutes on each side. Serve hot with a drizzle of orange juice. You could try experimenting with other berries such as blueberries and blackberries

NUTRITIONAL FACTS: Calories Fat Fiber Carbs Protein

137. STRAWBERRY & NUT GRANOLA

PREPARATION: 10'   **COOKING:** 50'   **SERVES:** 12

INGREDIENTS

- 200g (7oz) oats
- 250g (9oz) buckwheat flakes
- 100g (3½ oz.) walnuts, chopped
- 100g (3½ oz.) almonds, chopped
- 100g (3½ oz.) dried strawberries
- 1½ teaspoons ground ginger
- 1½ teaspoons ground cinnamon
- 120mls (4fl oz.) olive oil
- 2 tablespoon honey

DIRECTIONS

1. Combine the oats, buckwheat flakes, nuts, ginger and cinnamon. In a saucepan, warm the oil and honey. Stir until the honey has melted. Pour the warm oil into the dry ingredients and mix well. Spread the mixture out on a large baking tray (or two) and bake in the oven at 150C (300F) for around 50 minutes until the granola is golden. Allow it to cool. Add in the dried berries. Store in an airtight container until ready to use. Can be served with yogurt, milk or even dry as a handy snack.

NUTRITIONAL FACTS: Calories 391 Fat 0 Fiber 6 Carbs 3 Protein 8

138. CHILLED STRAWBERRY & WALNUT PORRIDGE

PREPARATION: 10'   **COOKING:** 0'   **SERVES:** 1

INGREDIENTS

- 100g (3½ oz.) strawberries
- 50g (2oz) rolled oats
- 4 walnut halves, chopped
- 1 teaspoon chia seeds
- 200mls (7fl oz.) unsweetened soya milk
- 100ml (3½ FL oz.) water

DIRECTIONS

1. Place the strawberries, oats, soya milk and water into a blender and process until smooth. Stir in the chia seeds and mix well. Chill in the fridge overnight and serve in the morning with a sprinkling of chopped walnuts. It's simple and delicious.

NUTRITIONAL FACTS: Calories 384 Fat 2 Fiber 5 Carbs 3 Protein 7

139. FRUIT & NUT YOGURT CRUNCH

PREPARATION: 5' **COOKING:** 0' **SERVES:** 1

INGREDIENTS
- 100g (3½ oz.) plain Greek yogurt
- 50g (2oz) strawberries, chopped
- 6 walnut halves, chopped
- Sprinkling of cocoa powder

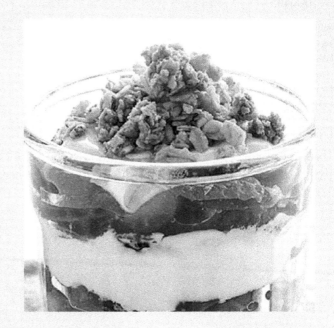

DIRECTIONS
1. Stir half of the chopped strawberries into the yogurt. Using a glass, place a layer of yogurt with a sprinkling of strawberries and walnuts, followed by another layer of the same until you reach the top of the glass. Garnish with walnuts pieces and a dusting of cocoa powder.

NUTRITIONAL FACTS: Calories 296 Fat 4 Fiber 2 Carbs 5 Protein 9

140. CHEESY BAKED EGGS

PREPARATION: 5' **COOKING:** 15' **SERVES:** 4

INGREDIENTS
- 4 large eggs
- 75g (3oz) cheese, grated
- 25g (1oz) fresh rocket (arugula) leaves, finely chopped
- 1 tablespoon parsley
- ½ teaspoon ground turmeric
- 1 tablespoon olive oil

DIRECTIONS
1. Grease each ramekin dish with a little olive oil. Divide the rocket (arugula) between the ramekin dishes then break an egg into each one. Sprinkle a little parsley and turmeric on top then sprinkle on the cheese. Place the ramekins in a preheated oven at 220C/425F for 15 minutes, until the eggs are set and the cheese is bubbling.

NUTRITIONAL FACTS: Calories 198 Fat 9 Fiber 3 Carbs 2 Protein 13

141. GREEN EGG SCRAMBLE

PREPARATION: 10' **COOKING:** 5' **SERVES:** 1

INGREDIENTS

- 2 eggs, whisked
- 25g (1oz) rocket (arugula) leaves
- 1 teaspoon chives, chopped
- 1 teaspoon fresh basil, chopped
- 1 teaspoon fresh parsley, chopped
- 1 tablespoon olive oil

DIRECTIONS

1. Mix the eggs together with the rocket (arugula) and herbs. Heat the oil in a frying pan and pour into the egg mixture. Gently stir until it's lightly scrambled. Season and serve.

NUTRITIONAL FACTS: Calories 250 Fat 5 Fiber 7 Carbs 8 Protein 11

142. SPICED SCRAMBLE

PREPARATION: 10' **COOKING:** 5' **SERVES:** 1

INGREDIENTS

- 25g (1oz) kale, finely chopped
- 2 eggs
- 1 spring onion (scallion) finely chopped
- 1 teaspoon turmeric
- 1 tablespoon olive oil
- Sea salt
- Freshly ground black pepper

DIRECTIONS

1. Crack the eggs into a bowl. Add the turmeric and whisk them. Season with salt and pepper. Heat the oil in a frying pan, add the kale and spring onions (scallions) and cook until it has wilted. Pour in the beaten eggs and stir until eggs have scrambled together with the kale.

NUTRITIONAL FACTS: Calories 259 Fat 3 Fiber 4 Carbs 3 Protein 9

143. POTATO BITES

PREPARATION: 10' **COOKING:** 20' **SERVES:** 3

INGREDIENTS
- 1 potato, sliced
- 2 bacon slices, already cooked and crumbled
- 1 small avocado, pitted and cubed
- Cooking spray

DIRECTIONS
1. Spread potato slices on a lined baking sheet, spray with cooking oil, introduce in the oven at 350 degrees F, bake for 20 minutes, arrange on a platter, top each slice with avocado and crumbled bacon and serve as a snack.

NUTRITIONAL FACTS: Calories 180 Fat 4 Fiber 1 Carbs 8 Protein 6

144. EGGPLANT SALSA

PREPARATION: 15' **COOKING:** 10' **SERVES:** 4

INGREDIENTS
- 1 and ½ cups tomatoes, chopped
- 3 cups eggplant, cubed
- A drizzle of olive oil
- 2 teaspoons capers
- 6 ounces' green olives, pitted and sliced
- 4 garlic cloves, minced
- 2 teaspoons balsamic vinegar
- 1 tablespoon basil, chopped
- Black pepper to the taste

DIRECTIONS
1. Heat a saucepan with the oil medium-high heat, add eggplant, stir and cook for 5 minutes.
2. Add tomatoes, capers, olives, garlic, vinegar, basil and black pepper, toss, cook for 5 minutes more, divide into small cups and serve cold.

NUTRITIONAL FACTS: Calories 120 Fat 6 Fiber 5 Carbs 9 Protein 7

145. CARROTS AND CAULIFLOWER SPREAD

PREPARATION: 10' **COOKING:** 40' **SERVES:** 4

INGREDIENTS

- 1 cup carrots, sliced
- 2 cups cauliflower florets
- ½ cup cashews
- 2 and ½ cups water
- 1 cup almond milk
- 1 teaspoon garlic powder
- ¼ teaspoon smoked paprika

DIRECTIONS

1. In a small pot, mix the carrots with cauliflower, cashews and water, stir, cover, bring to a boil over medium heat, cook for 40 minutes, drain and transfer to a blender.
2. Add almond milk, garlic powder and paprika, pulse well, divide into small bowls and serve

NUTRITIONAL FACTS: Calories 201 Fat 7 Fiber 4 Carbs 7 Protein 7

146. BLACK BEAN SALSA

PREPARATION: 15' **COOKING:** 0' **SERVES:** 6

INGREDIENTS

- 1 tablespoon coconut aminos
- ½ teaspoon cumin, ground
- 1 cup canned black beans, no-salt-added, drained and rinsed
- 1 cup salsa
- 6 cups romaine lettuce leaves, torn
- ½ cup avocado, peeled, pitted and cubed

DIRECTIONS

1. In a bowl, combine the beans with the aminos, cumin, salsa, lettuce and avocado, toss, divide into small bowls and serve as a snack.

NUTRITIONAL FACTS: Calories 181 Fat 4 Fiber 7 Carbs 14 Protein 7

147. MUNG SPROUTS SALSA

PREPARATION: 10' **COOKING:** 0' **SERVES:** 2

INGREDIENTS
- 1 red onion, chopped
- 2 cups Mung beans, sprouted
- A pinch of red chili powder
- 1 green chili pepper, chopped
- 1 tomato, chopped
- 1 teaspoon chaat masala
- 1 teaspoon lemon juice
- 1 tablespoon coriander, chopped
- Black pepper to the taste

DIRECTIONS
1. In a salad bowl, mix onion with Mung sprouts, chili pepper, tomato, chili powder, chaat masala, lemon juice, coriander and pepper, toss well, divide into small cups and serve.

NUTRITIONAL FACTS: Calories 100 Fiber Fat 3 Carbs 3 Protein 6

148. SPROUTS AND APPLES SNACK SALAD

PREPARATION: 10' **COOKING:** 0' **SERVES:** 4

INGREDIENTS
- 1-pound Brussels sprouts, shredded
- 1 cup walnuts, chopped
- 1 apple, cored and cubed
- 1 red onion, chopped

For the salad dressing:
- 3 tablespoons red vinegar
- 1 tablespoon mustard
- ½ cup olive oil
- 1 garlic clove, minced
- Black pepper to the taste

DIRECTIONS
1. In a salad bowl, mix sprouts with apple, onion and walnuts.
2. In another bowl, mix vinegar with mustard, oil, garlic and pepper, whisk really well, add this to your salad, toss well and serve as a snack.

NUTRITIONAL FACTS: Calories 120 Fat 2 Fiber 2 Carbs 8 Protein 6

149. DIJON CELERY SALAD

PREPARATION: 10'   **COOKING:** 0'   **SERVES:** 4

INGREDIENTS

- 5 teaspoons stevia
- ½ cup lemon juice
- 1/3 cup Dijon mustard
- 2/3 cup olive oil
- Black pepper to the taste
- 2 apples, cored, peeled and cubed
- 1 bunch celery and leaves, roughly chopped
- ¾ cup walnuts, chopped

DIRECTIONS

1. In a salad bowl, mix celery and its leaves with apple pieces and walnuts.
2. Add black pepper, lemon juice, mustard, stevia and olive oil, whisk well, add to your salad, toss, divide into small cups and serve as a snack.

NUTRITIONAL FACTS: Calories 125 Fat Fiber 2 Carbs 7 Protein 7

150. NAPA CABBAGE SLAW

PREPARATION: 10'   **COOKING:** 0'   **SERVES:** 4

INGREDIENTS

- ½ cup of red bell pepper, cut into thin strips
- 1 carrot, grated
- 4 cups Napa cabbage, shredded
- 3 green onions, chopped
- 1 tablespoon olive oil
- 2 teaspoons ginger, grated
- ½ teaspoon red pepper flakes, crushed
- 3 tablespoons balsamic vinegar
- 1 tablespoon coconut aminos
- 3 tablespoons low-fat peanut butter

DIRECTIONS

1. In a salad bowl, mix bell pepper with carrot, cabbage and onions and toss.
2. Add oil, ginger, pepper flakes, vinegar, aminos and peanut butter, toss, divide into small cups and serve.

NUTRITIONAL FACTS: Calories 160 Fat 10 Fiber 3 Carbs 10 Protein 5

151. DILL BELL PEPPER BOWLS

PREPARATION: 10' **COOKING:** 0' **SERVES:** 4

INGREDIENTS

- 2 tablespoons dill, chopped
- 1 yellow onion, chopped
- 1 pound multi colored bell peppers, cut into halves, seeded and cut into thin strips
- 3 tablespoons olive oil
- 2 and ½ tablespoons white vinegar
- Black pepper to the taste

DIRECTIONS

1. In a salad bowl, mix bell peppers with onion, dill, pepper, oil and vinegar, toss to coat, divide into small bowls and serve as a snack.

NUTRITIONAL FACTS: Calories 120 Fat 3 Fiber 4 Carbs 2 Protein 3

152. BAKED LEMON & PEPPER CHICKEN

PREPARATION: 20' **COOKING:** 25' **SERVES:** 4

INGREDIENTS

- 4 chicken breast fillets
- Salt to taste
- 1 tablespoon olive oil
- 1 lemon, sliced thinly
- 1 tablespoon maple syrup
- 2 tablespoons lemon juice
- 2 tablespoons butter
- Pepper to taste

DIRECTIONS

1. Preheat your oven to 425 degrees F.
2. Season chicken with salt.
3. Pour oil into a pan over medium heat.
4. Cook chicken for 5 minutes per side.
5. Transfer chicken to a baking pan.
6. Surround the chicken with the lemon slices.
7. Bake in the oven for 10 minutes.
8. Pour in maple syrup and lemon juice to the pan.
9. Put the butter on top of the chicken.
10. Sprinkle with pepper.
11. Bake for another 5 minutes.

NUTRITIONAL FACTS: Calories 286 Total Fat 13 g Saturated Fat 5 g Cholesterol 109 mg Sodium 448 mg Total Carbohydrate 7 g Dietary Fiber 1.4 g Protein 34.8 g Total Sugars 3 g Potassium 350 mg

153. SKILLET CHICKEN WITH WHITE WINE SAUCE

PREPARATION: 5'   COOKING: 30'   SERVES: 4

INGREDIENTS

- 4 boneless chicken thighs
- 1 tsp. garlic powder
- 1 tsp. dried thyme
- 1 tbsp. olive oil
- 1 tbsp. butter
- 1 yellow onion diced
- 3 garlic cloves minced
- 1 cup dry white wine
- ½ cup heavy cream
- fresh chopped parsley
- salt and pepper

DIRECTIONS

1. Heat your oil in a skillet. Season your chicken, add it to the skillet, and then cook it about 5-7 mins.
2. Flip the chicken and cook until looking golden brown.
3. Remove the chicken to a plate.
4. Add butter to the skillet. Then add onions and cook them until softened.
5. Stir in garlic salt and pepper, add wine and cook for 4-5 mins.
6. Stir in the thyme and the heavy cream.
7. Place the breasts back to the skillet and leave to simmer for 2-3 mins. Top them with the parsley.

NUTRITIONAL FACTS: Calories: 276 kcal Fats: 21 g Carbs: 6 g Protein: 25 g

154. STIR FRY KIMCHI AND PORK BELLY

PREPARATION: 10'   COOKING: 18'   SERVES: 3

INGREDIENTS

- 300 g pork belly
- 1 lb. kimchi
- 1 tbsp. soy sauce
- 1 tbsp. rice wine
- 1 tbsp. sesame seeds
- 1 stalk green onion

DIRECTIONS

1. Slice the pork as thin as possible and marinate it in soy sauce and rice wine for 8-10 mins.
2. Heat a pan. When very hot, add the pork belly and stir-fry until brown.
3. Add the kimchi to the pan and stir-fry for 2 mins to let the flavors completely mix.
4. Turn off heat and slice the green onion. Top with sesame seeds.

NUTRITIONAL FACTS: Calories: 790 kcal Fats: 68 g Carbs: 7 g Protein: 14 g

155. LEMON BUTTER SAUCE WITH FISH

PREPARATION: 10' **COOKING:** 10' **SERVES:** 2

INGREDIENTS

- 150 g thin white fish fillets
- 4 tbsps. butter
- 2 tbsps. white flour
- 2 tbsps. olive oil
- 1 tbsp. fresh lemon juice
- salt and pepper
- chopped parsley

DIRECTIONS

1. Place the butter in a small skillet over medium heat. Melt it and leave it, just stirring it casually. After 3 mins, pour into a small bowl.
2. Add lemon juice and season it and set it aside.
3. Dry the fish with paper towels, season it to taste, and sprinkle with flour.
4. Heat oil in a skillet over high heat: when shimmering, add the fish and cook around 2-3 mins.
5. Remove to a plate and serve with the sauce. Top with parsley.

NUTRITIONAL FACTS: Calories: 371 kcal Fats: 27 g Carbs: 3 g Protein: 30 g

156. PRESSURE COOKER CRACK CHICKEN

PREPARATION: 5' **COOKING:** 25' **SERVES:** 8

INGREDIENTS

- 2 lbs. boneless chicken thighs.
- 2 slices bacon
- 8 ozs. cream cheese
- 1 scallion sliced
- ½ cup shredded cheddar
- 1 ½ tsp. garlic and onion powder
- 1 tsp. red pepper flakes and dried dill
- salt and pepper
- 2 tbsps. apple cider vinegar
- 1 tbsp. dried chives

DIRECTIONS

1. On pressure cooker, use sauté mode and wait for it to heat up. Add the bacon and cook until crispy. Then set aside on a plate.
2. Add everything in the pot, except the cheddar cheese. On Manual high, pressure cook them for 15 mins and then release it.
3. On a large plate, shred the chicken and then return to the pot and the cheddar.
4. Top with the bacon and scallion.

NUTRITIONAL FACTS: Calories: 437 kcal Fats: 28 g Carbs: 5 g Protein: 41 g

157. BACON BLEU CHEESE FILLED EGGS

PREPARATION: 10' **COOKING:** 90-120' **SERVES:** 3

INGREDIENTS

- 8 eggs
- ¼ cup crumbled bleu cheese
- 3 slices of cooked bacon
- ¼ cup sour cream
- 1/3 cup mayo
- ¼ tsp. pepper and dill
- ½ tsp. salt
- 1 tbsp. mustard
- parsley

DIRECTIONS

1. Hard boil your eggs and then cut them half. Place the yolks in a bowl.
2. With a fork, mash the yolks, add the sour cream, mayo, bleu cheese, mustard, and the seasoning and mix until creamy enough for your taste. Slice up the bacon to small pieces. Stir in the rest of the ingredients and fill up the eggs.

NUTRITIONAL FACTS: Calories: 217 kcal Fats: 16 g Carbs: 1 g Protein: 6 g

158. SPINACH STUFFED CHICKEN BREASTS

PREPARATION: 25' **COOKING:** 15' **SERVES:** 4

INGREDIENTS

- 1 ½ lbs. chicken breasts
- 4 ozs. cream cheese
- ¼ cup frozen spinach
- ½ cup mozzarella
- 4 oz. artichoke hearts
- ¼ cup Greek yogurt
- salt and pepper
- 2 tbsps. olive oil

DIRECTIONS

1. Pound the breasts about 1 inch thick. Cut each chicken down the middle, but don't cut through it. Make a pocket for the filling: season the chicken.
2. In a bowl, combine the Greek yogurt, mozzarella, cream cheese, artichoke, and spinach. Next, season it. Mix until well-combined.
3. Fill all breasts equally with your mixture.
4. In a skillet over medium heat, add the oil and place your chicken. Cover the skillet and cook for 5-6 mins, turning the heat up in the last 1-2 mins.

NUTRITIONAL FACTS: Calories: 288 kcal Fats: 18 g Carbs: 3 g Protein: 31 g

159. CHICKEN WITH LEMON AND GARLIC

PREPARATION: 5'   **COOKING:** 20'   **SERVES:** 4

INGREDIENTS

- 4 boneless chicken thighs
- 2 garlic cloves minced
- Juice of 1 lemon
- ¼ tsp. smoked paprika, red chili flakes, garlic powder
- 2 tsps. Italian seasoning
- 1 tbsp. heavy cream
- fresh parsley
- ¼ small onion
- 1 tbsp. olive oil
- 1½ tbsp. butter
- salt and pepper

DIRECTIONS

1. Season your chicken with all spices.
2. In a skillet over medium heat, add the olive oil and cook for 5-6 mins on each side. Set aside on a plate.
3. Heat the skillet again and add in the butter. Stir in onion and garlic and add your lemon juice. Season them with everything left. After that, stir in your heavy cream. Once the sauce has thickened up, add the chicken back to the pot.
4. Serve it with lemon slices.

NUTRITIONAL FACTS: Calories: 279 kcal Fats: 15 g Carbs: 3 g Protein: 15 g

160. CHICKEN POT PIE IN A SLOW COOKER

PREPARATION: 3H   **COOKING:** 35'   **SERVES:** 6

INGREDIENTS

For the filling:
- 1 cup chicken broth
- ¾ cup heavy whipping cream
- 3 ½ oz. cooked chicken
- ½ cup mixed veggies
- ¼ onion
- 2 garlic cloves
- salt and pepper
- ¼ tsp. rosemary
- 1 tsp. poultry seasoning

For the crust:
- 4 eggs
- 4 ½ tbsps. butter
- 1/3 cup coconut flour
- 1 1/3 cup shredded cheddar
- 2 tsps. full-fat sour cream
- ¼ tsp. baking powder

DIRECTIONS

1. Cook 1-1 ½ lbs. chicken in the slow cooker for 3 hours on high.
2. Preheat your oven to 400°F.
3. Sauté your onion, veggies, garlic cloves and season with 2 tbsp. butter in a skillet for 5-6 mins.
4. Add in the whipping cream, chicken broth, poultry, thyme, and rosemary.
5. Simmer them covered for 5 mins and don't forget to use a lot of liquid; otherwise, it will be really dry. Add the diced chicken, too.
6. Make the breading by mixing melted butter, salt, sour cream, and eggs before whisking them.
7. Add coconut flour and baking powder and stir until well-combined.
8. Stir in the cheddar cheese.
9. Bake in a 400°F oven for 15-20 mins.
10. Set oven to broil and move the pie to the top shelf. Broil for 2-4 mins to brown nicely.

NUTRITIONAL FACTS: Calories: 301 kcal Carbs: 5 g Protein: 15 g Fats: 24 g

161. CHEESE CAULI BREADSTICKS

PREPARATION: 10' **COOKING:** 35' **SERVES:** 6

INGREDIENTS
- 4 eggs
- 4 cups cauli
- 3 cups mozzarella cheese
- 4 cloves garlic
- 3 tsps. oregano
- salt and pepper

DIRECTIONS
1. Preheat your oven 425°F. Prepare one baking sheet with paper on it.
2. Chop your cauli to florets. Add them to a food processor and then pulse.
3. Microwave it for 10 mins and then let it cool afterward. In a large bowl, add in the cauli, eggs, 2 cups of cheese, oregano, garlic and season it, while mixing it.
4. Place the mixture on your sheet while forming your desired shape. Bake it for 20-25 mins. Finally, top it with the rest of the cheese and bake for another 5 mins until golden and well melted.

NUTRITIONAL FACTS: Calories: 185 kcal Carbs: 4g Protein: 11 g Fats: 12 g

162. BAKED CRISPY CHICKEN

PREPARATION: 15' **COOKING:** 40' **SERVES:** 12

INGREDIENTS
- 4 oz. pork rinds
- Salt and pepper to taste
- 1 teaspoon oregano
- 1 ½ teaspoons thyme
- 1 teaspoon smoke paprika
- ½ teaspoon garlic powder
- 12 chicken legs
- 2 oz. mayonnaise
- 1 egg
- 3 tablespoons Dijon mustard

DIRECTIONS
1. Preheat your oven to 400 degrees F.
2. Grind pork rinds until they've turned into powdery texture.
3. Mix pork rinds with salt, pepper, oregano, thyme, paprika and garlic powder.
4. Spread mixture on a plate.
5. In a bowl, mix the mayo, egg and mustard.
6. Dip each chicken leg first into the egg mixture then coat with the pork rind mixture.
7. Bake in the oven for 40 minutes.

NUTRITIONAL FACTS: Calories 359 Total Fat 16.3g Saturated Fat 4.7g Cholesterol 158mg Sodium 391mg Total Carbohydrate 1.6g Dietary Fiber 0.3g Total Sugars 0.4g Protein 49g Potassium 370mg

KETO WOMEN over 50 **122**

163. BITALIAN CHICKEN

PREPARATION: 10' COOKING: 15' SERVES: 4

INGREDIENTS

- 2 tablespoons olive oil
- 1 ½ lb. chicken breast meat, sliced thinly
- ½ cup chicken broth
- 1 cup heavy cream
- 1 teaspoon Italian seasoning
- ½ cup Parmesan cheese
- 1 teaspoon garlic powder
- 1 cup spinach, chopped
- ½ cup sun dried tomatoes

DIRECTIONS

1. In a pan over medium heat, add olive oil.
2. Cook chicken for 4 to 5 minutes per side.
3. Transfer chicken on a plate.
4. Stir in the broth, cream, Italian seasoning, and Parmesan cheese and garlic powder.
5. Simmer until the sauce has thickened.
6. Add the tomatoes and spinach.
7. Cook until the spinach has wilted.
8. Put the chicken back to the pan and serve.

NUTRITIONAL FACTS: Calories 535 Total Fat 29.4g Saturated Fat 11g Cholesterol 199mg Sodium 317mg Total Carbohydrate 6.1g Dietary Fiber 1g Total Sugars 0.4g Protein 60.3g Potassium 783mg

164. CHICKEN & CARROTS

PREPARATION: 15' COOKING: 20' SERVES: 4

INGREDIENTS

- 1 ½ lb. carrots, peeled and sliced
- 1 onion, sliced into quarters
- 1 head garlic, top sliced off
- 4 tablespoons olive oil, divided
- Salt and pepper to taste
- 1 tablespoon fresh rosemary, chopped
- 4 chicken thighs

DIRECTIONS

1. Preheat your oven to 425 degrees F.
2. Arrange the onion and carrots on a single layer on a baking pan.
3. Place the garlic in the middle of the tray.
4. Drizzle half of the olive oil over the vegetables.
5. Season with salt, pepper and rosemary.
6. Coat the chicken with the remaining oil.
7. Season with salt and pepper.
8. Bake in the oven for 20 minutes.

NUTRITIONAL FACTS: Calories 532 Total Fat 25.2g Saturated Fat 5.1g Cholesterol 130mg Sodium 250mg Total Carbohydrate 31.1g Dietary Fiber 5.8g Total Sugars 9.9g Protein 46.1g Potassium 1083mg

165. LEMON & HERB CHICKEN

PREPARATION: 20' **COOKING:** 60' **SERVES:** 6

INGREDIENTS

- 1 whole chicken
- 4 tablespoons unsalted butter
- 3 lemons, sliced in half
- ½ bunch thyme
- ½ bunch rosemary
- Salt and pepper to taste

DIRECTIONS

1. Preheat your oven to 425 degrees F.
2. Cover the baking pan with foil.
3. Put a roasting rack on top.
4. Rub the chicken with butter.
5. Stuff the insides with lemon slices and herbs.
6. Season both inside and outside of chicken with salt and pepper.
7. Use twine to tie the chicken legs together.
8. Put the chicken on a roasting rack.
9. Roast for 40 minutes.
10. Reduce heat to 375 degrees F and roast until chicken is fully cooked.
11. Let chicken rest for 15 minutes before slicing and serving.

NUTRITIONAL FACTS: Calories 504 Total Fat 36.1g Saturated Fat 15g Cholesterol 180mg Sodium 216mg Total Carbohydrate 4.3g Dietary Fiber 1.8g Total Sugars 0.8g Protein 42.6g Potassium 65mg

166. CHICKEN & AVOCADO SALAD

PREPARATION: 5' **COOKING:** 15' **SERVES:** 4

INGREDIENTS

Chicken
- ¼ cup water
- 2 boneless chicken thigh fillets
- 2 tablespoons olive oil
- Salt and pepper to taste
- 1 teaspoon sweet chili powder
- 1 teaspoon dried thyme
- 4 cloves garlic

Salad
- 2 cups arugula
- 1 cup purslane leaves
- 1 cup basil leaves
- ½ cup fresh dill
- ½ cup cherry tomatoes, sliced in half
- 1 tablespoon olives
- 1 avocado, sliced
- 1 teaspoon sesame seeds
- ½ tablespoon olive oil
- 2 tablespoons avocado dressing

DIRECTIONS

1. Pour water into a skillet.
2. Cook chicken over medium low heat for 5 minutes.
3. Drizzle olive oil over the chicken
4. Season with the salt, pepper, thyme and chili powder.
5. Cook until golden, flipping several times to cook evenly.
6. Chop the chicken.
7. Arrange all the ingredients for the salad in a bowl.
8. Put the chicken on top of the salad.
9. Drizzle with the avocado dressing and olive oil.
10. Sprinkle sesame seeds on top.

NUTRITIONAL FACTS: Calories 517 Total Fat 38.6g Saturated Fat 6.4g Cholesterol 70mg Sodium 368mg Total Carbohydrate 27.3g Dietary Fiber 9.9g Total Sugars 7.2g Protein 22g Potassium 1102mg

167. VCHICKEN BOWL

PREPARATION: 10' **COOKING:** 20' **SERVES:** 4

INGREDIENTS

- Salt and pepper to taste
- 2 teaspoons basil
- 2 teaspoon rosemary
- 2 teaspoons thyme
- 1 teaspoon paprika
- 2 lb. chicken breast meat, sliced into bite sized pieces
- 1 ½ cups broccoli florets
- 1 onion, chopped
- 1 cup tomatoes
- 1 zucchini, chopped
- 2 teaspoons garlic, minced
- 2 tablespoons olive oil
- 2 cups cauliflower rice

DIRECTIONS

1. Preheat your oven to 450 degrees F.
2. Cover your baking pan with foil. Set aside.
3. In a bowl, mix salt, pepper and spices.
4. Put the chicken and vegetables on a baking pan.
5. Sprinkle the spice mixture and garlic over the vegetables and chicken.
6. Drizzle olive oil on top.
7. Bake in the oven for 20 minutes.
8. Broil the chicken for 2 minutes.
9. Serve the chicken and vegetables in a bowl on top of cauliflower rice.

NUTRITIONAL FACTS: Calories 558 Total Fat 19.1g Saturated Fat 4.4g Cholesterol 206mg Sodium 260mg Total Carbohydrate 14.2g Dietary Fiber 3.3g Total Sugars 5.9g Protein 80.3g Potassium 1039mg

168. BCHICKEN WITH BACON & RANCH SAUCE

PREPARATION: 10' **COOKING:** 20' **SERVES:** 4

INGREDIENTS

- 4 chicken breasts
- 1 teaspoon paprika
- 1 teaspoon garlic powder
- 1 teaspoon onion powder
- 1 tablespoon avocado oil
- 6 oz. cream cheese
- 1 tablespoon ranch seasoning powder
- 1 cup cheddar, grated
- 10 slices bacon, cooked and crumbled
- 2 tablespoons green onions, chopped

DIRECTIONS

1. Preheat your oven to 375 degrees F.
2. Season the chicken with the paprika, garlic powder and onion powder.
3. Pour the oil in a pan over medium heat.
4. Cook the chicken in a pan over medium heat.
5. Cook for 4 minutes per side.
6. In a bowl, mix the cream cheese and ranch seasoning.
7. Spread the cream cheese mixture on top of the chicken.
8. Top with the cheese.
9. Bake in the oven for 10 minutes.
10. Top with the bacon and green onion before serving.

NUTRITIONAL FACTS: Calories 743 Total Fat 48g Saturated Fat 20.2g Cholesterol 235mg Sodium 1523mg Total Carbohydrate 4.1g Dietary Fiber 0.5g Total Sugars 0.8g Protein 70.3g Potassium 738mg

169. CREAMY CHICKEN & MUSHROOM

PREPARATION: 10' **COOKING:** 20' **SERVES:** 4

INGREDIENTS

- 1 lb. chicken tenderloin
- Salt and pepper to taste
- 2 tablespoons butter, divided
- 2 tablespoons olive oil, divided
- ½ lb. mushrooms, sliced
- 2 cloves garlic, crushed
- ¼ cup fresh parsley, chopped
- 2 tablespoons fresh thyme
- 1 cup chicken broth
- ½ cup heavy cream
- ¼ cup sour cream

DIRECTIONS

1. Season chicken with salt and pepper.
2. Add 1 tablespoon each of butter and olive oil in a pan.
3. Sear the chicken until brown on both sides.
4. Set aside.
5. Add the remaining oil and butter.
6. Cook the mushrooms until crispy.
7. Add the garlic, parsley and thyme.
8. Pour in the broth.
9. Stir in the cream and sour cream.
10. Simmer until the sauce has thickened.
11. Put the chicken back to the sauce.

NUTRITIONAL FACTS: Calories 383 Total Fat 23g Saturated Fat 10.1g Cholesterol 122mg Sodium 611mg Carbohydrate 4.7g Dietary Fiber 1.2g Total Sugars 1.3g Protein 42.1g Potassium 304mg

170. MOZZARELLA CHICKEN

PREPARATION: 15' **COOKING:** 20' **SERVES:** 4

INGREDIENTS

- 4 chicken breasts (boneless, skinless)
- 1 tablespoon Italian seasoning, divided
- ½ teaspoon onion powder
- Salt and pepper to taste
- 1 teaspoon paprika
- 1 tablespoon olive oil
- 1 onion, chopped
- 4 cloves garlic, minced
- 1 fire roasted pepper, chopped
- 15 oz. tomato puree
- 2 tablespoons tomato paste
- ¾ cup mozzarella, shredded
- 1 tablespoons parsley, chopped

DIRECTIONS

1. Preheat your oven to 375 degrees F.
2. Season the chicken with 2 teaspoons Italian seasoning, onion powder, salt, pepper and paprika.
3. Pour the oil in a pan over medium heat.
4. Cook the chicken until brown on both sides.
5. Set aside.
6. Add the onion to the pan.
7. Cook for 3 minutes.
8. Add the garlic and pepper.
9. Cook for 1 minute.
10. Add the tomato puree and tomato paste. Mix well.
11. Stir in the remaining Italian sauce.
12. Simmer for 4 minutes.
13. Arrange the chicken on top of the sauce.
14. Add mozzarella on top.
15. Bake for 2 minutes.
16. Garnish with parsley before serving.

NUTRITIONAL FACTS: Calories 387 Total Fat 16.2g Saturated Fat 4.1g Cholesterol 130mg Sodium 193mg Total Carbohydrate 15.8g Dietary Fiber 3.3g Total Sugars 7.8g Protein 44.7g Potassium 963mg

KETO WOMEN over 50 126

171. CHICKEN PARMESAN

PREPARATION: 20'   **COOKING:** 8'   **SERVES:** 2

INGREDIENTS

- 2 chicken breast fillets
- 1 tablespoon heavy whipping cream
- 1 egg
- 1 ½ oz. pork rinds, crushed
- 1 oz. Parmesan cheese, grated
- Salt and pepper to taste
- ½ teaspoon garlic powder
- ½ teaspoon Italian seasoning
- 1 tablespoon ghee
- ½ cup tomato sauce
- ¼ cup mozzarella cheese, shredded

DIRECTIONS

1. Pound chicken fillet until flat.
2. In a bowl, mix the cream and egg.
3. Mix the pork rinds, Parmesan cheese, salt, pepper, garlic powder and Italian seasoning on another plate.
4. Dip the chicken fillet into the egg mixture.
5. Coat with the breading.
6. Add the ghee to a pan over medium heat.
7. Cook the chicken for 3 minutes per side.
8. Put the chicken to a baking pan.
9. Cover the top with tomato sauce and mozzarella cheese.
10. Broil for 2 minutes.

NUTRITIONAL FACTS: Calories 589 Total Fat 33.9g Saturated Fat 14.9g Cholesterol 282mg Sodium 1044mg Total Carbohydrate 5g Dietary Fiber 1g Total Sugars 3.1g Protein 65.3g Potassium 602mg

172. SPINACH FRITTATA

PREPARATION: 10'   **COOKING:** 35'   **SERVES:** 4

INGREDIENTS

- 5 ounces of diced bacon
- 2 tablespoons of butter
- 8 ounces of spinach that's fresh
- 8 eggs
- A single cup of heavy whipping cream
- 5 ounces of shredded cheese

DIRECTIONS

1. Preheat your oven to 350 and grease a 9 by 9 baking dishes.
2. Fry your bacon on a heat medium until it is crispy.
3. Add your spinach and stir until it has wilted.
4. Remove pan from heat.
5. Place it to the side.
6. Whisk cream and eggs together and pour into the baking dish.
7. Add the spinach and bacon and pour the cheese on top.
8. Put in the middle of the oven.
9. Bake a half hour.
10. It should be set in the middle. The color on top should be golden brown.

NUTRITIONAL FACTS: Calories: 661g Fat: 59g Fiber: 1g Protein: 27 grams Carbs: 4 grams

173. MUFFINS

PREPARATION: 15' **COOKING:** 10' **SERVES:** 12

INGREDIENTS
- 5 whisked medium eggs
- 2 cups of whole nuts

DIRECTIONS
1. Preheat oven to 350.
2. Grease a muffin tray (12 cups)
3. Process the nuts in a food processor.
4. Whisk eggs and nut flour, you made in a bowl.
5. Put in-tray.
6. Bake 25 minutes.
7. Stick should come out clean.
8. Let cool.

NUTRITIONAL FACTS: One muffin Calories: 117 Carbs: 4g Protein: 6g Fat: 10g

174. HALLOUMI TIME

PREPARATION: 5' **COOKING:** 15' **SERVES:** 2

INGREDIENTS
- 3 ounces of halloumi cheese that has been diced
- 2 chopped scallions
- 4 ounces of diced bacon
- 2 tablespoons of olive oil
- 4 tablespoons of chopped fresh parsley
- 4 eggs
- Half a cup of pitted olives

DIRECTIONS
1. In a frying pan on medium-high heat, heat the oil.
2. Fry the scallions, cheese, and bacon until they are nicely browned.
3. Get a bowl and whisk your eggs and parsley together.
4. Pour the egg mix into the pan over the bacon.
5. Lower heat.
6. Add olives.
7. Stir for 2 minutes.

NUTRITIONAL FACTS: Calories: 663g Protein: 28g Carbs: 4g Fat: 59g

175. HASH BROWNS

PREPARATION: 20' COOKING: 10' SERVES: 4

INGREDIENTS
- 3 eggs
- A pound of cauliflower
- Half a grated yellow onion
- 4 ounces of butter

DIRECTIONS
1. Rinse the cauliflower.
2. Trim it.
3. Grate it using a food processor.
4. Add it to a bowl.
5. Add everything and mix.
6. Set aside 10 minutes.
7. Melt a good amount of butter on medium heat.
8. You need a larger skillet.
9. Place the mix in the pan and flatten.
10. Fry for 5 minutes on each side.
11. Don't burn it.

NUTRITIONAL FACTS: Calories: 282 Carbs: 5g Protein: 7g Fat: 26g

176. MUSHROOM OMELET

PREPARATION: 5' COOKING: 10' SERVES: 1

INGREDIENTS
- 4 sliced large mushrooms
- A quarter chopped yellow onion
- A single ounce of shredded cheese
- An ounce of butter
- 3 eggs

DIRECTIONS
1. Crack the eggs and whisk them.
2. When smooth and frothy, they are good.
3. Melt butter over medium heat in a frying pan.
4. Add onions and mushrooms and stir until they become tender.
5. Pour the egg mix in. Surround the veggies.
6. When the omelet begins to get firm but is still a little raw on top, add cheese.
7. Carefully ease around the edges and fold in half.
8. When it's golden brown underneath (turning this color), remove and plate it.

NUTRITIONAL FACTS: Calories: 517g Protein: 26gFat: 4g Carbs: 5g

177. CRAB MELT

PREPARATION: 5' **COOKING:** 20' **SERVES:** 4

INGREDIENTS

- 2 zucchinis
- A single tablespoon olive oil
- 3 ounces of stalks from celery
- 3/4 cup of mayo
- 12 ounces of crab meat
- A single red bell pepper
- 7 ounces of cheese (use shredded cheddar)
- A single tablespoon of Dijon mustard

DIRECTIONS

1. Preheat your oven to 450.
2. Slice your zucchini lengthwise. Go for about a half-inch thick.
3. Add salt.
4. Let it sit for 15 minutes.
5. Pat it dries with a paper towel.
6. Place your slices on a baking sheet.
7. The baking sheet needs to be lined with parchment paper.
8. Brush olive oil on each side.
9. Finely chop the vegetables.
10. Mix with the other ingredients.
11. Apply mix to zucchini.
12. Bake for 20 minutes. Your top will be golden brown.

NUTRITIONAL FACTS: Calories-742 Fat-65 grams Fiber-3 grams Carbs-7 grams Protein-30 grams

178. POBLANO PEPPERS

PREPARATION: 5' **COOKING:** 15' **SERVES:** 2

INGREDIENTS

- A pound of grated cauliflower
- 3 ounces of butter
- 4 eggs
- 3 ounces of poblano peppers
- A single tablespoon of olive oil
- Half a cup of mayo

DIRECTIONS

1. Put your mayo in a bowl to the side.
2. Grate the cauliflower, including the stem.
3. Fry the cauliflower for 5 minutes in the butter.
4. Brush the oil on the peppers.
5. Fry them until you see the skin bubble a little.
6. Fry your eggs any way you like.
7. Serve with mayo.

NUTRITIONAL FACTS: Calories: 898 Fat: 87g Protein: 17g Carbs: 9g

179. SALAD WITH BUTTER

PREPARATION: 5' **COOKING:** 10' **SERVES:** 2

INGREDIENTS

- 10 ounces of goat cheese
- A quarter cup of pumpkin seeds
- 2 ounces of butter
- Tablespoons of balsamic vinegar
- 3 ounces of spinach (use baby spinach)

DIRECTIONS

1. Preheat oven to 400.
2. Put goat cheese in a baking dish that is greased.
3. Bake 10 minutes.
4. Toast pumpkin seeds in a frying pan that is dry. The temperature should be fairly high. They need some color, and they should start to pop.
5. Lower heat.
6. Add butter and simmer till it smells nutty and is golden brown.
7. Add vinegar and boil 3 minutes.
8. Turn off heat.
9. Spread the spinach on your plate and top with cheese and sauce.

NUTRITIONAL FACTS: Calories: 824 Fat: 73g Protein: 37g Carbs: 3g

179. TUNA CASSEROLE

PREPARATION: 7' **COOKING:** 20' **SERVES:** 4

INGREDIENTS

- A single green bell pepper
- 5 ? celery stalks
- 16 ounces of tuna in olive oil and drained
- A single yellow onion
- 2 ounces of butter
- A single cup of mayo
- 4 ounces of parmesan cheese freshly shredded
- A single teaspoon of chili flakes

DIRECTIONS

1. Preheat your oven to 400.
2. Chop all of the bell peppers, onions, and celery finely before frying it in butter in a frying pan. They should be slightly soft.
3. Mix mayo and tuna with the flakes and cheese.
4. This should be done in a greased baking dish.
5. Add the veggies.
6. Stir.
7. Bake 20 minutes.
8. It should be golden brown.

NUTRITIONAL FACTS: Calories: 953 Fat: 83g Protein: 43g Carbs: 5g

180. GOAT CHEESE FRITTATA

PREPARATION: 15' **COOKING:** 30' **SERVES:** 2

INGREDIENTS
- 4 ounces of goat cheese
- 5 ounces of mushrooms
- 3 ounces of fresh spinach
- 2 ounces of scallions
- 2 ounces of butter
- Half a dozen eggs

DIRECTIONS
1. Preheat your oven to 350.
2. Crack the eggs and whisk before crumbling cheese in the mix.
3. Cut mushrooms into wedge shapes.
4. Chop up the scallions.
5. Melt the butter in a skillet that is oven proof and cook scallions and mushrooms over medium heat for 10 minutes. They will be golden brown (or should be).
6. Add spinach and sauté two minutes.
7. Pour egg mixture into the skillet.
8. Place in the oven uncovered and bake 20 minutes.
9. It should be golden brown in the center.

NUTRITIONAL FACTS: Calories: 774 Fat: 67g Carbs: 6g Protein: 35g

181. PASTA

PREPARATION: 5' **COOKING:** 1' **SERVES:** 1

INGREDIENTS
- A single large egg yolk
- A single cup of mozzarella cheese that is part-skim low moisture and shredded

DIRECTIONS
1. In a bowl safe for the microwave, you will need to microwave the cheese for 60 seconds.
2. Stir until it's totally melted.
3. Allow to cool for 60 seconds.
4. Add in yolk and stir. It should make a yellow dough.
5. Place it on a flat surface that has been lined with parchment paper.
6. Place another paper over the dough.
7. Get a rolling pin and roll dough.
8. Remove the top piece when the dough is an eighth of an inch thick.
9. Cut the dough into half-inch wide strips.
10. Put in the fridge for 6 hours.
11. Put pasta in a pot of boiling water to cook and do not add salt.
12. Cook for 60 seconds.
13. Don't cook too long.
14. Remove and run under cold water.
15. Separate the strands.

NUTRITIONAL FACTS: Calories: 358 Fat: 22g Protein: 33g Carbs: 3g

182. MEATY SALAD

PREPARATION: 5' COOKING: 10' SERVES: 2

INGREDIENTS
- ounces of salami slices
- 2 cups of spinach
- A single avocado large and diced
- 2 tablespoons of olive oil
- A single teaspoon of balsamic vinegar

DIRECTIONS
1. Toss it all together.

NUTRITIONAL FACTS: Calories: 454 Carbs: 10g Protein: 9g Fat: 42g

183. SOUTHERN FRIED CHICKEN

PREPARATION: 15' COOKING: 15' SERVES: 6

INGREDIENTS
- 6 chicken thighs, skinless and boneless
- Avocado or canola oil for frying
- 3 large eggs
- 3 tablespoons heavy cream
- 1 cup almond flour
- 1 cup parmesan cheese
- Salt and pepper, to taste
- 1 teaspoon chili powder
- 1 teaspoon paprika powder

DIRECTIONS
1. Heat 2-inches of oil in a skillet over medium-high heat.
2. Beat eggs with heavy cream in a bowl.
3. Combine almond flour, parmesan paprika, and chili in a separate bowl.
4. Season chicken with salt and pepper.
5. Dip the chicken into the eggs and dredge through the almond flour mixture.
6. Fry the chicken in heated oil (up to 350F) for 5 minutes.
7. Drain the chicken on paper towels.
8. Serve while still warm.

NUTRITIONAL FACTS: Calories: 420 Fats: 23 Protein: 7 Carbohydrates: 0

184. LOW-CARB OKRA

PREPARATION: 10' **COOKING:** 40' **SERVES:** 4

INGREDIENTS

- 0.5lb. fresh okra
- Salt and pepper, to taste
- 1 tablespoon blanched almond flour
- 2 tablespoons grated Parmesan

DIRECTIONS

1. Preheat oven to 350F.
2. Wash and cut the okra into bite-size pieces.
3. Sprinkle the okra with salt and place in a colander for a few minutes.
4. Combine almond flour with parmesan cheese in a bowl.
5. Sprinkle with black pepper.
6. Add okra and toss to coat with the almond flour mixture.
7. Arrange the okra onto a baking sheet.
8. Bake the okra for 40 minutes, stirring halfway through the baking.
9. Serve warm.

NUTRITIONAL FACTS: Calories: 420 Fats: 13 Protein: 7 Carbohydrates: 0

185. CRAB SOUP

PREPARATION: 10' **COOKING:** 10' **SERVES:** 4

INGREDIENTS

- ½ tablespoon butter
- 1 teaspoon seafood seasoning
- 4oz. cream cheese
- 1 cup heavy cream
- ½ cup water
- ½ cup grated Pecorino Romano
- 0.5lb. crabmeat
- Salt and pepper, to taste
- 1 teaspoon dried dill

DIRECTIONS

1. Melt butter in a saucepot over medium-high heat.
2. Stir in seafood seasoning and cream cheese.
3. Let the cheese melt gently.
4. Add heavy cream, and water. Stir to combine.
5. Add parmesan cheese and puree the soup with an immersion blender.
6. Simmer for 5 minutes.
7. Add crab meat, dill, and stir gently. Cook for 3 minutes.
8. Season to taste with salt and pepper and remove from heat.
9. Serve warm.

NUTRITIONAL FACTS: Calories: 420 Fats: 23 Protein: 7 Carbohydrates: 0

186. SOUTHERN BEAN CASSEROLE

PREPARATION: 10'   **COOKING:** 40'   **SERVES:** 4

INGREDIENTS

- 0.5lb. frozen green beans, thawed
- 5oz. cooked and chopped bacon
- ½ onion, diced
- 1 small clove garlic, minced
- 2 tablespoons dry white wine
- ½ teaspoon finely grated lemon zest
- 1 tablespoon chopped parsley
- 1 tablespoon bacon fat
- 3oz. cream cheese
- 1oz. grated sharp cheddar cheese
- Salt and pepper, to taste
- ½ cup chicken stock
- 1 teaspoon whole-grain mustard

For topping:
- 2 tablespoons crushed pork rinds
- 1 good pinch garlic powder
- 1 teaspoon olive oil

DIRECTIONS

1. Preheat oven to 350F.
2. Cook the beans in simmering water for 1 minute. Rinse the beans under cold water and drain.
3. In a bowl, combine onion, garlic. and parsley.
4. Heat bacon fat in a skillet.
5. Add onion mixture and cook for 5 minutes.
6. Add lemon zest and cook for 1 minute.
7. Add the cream cheese and cook until melted.
8. Gradually add in the chicken stock and bring to a simmer.
9. Add sharp cheddar cheese, whole-grain mustard, and salt and pepper. Remove from the heat.
10. Pour the sauce over cooked beans.
11. Transfer the beans into greased baking dish.
12. Combine the pork rinds with garlic powder and sprinkle on top of the green beans.
13. Drizzle with olive oil and bake for 20 minutes.
14. Serve warm.

NUTRITIONAL FACTS: Calories: 410 Fats: 23 Protein: 7 Carbohydrates: 0

187. STUFFED CHICKEN BREASTS

PREPARATION: 30'   **COOKING:** 30'   **SERVES:** 4

INGREDIENTS

- 1 tablespoon butter
- ¼ cup chopped sweet onion
- ½ cup goat cheese, at room temperature
- ¼ cup Kalamata olives, chopped
- ¼ cup chopped roasted red pepper
- 2 tablespoons chopped fresh basil
- 4 (5-ounce) chicken breasts, skin-on
- 2 tablespoons extra-virgin olive oil

DIRECTIONS

1. Preheat the oven to 400°F.
2. In a small skillet over medium heat, melt the butter and add the onion. Sauté until tender, about 3 minutes.
3. Transfer the onion to a medium bowl and add the cheese, olives, red pepper, and basil. Stir until well blended, then refrigerate for about 30 minutes.
4. Cut horizontal pockets into each chicken breast, and stuff them evenly with the filling. Secure the two sides of each breast with toothpicks.
5. Place a large ovenproof skillet over medium-high heat and add the olive oil.
6. Brown the chicken on both sides, about 10 minutes in total.
7. Place the skillet in the oven and roast until the chicken is just cooked through, about 15 minutes. Remove the toothpicks and serve.

NUTRITIONAL FACTS: Calories: 389 Fat: 30g Protein: 25g Carbohydrates: 3g Fiber: 0g

188. CAULI RICE

PREPARATION: 10' COOKING: 15' SERVES: 4

INGREDIENTS

- 1 tablespoon olive oil
- 1 yellow bell pepper, seeded, chopped
- 1 onion, diced
- 1 clove garlic, minced
- 0.75lb. pork sausage, sliced
- 1 large head cauliflower, riced
- 2 tablespoon Cajun seasoning
- Salt and pepper, to taste
- Chopped parsley, for garnish

DIRECTIONS

1. Heat olive oil in a large skillet.
2. Add bell pepper and onion. Cook stirring for 5 minutes.
3. Add garlic and cook for 1 minute,
4. Add sliced sausage and cook for 5-7 minutes or until the sausage begins to brown.
5. Stir in "riced" cauliflower and spices.
6. Cook until the mixture us dry.
7. Serve warm, topped with chopped parsley.

NUTRITIONAL FACTS: Calories: 420 Fats: 23 Protein: 7 Carbohydrates: 5

189. LOW-CARB LASAGNA

PREPARATION: 15' COOKING: 50' SERVES: 4

INGREDIENTS

Lasagna noodles:
- 2 large eggs, room temperature
- 4oz. softened cream cheese
- 1 ¼ cup whole milk shredded mozzarella
- ¼ cup grated Parmesan
- ½ teaspoon onion powder
- ¼ teaspoon garlic powder
- ½ teaspoon dried basil

Filling:
- 1lb. ground beef
- 1 ½ cups sugar-free tomato sauce

- ¾ cup whole milk shredded mozzarella
- ½ cup ricotta cheese
- 1 tablespoon dried onion flakes
- 1 tablespoon Italian seasoning
- Salt and pepper, to taste

DIRECTIONS

1. Preheat oven to 375F. Line a baking sheet with parchment paper.
2. Make the noodles; cream eggs and cream cheese in a bowl.
3. Fold in remaining ingredients and stir until smooth. Spread the cheese mixture into the 9-inch baking dish. Bake the noodles for 25 minutes.
4. Cool the noodles on a wire rack and place in a fridge for 30 minutes. Cut the noodles into three equal parts.
5. Make the filling; cook the beef in a skillet until browned.
6. Stir in tomato sauce, and seasonings. Simmer for 10 minutes.
7. Assemble; Pour a ¼ cup of prepared sauce into the bottom of a baking dish.
8. Top with one piece of prepared noodle.
9. Top the noodle with 1/3 of the beef mixture, 1/3 mozzarella and 1/3 of ricotta.
10. Repeat layers until you have used all ingredients.
11. Bake the lasagna for 20-25 minutes.
12. Cool for 5 minutes before slicing and serving.

NUTRITIONAL FACTS: Calories: 420 Fats: 23 Protein: 7 Carbohydrates: 0

190. LOW-CARB SPAGHETTI BOLOGNESE

PREPARATION: 10' **COOKING:** 15' **SERVES:** 4

INGREDIENTS

- 1.5lb. ground beef
- 1 cup sugar-free tomato sauce
- 1 cup chopped tomatoes
- 2 teaspoons Worcestershire sauce
- 2 cloves garlic, minced
- 1 teaspoon dried basil
- 1 teaspoon dried oregano
- 2 packages Zero-Carb noodles
- 2 tablespoons grated parmesan
- Salt, to taste

DIRECTIONS

1. Cook the beef in a skillet until browned.
2. Add the Worcestershire sauce, garlic, and herbs.
3. Cook for 1 minute.
4. Stir in tomato sauce and tomatoes. Simmer for 10 minutes.
5. Prepare the noodles; prepare the noodles according to package directions.
6. Serve noodles on a plate.
7. Top with Bolognese sauce and parmesan.
8. Serve.

NUTRITIONAL FACTS: Calories: 220 Fats: 33 Protein: 6 Carbohydrates: 0

191. RANCH CASSEROLE

PREPARATION: 10' **COOKING:** 50' **SERVES:** 6

INGREDIENTS

- 1.5lb. chicken breasts, boneless and skinless, chopped
- Salt and pepper, to taste
- 2 tablespoons olive oil
- 1 12oz. can chopped tomatoes with green chiles
- 8oz. sliced mushrooms
- 1 cup sour cream
- 2 cups shredded cheese, like Monterey Jack

DIRECTIONS

1. Preheat oven to 350F.
2. Cut the chicken into small pieces.
3. Heat olive oil in a skillet. Add chicken and season to taste.
4. Cook the chicken for 7-8 minutes or until cooked through.
5. Stir in chopped tomatoes, mushrooms, and sour cream. Cook for 2 minutes.
6. Drain and excess liquid and transfer the mixture into the baking dish.
7. Top the chicken with cheese.
8. Bake the casserole for 40 minutes.
9. Serve warm.

NUTRITIONAL FACTS: Calories: 120 Fats: 25 Protein: 7 Carbohydrates: 0

CHAPTER 12.
SIDE DISHES

192. CHILI CAULIFLOWER MIX

PREPARATION: 10' **COOKING:** 35' **SERVES:** 4

INGREDIENTS

- 2 tablespoons sweet chili sauce
- 3 tablespoons olive oil
- 3 garlic cloves, minced
- Juice of 1 lime
- 1 cauliflower head, florets separated
- 1 teaspoon cilantro, chopped
- A pinch of salt and black pepper

DIRECTIONS

1. In a bowl, the chili sauce with the oil, garlic, lime juice, salt, pepper, cilantro and the cauliflower, toss well, spread on a lined baking sheet, introduce in the oven and cook at 425 degrees F for 35 minutes.
2. Divide the cauliflower between plates and serve as a side dish.

NUTRITIONAL FACTS: Calories: 271 Fat: 4 Fiber: 7, Carbohydrates: 11 Protein: 7

193. MOZZARELLA BRUSSELS SPROUTS

PREPARATION: 10' **COOKING:** 30' **SERVES:** 6

INGREDIENTS

- 2 tablespoons olive oil
- 2 pounds Brussels sprouts
- 2 garlic cloves, minced
- 1 teaspoon thyme, chopped
- A pinch of salt and black pepper
- 1 cup mozzarella, shredded
- ¼ cup parmesan, grated
- 1 tablespoon parsley, chopped

DIRECTIONS

1. Put some water in a pot, bring to a boil over medium-high heat, add sprouts, cook them for 10 minutes, transfer them to a bowl filled with ice water, cool them down and drain them well.
2. In a bowl, combine the Brussels sprouts with salt, pepper, oil, garlic and thyme, toss and smash them a bit.
3. Spread smashed Brussels sprouts on a lined baking sheet, sprinkle mozzarella and parmesan on top, introduce in the oven and bake them at 425 degrees F for 20 minutes.
4. Sprinkle parsley on top, divide between plates and serve as a side dish.

NUTRITIONAL FACTS: Calories: 288 Fat: 4 Fiber: 6 Carbohydrates: 13 Protein: 6

194. MOZZARELLA BROCCOLI MIX

PREPARATION: 10' **COOKING:** 15' **SERVES:** 4

INGREDIENTS

- 2 tablespoons olive oil
- 1 broccoli head, florets separated
- 2 garlic cloves, minced
- ½ cup mozzarella, shredded
- ¼ cup parmesan, grated
- ½ cup coconut cream
- 1 tablespoon parsley, chopped

DIRECTIONS

1. Heat up a pan with the oil over medium-high heat add broccoli, salt, pepper and garlic, stir and cook for 6 minutes.
2. Add parmesan, mozzarella and cream, toss, introduce the pan in the oven and cook at 375 degrees F for 10 minutes.
3. Add parsley, toss, divide between plates and serve as a side dish.

NUTRITIONAL FACTS: Calories: 261 Fat: 4 Fiber: 4 Carbohydrates: 13 Protein: 8

195. PARSLEY BACON BRUSSELS SPROUTS

PREPARATION: 10' **COOKING:** 20' **SERVES:** 6

INGREDIENTS

- 1-pound Brussels sprouts, halved
- A pinch of salt and black pepper
- 7 bacon slices, chopped
- 1 yellow onion, chopped
- 2 tablespoons stevia
- 2 tablespoons olive oil
- 1 tablespoon parsley, chopped
- 2 teaspoons sweet paprika

DIRECTIONS

1. Heat up a pan with the oil over medium-high heat, add the onion, stir and sauté for 4-5 minutes.
2. Add the bacon, stir and cook for 3 minutes more.
3. Add the sprouts, salt, pepper, stevia, paprika and parsley, toss, cook for 10 minutes more, divide between plates and serve as a side dish.

NUTRITIONAL FACTS: Calories: 261 Fat: 4 Fiber: 8 Carbohydrates: 12 Protein: 8

196. MEDITERRANEAN SIDE SALAD

PREPARATION: 10' **COOKING:** 0' **SERVES:** 4

INGREDIENTS

- 1-pint cherry tomatoes, halved
- 1 cup kalamata olives, pitted and sliced
- 1 cucumber, sliced
- ½ red onion, sliced
- 1 cup feta cheese, crumbled
- Juice of ½ lemon
- 2 tablespoons red vinegar
- A pinch of salt and black pepper
- 1 teaspoon oregano, dried
- ¼ cup olive oil

DIRECTIONS

1. In a salad bowl, combine the tomatoes with the olives, cucumber and onion.
2. In a separate bowl, combine the lemon juice with the vinegar, salt, pepper, oregano and oil and whisk well.
3. Pour this over your salad, toss, sprinkle cheese at the end and serve as a side dish.

NUTRITIONAL FACTS: Calories: 200 Fat: 3 Fiber: 6 Carbohydrates: 12 Protein: 8

197. MOZZARELLA AND ARTICHOKE MIX

PREPARATION: 10' **COOKING:** 10' **SERVES:** 4

INGREDIENTS

- 14 ounces canned artichoke hearts, drained
- A pinch of salt and black pepper
- 2 cups baby spinach
- 2 tablespoons parsley, chopped
- 1 cup mozzarella, shredded
- Juice of 1 lemon
- 1 and ¾ cup coconut milk
- ½ cup chicken stock
- 2 garlic cloves, minced
- 3 tablespoons ghee, melted
- A pinch of red pepper flakes

DIRECTIONS

1. Heat up a pan with the ghee over medium-high heat, add the garlic, stir and cook for 2 minutes.
2. Add lemon juice, coconut milk, stock, artichokes, salt and pepper, stir and cook for 5 minutes.
3. Add spinach, pepper flakes and mozzarella, toss, cook for 3 minutes more, and divide between plates, sprinkle parsley on top and serve as a side dish.

NUTRITIONAL FACTS: Calories: 277 Fat: 3 Fiber: 6 Carbohydrates: 12 Protein: 8

198. ROASTED BRUSSELS SPROUTS

PREPARATION: 10' **COOKING:** 25' **SERVES:** 4

INGREDIENTS

- 1-pound Brussels sprouts, halved
- 2 tablespoons olive oil
- A pinch of salt and black pepper

DIRECTIONS

1. Spread the sprouts on a lined baking sheet, add the oil, salt and pepper, toss, introduce in the oven and bake at 425 degrees F for 25 minutes.
2. Divide between plates and serve as a side dish.

NUTRITIONAL FACTS: Calories: 200 Fat: 2 Fiber: 6 Carbohydrates: 11 Protein: 8

199. ROSEMARY VEGGIE MIX

PREPARATION: 10' **COOKING:** 20' **SERVES:** 4

INGREDIENTS

- 1-pound Brussels sprouts, halved
- 2 tablespoons olive oil
- 1 teaspoon rosemary, chopped
- 1 tablespoon balsamic vinegar
- 1 teaspoon thyme, chopped
- ½ cup cranberries, dried

DIRECTIONS

1. Spread the sprouts on a lined baking sheet, add rosemary, vinegar, oil and thyme, toss, introduce in the oven and cook at 400 degrees F for 20 minutes.
2. Divide between plates, sprinkle cranberries on top and serve as a side dish.

NUTRITIONAL FACTS: Calories: 199 Fat: 3 Fiber: 5 Carbohydrates: 12 Protein: 7

200. CITRIC CAULIFLOWER RICE

PREPARATION: 10' **COOKING:** 15' **SERVES:** 4

INGREDIENTS

- 1 tablespoon ghee, melted
- Juice of 2 limes
- A pinch of salt and black pepper
- 1 cup cauliflower rice
- 1 and ½ cups veggie stock
- 1 tablespoon cilantro, chopped

DIRECTIONS

1. Heat up a pan with the ghee over medium-high heat, add the cauliflower rice, stir and cook for 5 minutes.
2. Add lime juice, salt, pepper and stock, stir, bring to a simmer and cook for 10 minutes.
3. Add cilantro, toss, divide between plates and serve as a side dish.

NUTRITIONAL FACTS: Calories: 200 Fat: 3 Fiber: 6 Carbohydrates: 9 Protein: 6

201. ZOODLES SIDE DISH

PREPARATION: 10' **COOKING:** 0' **SERVES:** 4

INGREDIENTS

- 4 zucchinis, cut with a spiralizer
- 2 tablespoons olive oil
- A pinch of salt and black pepper
- 1 cup mozzarella, shredded
- 2 cups cherry tomatoes, halved
- ¼ cup basil, torn
- 2 tablespoons balsamic vinegar

DIRECTIONS

1. In a bowl, combine the zucchini noodles with salt, pepper and the oil, toss and leave aside for 10 minutes.
2. Add mozzarella, tomatoes, basil and vinegar, toss, divide between plates and serve as a side dish.

NUTRITIONAL FACTS: Calories: 188 Fat: 6 Fiber: 8 Carbohydrates: 8 Protein: 6

202. COCONUT CAULIFLOWER MASH

PREPARATION: 10' **COOKING:** 10' **SERVES:** 6

INGREDIENTS
- 2 cauliflower heads, florets separated
- 1/3 cup coconut cream
- 1/3 cup coconut milk
- 1 tablespoon chives, chopped
- A pinch of salt and black pepper

DIRECTIONS
1. Put some water in a pot, bring to a boil over medium-high heat, add cauliflower florets, cook them for 10 minutes, drain them well, mash using a potato masher and stir.
2. Add the cream, the coconut milk, salt, pepper and chives, stir well, divide between plates and serve as a side dish.

NUTRITIONAL FACTS: Calories: 200 Fat: 3 Fiber: 3 Carbohydrates: 12 Protein: 5

203. PARMESAN BRUSSELS SPROUTS

PREPARATION: 10' **COOKING:** 30' **SERVES:** 4

INGREDIENTS
- 1-pound Brussels sprouts, halved
- 1 teaspoon oregano, dried
- 1 tablespoon olive oil
- 3 garlic cloves, minced
- ½ teaspoon hot paprika
- A pinch of salt and black pepper
- 2 tablespoons keto ranch dressing
- 1 tablespoon parmesan, grated

DIRECTIONS
1. Spread the sprouts on a lined baking sheet, add oregano, oil, garlic, paprika, salt and pepper, toss, bake them in the oven at 425 degrees F for 30 minutes, add parmesan and keto ranch dressing, toss well, divide between plates and serve as a side dish.

NUTRITIONAL FACTS: Calories: 222 Fat: 4 Fiber: 6 Carbohydrates: 12 Protein: 8

204. FRIED CAULIFLOWER RICE

PREPARATION: 10' **COOKING:** 15' **SERVES:** 4

INGREDIENTS

- 1 tablespoon ghee, melted
- 1 small yellow onion, chopped
- 2 hot dogs, sliced
- 1 tablespoon avocado oil
- 1 garlic clove, minced
- 2 and ½ cups cauliflower rice, steamed
- 2 eggs, whisked
- 2 tablespoons coconut amino
- 2 scallions, sliced

DIRECTIONS

1. Heat up a pan with the ghee over medium-high heat, add onion, garlic and hot dogs, stir and cook for 5 minutes.
2. Add cauliflower rice and avocado oil, stir and cook for 5 minutes more.
3. Add the eggs, toss everything, and cook for 5 more minutes until the eggs are scrambled, add the amino and the scallions, toss, divide between plates and serve as a side dish.

NUTRITIONAL FACTS: Calories: 200 Fat: 3 Fiber: 6 Carbohydrates: 12 Protein: 8

205. CHEESY ASPARAGUS DISH

PREPARATION: 10' **COOKING:** 30' **SERVES:** 6

INGREDIENTS

- 3 garlic cloves, minced
- ¾ cup coconut cream
- 2 pounds asparagus, trimmed
- 1 cup parmesan, grated
- A pinch of salt and black pepper
- 1 cup mozzarella, shredded

DIRECTIONS

1. In a baking dish, combine the asparagus with the garlic, cream, salt, pepper, mozzarella and top with the parmesan, introduce in the oven and bake at 400 degrees F for 30 minutes.
2. Divide between plates and serve as a side dish.

NUTRITIONAL FACTS: Calories: 200 Fat: 3 Fiber: 6 Carbohydrates: 12 Protein: 9

206. ROASTED CAULIFLOWER WITH PROSCIUTTO, CAPERS, AND ALMONDS.

PREPARATION: 10' COOKING: 25' SERVES: 2

INGREDIENTS

- 12 ounces cauliflower florets (I get precut florets at Trader Joe's)
- 2 tablespoons leftover bacon grease, or olive oil
- Pink Himalayan salt
- Freshly ground black pepper
- 2 ounces sliced prosciutto, torn into small pieces
- ¼ cup slivered almonds
- 2 tablespoons capers
- 2 tablespoons grated Parmesan cheese

DIRECTIONS

1. Preheat the oven to 400 degrees F. Line a baking pan with a silicone baking mat or parchment paper.
2. Put the cauliflower florets in the prepared baking pan with the bacon grease, and season with pink Himalayan salt and pepper. Or if you are using olive oil instead, drizzle the cauliflower with olive oil and season with pink Himalayan salt and pepper.
3. Roast the cauliflower for 15 minutes.
4. Stir the cauliflower so all sides are coated with the bacon grease.
5. Distribute the prosciutto pieces in the pan. Then add the slivered almonds and capers. Stir to combine. Sprinkle the Parmesan cheese on top, and roast for 10 minutes more.
6. Divide between two plates, using a slotted spoon so you don't get excess grease in the plates, and serve.

NUTRITIONAL FACTS: Calories: 288 Fat: 24g Carbohydrates: 7 Fiber: 3 Protein: 14

207. KETO JALAPENO POPPERS

PREPARATION: 10' COOKING: 20' SERVES: 16

INGREDIENTS

- 8 oz. cream cheese
- 1/2 cup shredded sharp cheddar cheese
- 1 tsp pink himalayan salt
- 1/2 tsp black pepper
- 8 jalapenos, halved, de-seeded
- 8 slices of bacon, cut in half

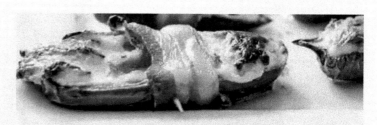

DIRECTIONS

1. Preheat stove to 375 degrees and line heating sheet with material paper.
2. Spot bacon cuts on paper towel-lined plate and microwave for 3 minutes. Put aside to somewhat cool.
3. In a medium bowl, include cream cheddar, destroyed sharp cheddar, salt, and pepper and microwave for 15 seconds. Mix together
4. Cautiously scoop cream cheddar blend into a plastic baggie
5. Wrap bacon cuts around jalapenos and stick with a toothpick.
6. Spot jalapenos on arranged heating sheet and prepare for 15 minutes.
7. Increment broiler warmth to cook and sear for 2-3 minutes, watching to guarantee cream cheddar doesn't consume.
8. Remove from broiler and permit cooling marginally before eating.

NUTRITIONAL FACTS: Calories 79 Fat 6.6g, Carbs 2.1g, Protein 8g

208. BARBECUE FAT BALLS

PREPARATION: 5' COOKING: 0' SERVES: 6

INGREDIENTS
- 4 ounces cream cheese
- 4 tbsp. bacon fat
- ½ tsp smoke flavor
- 2 drops stevia
- 1/8 tsp apple cider vinegar
- 1 tbsp. sweet smoked chili powder

DIRECTIONS
1. In a food processor, process all ingredients except chili powder until they form a smooth cream.
2. Scrap mixture and transfer into a small bowl, then refrigerate for 2 hours.
3. Form into 6 balls.
4. Sprinkle balls with chili powder, roll to coat well.
5. Serve.

NUTRITIONAL FACTS: Calories 146 Fat 14g Carbs 1.5g Protein 1.3g

209. BACON-WRAPPED SCALLOPS

PREPARATION: 10' COOKING: 15' SERVES: 4

INGREDIENTS
- 16 sea scallops
- 8 slices bacon
- 16 toothpicks
- olive oil for drizzling
- black pepper and kosher salt to taste

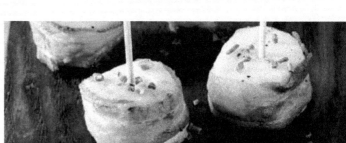

DIRECTIONS
1. Preheat broiler to 425°F.
2. Line a heating sheet with material paper. Put in a safe spot.
3. Envelop one scallop by using a half-reduce of bacon and comfortable with a toothpick.
4. Shower olive oil over every scallop and season with pepper and valid salt.
5. Orchestrate scallops in a solitary layer on a readied preparing sheet, giving every scallop some space to permit the bacon to clean.
6. Heat 12 to 15mins until scallop is sensitive and bacon is cooked through. Serve hot.

NUTRITIONAL FACTS: Calories 224 Fat 17g, Carbs 2g, Protein 12g

210. LOW CARB TORTILLA PORK RIND WRAPS

PREPARATION: 10' COOKING: 30' SERVES: 8

INGREDIENTS
- 4 large eggs
- 3 ounces pork rinds
- ½ tsp garlic powder
- ¼ tsp ground cumin
- ¼ to ½ cup water
- avocado oil or coconut oil

DIRECTIONS
1. In a powerful blender or nourishment processor, consolidate the eggs, pork skins, garlic powder, and cumin. Mix until smooth and very much joined. Include 1/4 cup of the water and mix once more. On the off chance that the blend is extremely thick, keep on including water until it is the consistency of hotcake hitter.
2. Warmth a sparse 1/2 teaspoon of oil in an 8-inch nonstick skillet over medium-low warmth, include around 3 tablespoons of the hitter and utilize an elastic spatula to spread it meagerly over the base of the dish, nearly to the edges.
3. Cook for about a moment, until the base is starting to dark-colored.
4. Rehash with the rest of the player, adding oil to the skillet just as essential
5. Add more water to the player as required; it will thicken as it sits.

NUTRITIONAL FACTS: Calories 194, Fat 5.6g, Carbs 5.4g, Protein 9.7g

211. AVOCADO CHICKEN SALAD

PREPARATION: 18' COOKING: 20' SERVES: 3

INGREDIENTS
- 3 avocados
- 1 lb. chicken (cooked in any way from this book)
- 1 medium tomato
- 1 onion
- 4 limes
- sea salt and fresh ground black pepper

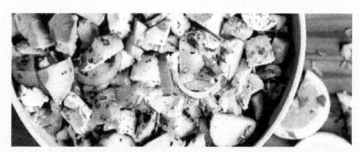

DIRECTIONS
1. In an enormous bowl pound the avocados until smooth.
2. Include the chicken, onions, tomatoes, lime squeeze, salt, and pepper.
3. Blend well.

NUTRITIONAL FACTS: Calories 465, Fat 38g, Carbs 6.7g, Protein 55g

212. PALEO-ITALIAN CARPACCIO

PREPARATION: 1H 30'   COOKING: 1H   SERVES: 4

INGREDIENTS

- 8 ounces of grass-fed, grass-finished filet mignon
- 1 bunch fresh organic Arugula
- 4 tsp truffle infused extra virgin olive oil
- 1 tsp unrefined sea salt
- freshly ground black pepper to taste

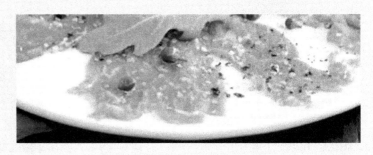

DIRECTIONS

1. Spot the meat in the cooler for around 2 hours. This will make it firm enough to cut with a sharp gourmet specialist's blade or with a meat slicer.
2. Cut meagerly and isolate the individual cuts laying them on 4 individual plates.
3. Organize the arugula over the meat, separating it similarly
4. Shower the oil on the plates, at that point sprinkle with salt and pepper
5. In the event that you are utilizing cheddar, mastermind the shaved parmesan on top
6. You can include extra naturally ground dark pepper to decorate the top.
7. Plates can be chilled in the icebox for 30 minutes before serving.

NUTRITIONAL FACTS: Calories 437, Fat 28g, Carbs 4g, Protein 31g

213. MEAT-LOVER PIZZA CUPS

PREPARATION: 15'   COOKING: 11'   SERVES: 12

INGREDIENTS

- 12 deli ham slices
- 1 lb. bulk Italian sausages
- 12 tbsp. sugar-free pizza sauce
- 3 cups grated mozzarella cheese
- 24 pepperoni slices
- 1 cup cooked and crumbled bacon

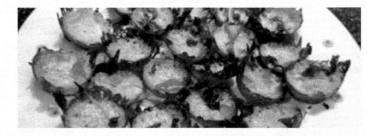

DIRECTIONS

1. Preheat broiler to 375 F. Fry Italian frankfurters in a skillet, depleting abundance oil.
2. Line 12-cup biscuit tin with ham cuts. Italian sausages, ham slices, pizza sauce, mozzarella cheese, pepperoni cuts, and bacon disintegrate between each cup, in a specific order.
3. Heat at 375 F for 10 minutes, cook for 1 moment until cheese air pockets and tans and the edges of the meat ingredients look firm.
4. Remove pizza cups from biscuit tin and set on paper towels to keep the bottoms from getting wet.
5. Serve.

NUTRITIONAL FACTS: Calories 165, Fat 14g, Carbs 6.1g, Protein 2g

214. BACON ONION BUTTER

PREPARATION: 15' COOKING: 35' SERVES: 6

INGREDIENTS

- 9 tbsp. butter
- 4 strips bacon sliced into small strips
- 90 grams onion
- 2 tsp spicy brown mustard
- 1/2 tsp black pepper

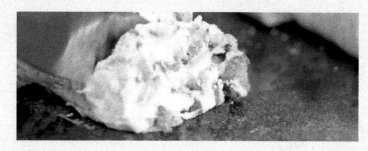

DIRECTIONS

1. Dissolve 1 tablespoon margarine in a skillet on medium warmth and include bacon pieces.
2. When the bacon fat is beginning to cook include diced onion and fry until onion and bacon are fresh yet not overcooked.
3. Put aside bacon/onion blend in a bowl and cool to room temp.
4. Include mellowed margarine, 8 tablespoons, to an enormous blending bowl.
5. Include bacon and onions, yellow mustard, and pepper.
6. Cream together ingredients or utilize an electric blender.
7. Spoon into a smaller than normal biscuit tin, place in cooler until margarine is strong again.

NUTRITIONAL FACTS: Calories 830, Fat 117g, Carbs 7.0g, Protein 15g

215. CAESAR EGG SALAD LETTUCE WRAPS

PREPARATION: 10' COOKING: 15' SERVES: 4

INGREDIENTS

- 6 large hard-boiled eggs
- 3 tbsp. creamy Caesar dressing
- 3 tbsp. mayonnaise
- 1/2 cup Parmesan cheese
- cracked black pepper
- 4 large romaine lettuce leaves

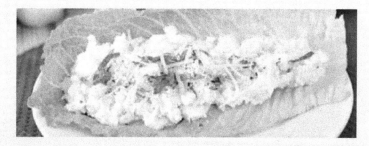

DIRECTIONS

1. In a blending bowl, join hacked eggs, velvety Caesar dressing, mayonnaise, and 1/4 cup Parmesan cheddar and broke dark pepper.
2. Spoon blend onto romaine leaves and top with residual Parmesan cheddar.

NUTRITIONAL FACTS: Calories 254, Fat 22g, Carbs 2.7g, Protein 13.5g

216. BEST KETO POPCORN CHEESE PUFFS

PREPARATION: 5'   COOKING: 5'   SERVES: 4

INGREDIENTS
- 4 ounces cheddar cheese sliced

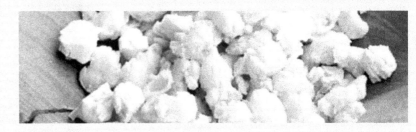

DIRECTIONS
1. Cut the cheddar into little ¼ inch squares.
2. Prior to heating, this formula must be readied 24 hours in advance
3. Cover the pan with baking parchment.
4. Leave the cheddar to dry out for in any event 24 hours.
5. The following day preheat your stove to 200C/390F and heat the cheddar for 3-5 minutes until it is puffed up.
6. Leave to cool for 10 minutes before getting a charge out of.

NUTRITIONAL FACTS: Calories 114, Fat 9g, Carbs 2.2g, Protein 7g

217. KETO BACON WRAPPED SALMON WITH PESTO

PREPARATION: 5'   COOKING: 15'   SERVES: 1

INGREDIENTS
- 170g salmon fillet
- 1 slice streaky bacon
- 2 tbsp. pesto

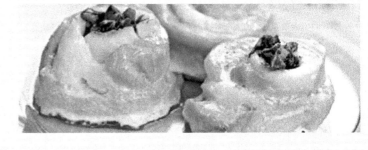

DIRECTIONS
1. Spot the streaky bacon on a hacking board.
2. Spot the salmon filet over the bacon. Move up firmly and comfy with a wooden stick.
3. Spot 1-2 tbsp. pesto inside the center.
4. Spot in the skillet, unfold, and fry tenderly for 10 minutes until the salmon and bacon are cooked. There is not any compelling motive to show the keto bacon-wrapped salmon. At the factor when you prepare dinner it in the griddle with the top, on medium warm temperature, it'll permit the steam internal to cook dinner the salmon from above.
5. Then again, region the bacon-wrapped salmon on a covered making ready plate/sheet container within the stove at 180C/350F for 15mins

NUTRITIONAL FACTS: Calories 449, Fat 31g, Carbs 3g, Protein 38g

218. DELI FAT BOMBS

PREPARATION: 5' COOKING: 0' SERVES: 2

INGREDIENTS
- 8 (1-ounce) slices sugar-free deli ham
- 4 ounces chive cream cheese
- 1 cup chopped baby spinach
- 1 medium red bell pepper, seeded and sliced

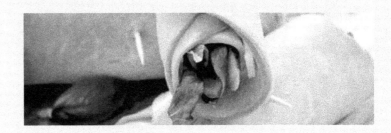

DIRECTIONS
1. Lay out each slice of ham flat. Spread 1 tbsp. cream cheese on each slice.
2. Put 2 tbsp. chopped spinach on top of the cream cheese on each slice.
3. Divide bell pepper into 8 portions and put the portions on top of spinach.
4. Roll up the ham and secure with a toothpick.
5. Serve.

NUTRITIONAL FACTS: Calories 399, Fat 25.9g, Carbs 6.7g, Protein 23.2g

219. KETO LOW CARB TORTILLA CHIPS

PREPARATION: 10' COOKING: 7' SERVES: 8

INGREDIENTS
- 2 cups mozzarella
- 3/4 cup almond flour
- 1/4 tsp onion, garlic and paprika
- 2 tbsp. psyllium husk Pinch salt

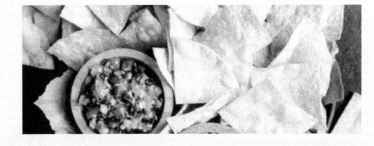

DIRECTIONS
1. Warmth you're stove to 350F.
2. Dissolve the mozzarella in the microwave. On the other hand, heat delicately in a non-stick pot.
3. Include the almond flour/ground almonds and psyllium husk in addition to the salt and flavors, if utilizing. Mix until consolidated, at that point ply until you have a smooth mixture.
4. Separate the batter into 2 balls and turn out between 2 sheets of preparing/material paper. Turn out as meagerly as could be expected under the circumstances! The more slender, the crispier your tortilla chips will turn out.
5. Cut into triangles and spread out on a sheet of preparing paper so the tortilla chips don't contact.
6. Prepare 6-8 minutes or until sautéed on the edges. Heating time will rely upon the thickness of your tortilla chips. I heated mine in 2 rounds, in addition to a third-round for the off-cuts.

NUTRITIONAL FACTS: Calories 143, Fat 9.2g, Carbs 4.8g, Protein 8.3g

CHAPTER 13. VEGETABLES

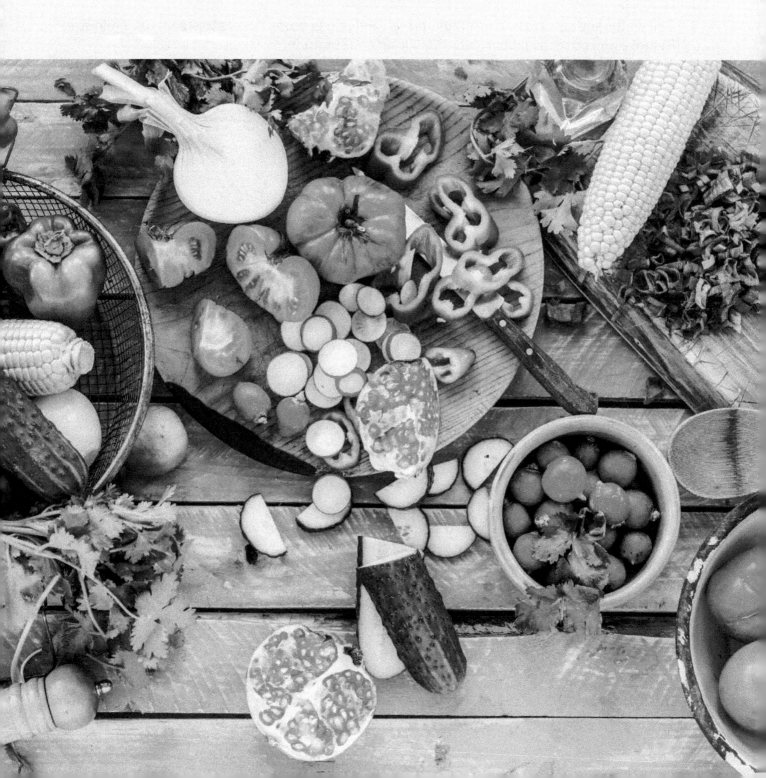

220. TOMATO AND BROCCOLI SOUP

PREPARATION: 50' **COOKING:** 55' **SERVES:** 4

INGREDIENTS
- A drizzle of olive oil
- Canned sugar-free tomatoes- 28 oz.
- Crushed red pepper- ¼ tsp.
- Broccoli head: into florets- 1
- Small ginger: chopped- 1
- Onion: chopped – 1
- Garlic clove: minced- 1
- Coriander seeds- 2 tsp.
- Black pepper
- Salt

DIRECTIONS
1. Boil water and salt in a pan on medium-high and add broccoli florets to steam for 2 minutes.
2. Remove and put in a bowl of ice water. Drain and set aside.
3. Heat pan and put in coriander seeds to toast for 4 minutes. Blend in a blender and set aside.
4. Pour olive oil in a pot and set to medium and add red pepper, salt, pepper and onions and cook for 7 minutes.
5. Mix in coriander seeds and garlic and let it cook for 3 minutes.
6. Pour in tomatoes and let simmer for 10 minutes.
7. Mix in broccoli and cook for 12 minutes.
8. Serve

NUTRITIONAL FACTS: Calories- 152, carbs- 1, protein- 9, fiber- 8, fats- 9

221. BOK CHOY STIR FRY WITH FRIED BACON SLICES

PREPARATION: 17' **COOKING:** 15' **SERVES:** 2

INGREDIENTS
- Bok choy; chopped - 2 cup.
- Garlic cloves; minced - 2
- Bacon slices; chopped - 2
- A drizzle of avocado oil
- Salt and black pepper to the taste.

DIRECTIONS
1. Take a pan and heat it with oil over medium heat.
2. When the oil is hot, add bacon and keep stirring it until it's brown and crispy.
3. Transfer them to paper towels to drain out the excess oil.
4. Now bring the pan to medium heat and in it add garlic and bok choy.
5. Again give it a stir and cook it for 5 minutes.
6. Now drizzle and add some salt, pepper and the fried bacon and stir them for another 1 minute.
7. Turn off the heat and divide them in plates to serve.

NUTRITIONAL FACTS: Calories: 50; Fat: 1; Fiber: 1; Carbs: 2; Protein: 2

222. BROCCOLI-CAULIFLOWER STEW

PREPARATION: 25' **COOKING:** 15' **SERVES:** 5

INGREDIENTS
- Bacon slices: chopped -2
- Cauliflower head: separated into florets- 1
- Broccoli head: separated into florets- 1
- Butter- 2 tbsp.
- Garlic cloves: minced- 2
- Salt
- Black pepper

DIRECTIONS
1. Put a pan on medium heat and dissolve the butter and the garlic. Add the bacon slices to brown for 3 minutes all over.
2. Mix in broccoli and cauliflower florets to cook for 2 minutes.
3. Pour water over it and cover the lid and let cook for 10 minutes.
4. Season with pepper and salt and puree soup with a dipping blend.
5. Let boil slowly for some minutes on medium heat.
6. Serve into bowls.

NUTRITIONAL FACTS: Calories- 128, carbs- 4, protein- 6, fiber- 7, fats- 2

223. CREAMY AVOCADO SOUP

PREPARATION: 20' **COOKING:** 15' **SERVES:** 4

INGREDIENTS
- Chicken stock, 3 c.
- Black pepper
- Chopped scallions, 2
- Salt
- Heavy cream, 2/3 c.
- Butter, 2 tbsps.
- Chopped avocados, 2

DIRECTIONS
1. Over a medium source of heat, set the saucepan and cook the scallions for 2 minutes
2. Stir in 2 ½ cups stock to simmer for 3 minutes
3. Set the blender in position to blend avocados, heavy cream, the remaining stock, and seasonings.
4. Return to a pan to cook for 2 minutes as you adjust the seasoning
5. Serve in soup bowls

NUTRITIONAL FACTS: Calories: 335, Fat: 32, Fiber: 9, Carbs: 13, Protein: 3

224. BOK CHOY MUSHROOM SOUP

PREPARATION: 25'   **COOKING:** 15'   **SERVES:** 4

INGREDIENTS

- Bacon strips: chopped- 2
- Beef stock- 3 cups
- Bok choy: chopped- 1 bunch
- Onion: chopped- 1
- Parmesan cheese: grated- 3 tbsp.
- Coconut aminos- 3 tbsp.
- Worcestershire sauce- 2 tbsp.
- Red pepper flakes- ½ tbsp.
- Mushrooms: chopped- 1½ cups
- Black Pepper
- Salt

DIRECTIONS

1. Put bacon in a saucepan over medium-high heat to brown until crispy then remove to paper towels to drain.
2. To medium heat, add the mushrooms and onions in the pan and cook for 15 minutes.
3. Pour in the stock, pepper flakes, aminos, bok choy, Worcestershire sauce, salt and pepper and mix.
4. Cook until bok choy is tender.
5. Serve into bowls and sprinkle with Parmesan cheese and bacon.

NUTRITIONAL FACTS: Calories- 100, carbs- 1, protein- 5, fiber- 9, fats- 5

225. TASTY RADISH SOUP

PREPARATION: 30'   **COOKING:** 45'   **SERVES:** 4

INGREDIENTS

- Chopped onion, 1
- Salt
- Chopped celery stalk, 2
- Chicken stock, 6 c.
- Coconut oil, 3 tbsps.
- Quartered radishes, 2 bunches
- Black pepper
- Minced garlic cloves, 6

DIRECTIONS

1. Set the pan over medium heat and melt the oil
2. Stir in the celery, onion, and garlic to cook until soft, about 5 minutes
3. Stir in the stock, radishes, and seasonings.
4. Cover and simmer to boil for 15 minutes
5. Enjoy while still hot

NUTRITIONAL FACTS: Calories: 131, Fat: 12, Fiber: 8, Carbs: 4, Protein: 1

226. NFRIED GARLICY BACON AND BOK CHOY BROTH

PREPARATION: 17'   **COOKING:** 15'   **SERVES:** 2

INGREDIENTS
- Bok choy: chopped- 2 cups
- A drizzle of avocado oil
- Bacon slices: chopped- 2
- Garlic cloves: minced- 2
- Black pepper
- Salt

DIRECTIONS
1. Put bacon in a pan on medium heat and let crisp. Remove and let drain on paper towels.
2. Add bok choy and garlic to the pan and let cook for 4 minutes.
3. Season with pepper and salt and put the bacon back into the pan.
4. Let cook for 1 minute and serve.

NUTRITIONAL FACTS: Calories- 116, carbs- 8, protein- 3, fiber- 8, fats- 1

227. NUTRITIONAL MUSTARD GREENS AND SPINACH SOUP

PREPARATION: 25'   **COOKING:** 15'   **SERVES:** 6

INGREDIENTS
- Spinach; torn - 5 cups.
- Fenugreek seeds - 1/2 teaspoon.
- Cumin seeds - 1 teaspoon.
- Jalapeno; chopped - 1 tablespoon.
- Mustard greens; chopped - 5 cups.
- Ghee - 2 teaspoons.
- Paprika - 1/2 teaspoon.
- Avocado oil - 1 tablespoon.
- Coriander seeds - 1 teaspoon.
- Yellow onion; chopped - 1 cup.
- Garlic; minced - 1 tablespoon.
- Ginger; grated - 1 tablespoon.
- Turmeric; ground - 1/2 teaspoon.
- Coconut milk - 3 cups.
- Salt and black pepper to the taste.

DIRECTIONS
1. Add coriander, fenugreek and cumin seed in a heated pot with oil over medium high heat.
2. Now stir and brow them for 2 minutes.
3. In the same pot, add onions and again stir them for 3 minutes.
4. Now after the onion's cooked, add half of the garlic, jalapenos, ginger and turmeric.
5. Again, give it a good stir and cook for another 3 minutes.
6. Add some more mustard greens, spinach and saute everything for 10 minutes.
7. After it's done add milk, salt, pepper before blending the soup with an immersion blender.
8. Now take another pan and heat it up over medium heat with some ghee drizzled on it.
9. In it, add garlic, paprika, and give it a good stir before turning off the heat.
10. Bring the soup to heat over medium heat and transfer them into soup bowls.
11. Top it with some drizzles of ghee and paprika. Now it's ready to serve hot.

NUTRITIONAL FACTS: Calories: - 143; Fat: 6; Fiber: 3; Carbs: 7; Protein: 7

228. HASH BROWNS WITH RADISH

PREPARATION: 20' **COOKING:** 15' **SERVES:** 4

INGREDIENTS
- Shredded Parmesan cheese, 1/3 c.
- Garlic powder, ½ tsp.
- Salt
- Shredded radishes, 1 lb.
- Black pepper
- Onion powder, ½ tsp.
- Medium eggs, 4

DIRECTIONS
1. Set a large mixing bowl in a working surface.
2. Combine the seasonings, radishes, eggs, onion, and parmesan cheese
3. Arrange the mixture in a well-lined baking tray.
4. Set the oven for 10 minutes at 375oF. Allow to bake
5. Enjoy while still hot
6. v

NUTRITIONAL FACTS: Calories: 104, Fat: 6, Fiber: 8, Carbs: 5, Protein: 6

229. BAKED RADISHES

PREPARATION: 30' **COOKING:** 35' **SERVES:** 4

INGREDIENTS
- Chopped chives, 1 tbsp.
- Sliced radishes, 15
- Salt
- Vegetable oil cooking spray
- Black pepper

DIRECTIONS
1. Line your baking sheet well then spray with the cooking spray
2. Set the sliced radishes on the baking tray then sprinkle with cooking oil
3. Add the seasonings then top with chives
4. Set the oven for 10 minutes at 375oF, allow to bake
5. Turn the radishes to bake for 10 minutes
6. Serve cold

NUTRITIONAL FACTS: Calories: 63, Fat: 8, Fiber: 3, Carbs: 6, Protein: 1

230. COLESLAW AVOCADO SALAD

PREPARATION: 10' COOKING: 15' SERVES: 4

INGREDIENTS

- White vinegar, 1 tbsp.
- Salt
- Olive oil, 2 tbsps.
- Black pepper
- Lemon stevia, ¼ tsp.
- Juice from 2 limes
- Mashed avocados, 2
- Chopped onion, ¼ c.
- Chopped cilantro, ¼ c.
- For coleslaw mix
- Salt, 1 tsp.
- Small red cabbage, ¼
- Shredded carrot, ½
- Lemon juice, ¼ c.
- Small green cabbage, ½
- Olive oil, ¼ c.
- Stevia, 1 tbsp.
- Zest of ½ lemon

DIRECTIONS

1. Set the mixing bowl in place to make the coleslaw salad
2. Add the mashed avocado and onions to coat well
3. Combine the seasonings, lime juice, vinegar, stevia, and oil in another bowl.
4. Add the mixture to the salad, mix to coat evenly
5. Enjoy

NUTRITIONAL FACTS: Calories: 481, Fat: 42, Fiber: 12, Carbs: 26, Protein: 6

231. SHERRY WATERCRESS BROTH

PREPARATION: 20' COOKING: 15' SERVES: 4

INGREDIENTS

- Sherry - ¼ cup
- Watercress - 6½ cups
- Chicken stock - 6 cups
- Coconut aminos - 2 tsp.
- Whisked egg whites of 3 eggs
- Shallots: chopped - 3
- Sesame seeds - 2 tsp.
- Salt and pepper

DIRECTIONS

1. Pour the stock into the pot and add sherry, coconut amino, salt and pepper and mix. Boil on medium heat.
2. Mix in watercress, shallots, and whisked whites and let boil.
3. Serve sprinkled with sesame seeds.

NUTRITIONAL FACTS: Calories - 73, carbs - 7, protein - 9, fiber - 2, fats - 7

232. CREAMED CHEDDAR RADISHES

PREPARATION: 35' **COOKING:** 15' **SERVES:** 1

INGREDIENTS
- Black pepper
- Halved radishes, 7 oz.
- Bacon slices, 2
- Chopped green onion, 1 tbsp.
- Sour cream, 2 tbsps.
- Cayenne pepper powder
- Salt
- Grated cheddar cheese, 1 tbsp.

DIRECTIONS
1. Set the radishes in a saucepan then add water.
2. Let it boil for 10 minutes over medium heat then drain the water
3. Set your pan over medium-high heat to cook the bacon to a crispy texture.
4. Drain the excess grease in a paper towel and reserve
5. Set the same pan again over medium heat then stir-fry the radishes for seven minutes
6. Stir in the seasonings, sour cream, and cayenne pepper powder for 7 minutes
7. Serve with crumbled bacon topped with cheddar cheese

NUTRITIONAL FACTS: Calories: 319, Fat: 25, Fiber: 3, Carbs: 8, Protein: 11

233. MUSTARD EGG AND AVOCADO SALAD

PREPARATION: 17' **COOKING:** 15' **SERVES:** 4

INGREDIENTS
- Salt
- Mayonnaise, ¼ c.
- Medium eggs, 4
- Sliced avocado, 1
- Mustard, 2 tsps.
- Mixed lettuce leaves, 4 c.
- Chopped chives, 1 tbsp.
- Black pepper
- Minced garlic cloves, 2

DIRECTIONS
1. Set the cooking pan over medium-high heat.
2. Add water, eggs, and salt then allow to boil for about 7minutes.
3. Once boiled, drain the liquid, let cool then chop them.
4. Set a salad bowl in position to mix lettuce eggs and avocado
5. Toss with garlic, seasonings, and chives to coat
6. Combine the seasonings, mustard, and mayonnaise in another bowl
7. Add to the salad, toss and serve.

NUTRITIONAL FACTS: Calories: 278, Fat: 16, Fiber: 7, Carbs: 13, Protein: 12

234. CUCUMBER AVOCADO SALAD MIX

PREPARATION: 10' **COOKING:** 0' **SERVES:** 4

INGREDIENTS

- Salt
- Sliced cucumber, 1
- Chopped avocados, 2
- Olive oil, 2 tbsps.
- Sliced onion, 1
- Chopped cilantro, ¼ c.
- Lemon juice, 2 tbsps.
- Black pepper
- Halved cherry tomatoes, 1 lb.

DIRECTIONS

1. Stir together cucumber, tomatoes, avocado, and onion in a salad bowl
2. Add the seasonings, lemon juice, and oil. Mix to coat well.
3. Serve cold topped with cilantro

NUTRITIONAL FACTS: Calories: 310, Fat: 27, Fiber: 1, Carbs: 16, Protein: 8

235. FRIED EGGS WITH KALE AND BACON

PREPARATION: 5' **COOKING:** 15' **SERVES:** 2

INGREDIENTS

- 4 slices of turkey bacon, chopped
- 1 bunch of kale, chopped
- 3 oz. butter, unsalted
- 2 eggs
- 2 tbsp. chopped walnuts

Seasoning:
- 1/3 tsp salt
- 1/3 tsp ground black pepper

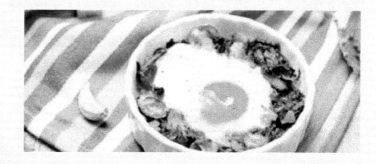

DIRECTIONS

1. Take a frying pan, place it over medium heat, add two-third of the butter in it, and let it melt, then add kale, switch heat to medium-high level and cook for 4 to 5 minutes until edges have turned golden brown.
2. When done, transfer kale to a plate, set aside until required, add bacon into the pan and cook for 4 minutes until crispy.
3. Return kale into the pan, add nuts, stir until mixed and cook for 2 minutes until thoroughly warmed.
4. Transfer kale into the bowl, add remaining butter into the pan, crack eggs into the pan and fry them for 2 to 3 minutes until cooked to the desired level.
5. Distribute kale between two plates, add fried eggs on the side, sprinkle with salt and black pepper, and then serve.

NUTRITIONAL FACTS: 525 Calories; 50 g Fats; 14.4 g Protein; 1.1 g Net Carb; 2.8 g Fiber;

236. EGGS WITH GREENS

PREPARATION: 5' **COOKING:** 10' **SERVES:** 2

INGREDIENTS

- 3 tbsp. chopped parsley
- 3 tbsp. chopped cilantro
- ¼ tsp cayenne pepper
- 2 eggs
- 1 tbsp. butter, unsalted

Seasoning:
- ¼ tsp salt
- 1/8 tsp ground black pepper

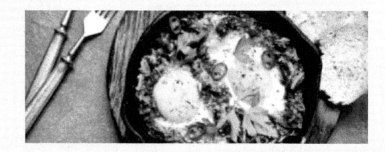

DIRECTIONS

1. Take a medium skillet pan, place it over medium-low heat, add butter and wait until it melts.
2. Then add parsley and cilantro, season with salt and black pepper, stir until mixed and cook for 1 minute.
3. Make two space in the pan, crack an egg into each space, and then sprinkle with cayenne pepper, cover the pan with the lid and cook for 2 to 3 minutes until egg yolks have set.
4. Serve.

NUTRITIONAL FACTS: : 135 Calories; 11.1 g Fats; 7.2 g Protein; 0.2 g Net Carb; 0.5 g Fiber;

237. SPICY CHAFFLE WITH JALAPENO

PREPARATION: 5' **COOKING:** 10' **SERVES:** 2

INGREDIENTS

- 2 tsp coconut flour
- ½ tbsp. chopped jalapeno pepper
- 2 tsp cream cheese
- 1 egg
- 2 oz. shredded mozzarella cheese

Seasoning:
- ¼ tsp salt
- 1/8 tsp ground black pepper

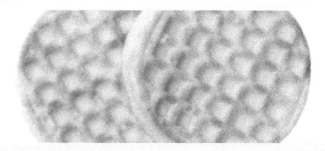

DIRECTIONS

1. Switch on a mini waffle maker and let it preheat for 5 minutes.
2. Meanwhile, take a medium bowl, place all the ingredients in it and then mix by using an immersion blender until smooth.
3. Ladle the batter evenly into the waffle maker, shut with lid, and let it cook for 3 to 4 minutes until firm and golden brown.
4. Serve.

NUTRITIONAL FACTS: 153 Calories; 10.7 g Fats; 11.1 g Protein; 1 g Net Carb; 1 g Fiber;

238. BULLETPROOF TEA

PREPARATION: 5'   COOKING: 0'   SERVES: 2

INGREDIENTS
- ¼ tsp cinnamon
- 2 cups strong tea
- 2 tbsp. coconut oil
- 2 tbsp. coconut milk

DIRECTIONS
1. Distribute tea between two mugs, add remaining ingredients evenly and then stir until blended.
2. Serve.

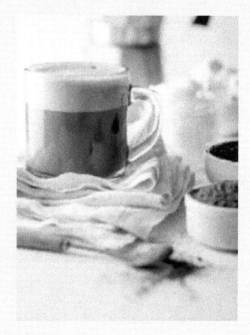

NUTRITIONAL FACTS: 151 Calories; 17 g Fats; 0 g Protein; 1 g Net Carb; 0 g Fiber;

239. TEA WITH COCONUT

PREPARATION: 10'   COOKING: 0'   SERVES: 2

INGREDIENTS
- 2 tea bags, cinnamon-flavored
- 2 tbsp. MCT oil
- ¼ cup coconut milk, unsweetened
- 2 cups boiling water

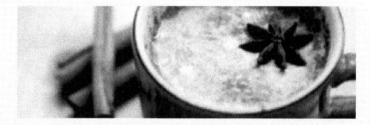

DIRECTIONS
1. Pour boiling water between two mugs, add a tea into each mug and let them steep for 5 minutes.
2. Meanwhile, take a small saucepan, place it over medium heat, pour in milk and heat for 3 minutes or more until hot.
3. After 5 minutes, remove tea bags from mugs, stir in milk, and MCT oil by using a milk frother until combined and then serve.

NUTRITIONAL FACTS: 191 Calories; 16 g Fats; 11 g Protein; 2 g Net Carb; 0 g Fiber;

240. CAULIFLOWER AND EGG PLATE

PREPARATION: 5'   COOKING: 12'   SERVES: 2

INGREDIENTS

- 4 oz. cauliflower florets, chopped
- 1 jalapeno pepper, sliced
- 2 eggs
- 1 ½ tbsp. avocado oil

Seasoning:
- ¼ tsp salt
- 1/8 tsp ground black pepper

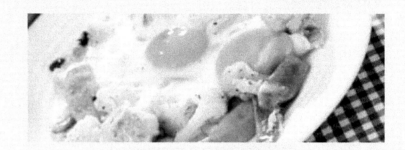

DIRECTIONS

1. Take a skillet pan, place it over medium heat, add oil and when hot, add cauliflower florets and jalapeno and then cook for 5 to 7 minutes until tender.
2. Make two spaces in the pan, crack an egg in each space, and then cook for 3 to 4 minutes until eggs have cooked to the desired level.
3. When done, sprinkle salt and black pepper over eggs and then serve.

NUTRITIONAL FACTS: 191 Calories; 16 g Fats; 11 g Protein; 2 g Net Carb; 0 g Fiber

241. BUTTERNUT SQUASH AND GREEN ONIONS WITH EGGS

PREPARATION: 5'   COOKING: 8'   SERVES: 2

INGREDIENTS

- 4 oz. butternut squash pieces
- 1 green onion, sliced
- ½ tbsp. butter, unsalted
- 2 tsp grated parmesan cheese
- 2 eggs

Seasoning:
- ¼ tsp salt
- ¼ tsp ground black pepper
- 1 tsp avocado oil

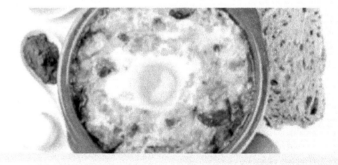

DIRECTIONS

1. Take a skillet pan, place it over medium heat, add butter and oil and when hot, add butternut squash and green onion, season with 1/8 tsp of each salt and black pepper, stir until mixed and cook for 3 to 5 minutes until tender.
2. Make two space in the pan, crack an egg in each space, and sprinkle with cheese, season with remaining salt and black pepper, cover with the lid and cook for 2 to 3 minutes until the egg has cooked to the desired level.
3. Serve.

NUTRITIONAL FACTS: 191 Calories; 16 g Fats; 11 g Protein; 2 g Net Carb; 0 g Fiber

242. BROCCOLI, ASPARAGUS AND CHEESE FRITTATA

PREPARATION: 5' **COOKING:** 16' **SERVES:** 2

INGREDIENTS

- ¼ cup chopped broccoli florets
- 1-ounce asparagus spear cuts
- ½ tsp garlic powder
- 2 tbsp. whipping cream
- 2 eggs

Seasoning:
- 2 tsp tbsp. avocado oil
- 1/8 tsp salt
- 1/8 tsp ground black pepper

DIRECTIONS

1. Turn on the oven, then set it to 350 degrees F and let it preheat.
2. Take a medium bowl, crack eggs in it, add salt, black pepper and cream, whisk until combined and then stir in cheese, set aside until required.
3. Take a medium skillet pan, place it over medium heat, add oil and when hot, add broccoli florets and asparagus, sprinkle with garlic powder, stir until mixed and cook for 3 to 4 minutes until tender.
4. Spread the vegetables evenly in the pan, pour egg mixture over them and cook for 1 to 2 minutes until the mixture begins to firm.
5. Transfer the pan into the oven and then cook for 10 to 12 minutes until frittata has cooked and the top has turned golden brown.
6. When done, cut the frittata into slices and then serve.

NUTRITIONAL FACTS: 206 Calories; 17 g Fats; 10 g Protein; 2 g Net Carb; 1 g Fiber;

243. BROCCOLI AND EGG PLATE

PREPARATION: 5' **COOKING:** 5' **SERVES:** 2

INGREDIENTS

- 3 oz. broccoli florets, chopped
- 2 eggs
- 1 tbsp. avocado oil
- ¼ tsp salt
- 1/8 tsp ground black pepper

DIRECTIONS

1. Take a heatproof bowl, place broccoli florets in it, cover with a plastic wrap, microwave for 2 minutes, and then drain well.
2. Take a medium skillet pan, place it over medium heat, add oil and when hot, add broccoli florets and cook for 2 minutes until golden brown.
3. Spread broccoli florets evenly in the pan crack eggs in the pan, sprinkle with salt and black pepper, cover with the lid and cook for 2 to 3 minutes until eggs have cooked to the desired level.
4. Serve.

NUTRITIONAL FACTS: 155 Calories; 12 g Fats; 8 g Protein; 1.6 g Net Carb; 1 g Fiber;

244. RADISH WITH FRIED EGGS

PREPARATION: 5' COOKING: 10' SERVES: 2

INGREDIENTS
- ½ bunch of radish, diced
- ½ tsp garlic powder
- 1 tbsp. butter
- 1 tbsp. avocado oil
- 2 eggs

Seasoning:
- 1/3 tsp salt
- ¼ tsp ground black pepper

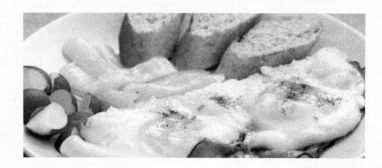

DIRECTIONS
1. Take a medium skillet pan, place it over medium heat, add butter and when it melts, add radish, sprinkle with garlic powder and ¼ tsp salt and cook for 5 minutes until tender.
2. Distribute radish between two plates, then return pan over medium heat, add oil and when hot, crack eggs in it and fry for 2 to 3 minutes until cooked to desired level.
3. Add eggs to the radish and then serve.

NUTRITIONAL FACTS: 187 Calories; 17 g Fats; 7 g Protein; 0.4 g Net Carb; 0.5 g Fiber;

245. SUNNY SIDE UP EGGS ON CREAMED SPINACH

PREPARATION: 5' COOKING: 10' SERVES: 2

INGREDIENTS
- 4 oz. of spinach leaves
- 1 tbsp. mustard paste
- 4 tbsp. whipping cream
- 2 eggs
- 1 tbsp. avocado oil

Seasoning:
- ¼ tsp salt
- ¼ tsp ground black pepper
- ½ tsp dried thyme

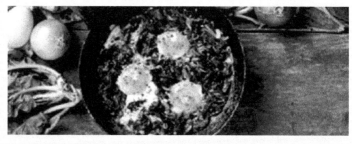

DIRECTIONS
1. Take a medium skillet pan, place it over high heat, pour in water to cover its bottom, then add spinach, toss until mixed and cook for 2 minutes until spinach wilts.
2. Then drain the spinach by passing it through a sieve placed on a bowl and set it aside.
3. Take a medium saucepan, place it over medium heat, add spinach, mustard, thyme, and cream, stir until mixed and cook for 2 minutes.
4. Then sprinkle black pepper over spinach, stir until mixed and remove the pan from heat.
5. Take a medium skillet pan, place it over medium-high heat, add oil and when hot, crack eggs in it and fry for 3 to 4 minutes until eggs have cooked to the desired level.
6. Divide spinach mixture evenly between two plates, top with a fried egg and then serve.

NUTRITIONAL FACTS: 280 Calories; 23.3 g Fats; 10.2 g Protein; 2.7 g Net Carb; 2.8 g Fiber;

246. CREAMY KALE BAKED EGGS

PREPARATION: 10' **COOKING:** 20' **SERVES:** 2

INGREDIENTS

- 1 bunch of kale, chopped
- 1-ounce grape tomatoes, halved
- 3 tbsp. whipping cream
- 2 tbsp. sour cream
- 2 eggs

Seasoning:
- ½ tsp salt
- ½ tsp ground black pepper
- ½ tsp Italian seasoning
- 1 ½ tbsp. butter, unsalted

DIRECTIONS

1. Turn on the oven, then set it to 400 degrees F and let it preheat.
2. Meanwhile, take a medium skillet pan, place butter in it, add butter and when it melts, add kale and cook for 2 minutes until wilted
3. Add Italian seasoning, 1/3 tsp each of salt and black pepper, cream and sour cream, then stir until mixed and cook for2 minutes until cheese has melted and the kale has thickened slightly.
4. Take two ramekins, divide creamed kale evenly between them, then top with cherry tomatoes and carefully crack an egg into each ramekin.
5. Sprinkle remaining salt and black pepper on eggs and then bake for 15 minutes until eggs have cooked completely.
6. Serve.

NUTRITIONAL FACTS: 301.5 Calories; 25.5 g Fats; 9.8 g Protein; 4.3 g Net Carb; 4 g Fiber;

247. BUTTER ASPARAGUS WITH CREAMY EGGS

PREPARATION: 5' **COOKING:** 8' **SERVES:** 2

INGREDIENTS

- 4 oz. asparagus
- 2 eggs, blended
- oz. grated parmesan cheese
- 1-ounce sour cream
- 2 tbsp. butter, unsalted

Seasoning:
- 1/3 tsp salt
- 1/8 tsp ground black pepper
- ¼ tsp cayenne pepper
- ½ tbsp. avocado oil

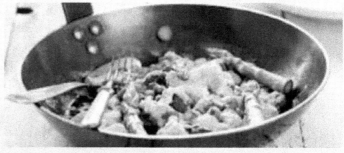

DIRECTIONS

1. Take a medium skillet pan, place it over medium heat, add butter and when it melts, add blended eggs and then cook for 2 to 3 minutes until scrambled to the desired level; don't overcook.
2. Spoon the scrambled eggs into a food processor, add 1/8 tsp salt, cayenne pepper, sour cream and cheese and then pulse for 1 minute until smooth.
3. Return skillet pan over medium heat, add oil and when hot, add asparagus, season with black pepper and remaining salt, toss until mixed and cook for 3 minutes or more until roasted.
4. Distribute asparagus between two plates, add egg mixture, and then serve.

NUTRITIONAL FACTS: 338 Calories; 28.5 g Fats; 14.4 g Protein; 4.7 g Net Carb; 1.2 g Fiber;

248. SPINACH EGG MUFFINS

PREPARATION: 5' COOKING: 10' SERVES: 2

INGREDIENTS

- ½ cups chopped spinach
- 1/8 tsp dried basil
- 1/8 tsp garlic powder
- 2 large eggs
- 3 tbsp. grated Parmesan cheese

Seasoning:
- ¼ tsp of sea salt
- 1/8 tsp ground black pepper

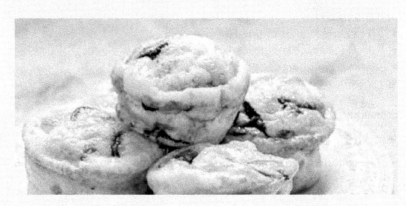

DIRECTIONS

1. Turn on the oven, then set it to 400 degrees F, and let preheat.
2. Meanwhile, place eggs in a bowl, season with salt and black pepper and whisk until blended.
3. Add garlic and basil, whisk in mixed and then stir in spinach and cheese until combined.
4. Take two silicone muffin cups, grease them with reserved bacon greased, fill them evenly with prepared egg mixture and bake for 8 to 10 minutes until the top has nicely browned.
5. Serve.

NUTRITIONAL FACTS: 55 Calories; 3.5 g Fats; 4.5 g Protein; 0.4 g Net Carb; 0.2 g Fiber;

249. BROCCOLI AND EGG MUFFIN

PREPARATION: 10' COOKING: 10' SERVES: 2

INGREDIENTS

- ¼ cup broccoli florets, steamed, chopped
- 2 tbsp. grated cheddar cheese
- 1/16 tsp dried thyme
- 1/16 tsp garlic powder
- 1 egg
- t¼ tsp salt
- 1/8 tsp ground black pepper

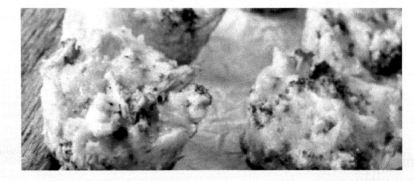

DIRECTIONS

1. Turn on the oven, then set it to 400 degrees F and let it preheat.
2. Meanwhile, take two silicone muffin cups, grease them with oil, and evenly fill them with broccoli and cheese.
3. Crack the egg in a bowl, add garlic powder, thyme, salt, and black pepper, whisk well, then evenly pour the mixture into muffin cups and bake for 8 to 10 minutes until done.
4. Serve.

NUTRITIONAL FACTS: 76 Calories; 5.1 g Fats; 5.7 g Protein; 1.2 g Net Carb; 0.7 g Fiber;

250. JALAPENO AND CHEESE EGG MUFFINS

PREPARATION: 10' COOKING: 15' SERVES: 2

INGREDIENTS

- 1 jalapeno pepper, diced
- 2 tbsp. sliced green onions
- 2 tbsp. grated parmesan cheese
- 1 tsp all-purpose seasoning
- 2 eggs

Seasoning:
- 1/3 tsp salt
- ¼ tsp ground black pepper

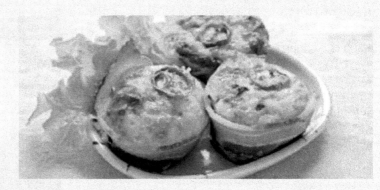

DIRECTIONS

1. Turn on the oven, then set it to 375 degrees F, and let it preheat.
2. Meanwhile, take two silicone muffin cups, grease with oil, and evenly fill them with cheese, jalapeno pepper, and green onion.
3. Crack eggs in a bowl, season with salt, black pepper, and all-purpose seasoning, whisk well, then evenly pour the mixture into muffin cups and bake for 15 to 20 minutes or until the top is slightly brown and muffins have puffed up.
4. Serve.

NUTRITIONAL FACTS: 108 Calories; 7.1 g Fats; 8.9 g Protein; 1.8 g Net Carb; 0.4 g Fiber;

251. CHEESY TOMATO AND OLIVE MUFFINS

PREPARATION: 10' COOKING: 12' SERVES: 2

INGREDIENTS

- 4 1/3 tbsp. almond flour
- ½ tbsp. coconut flour
- 1/3 tbsp. chopped tomato
- 1/3 tbsp. sliced green olives
- 2 tbsp. sour cream
- ½ of egg

Seasoning:
- 1/8 tsp baking powder
- 2/3 tbsp. avocado oil
- 3 tbsp. grated parmesan cheese

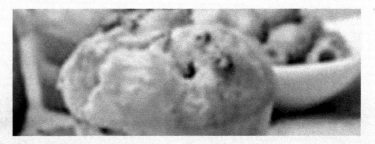

DIRECTIONS

1. Turn on the oven, then set it to 320 degrees F and let it preheat.
2. Meanwhile, take a medium bowl, place flours in it, and stir in the baking powder until mixed.
3. Add eggs along with sour cream and oil, whisk until blended and then fold in cheese, tomato, and olives until just mixed.
4. Take two silicone muffin cups, add the prepared batter in it evenly and then bake for 10 to 12 minutes until cooked but slightly moist in the middle.
5. When done, let muffin cools for 5 minutes, then take them out and serve.

NUTRITIONAL FACTS: 256 Calories; 23.5 g Fats; 8.7 g Protein; 1 g Net Carb; 1.8 g Fiber;

252. BUTTERY BROCCOLI AND BACON

PREPARATION: 5' **COOKING:** 12' **SERVES:** 2

INGREDIENTS
- 1 slice of turkey bacon
- 1 cup chopped broccoli florets
- 1/8 tsp garlic powder
- ¼ tsp Italian seasoning
- ¼ tbsp. unsalted butter

Seasoning:
- 1/8 tsp salt
- 1/8 tsp ground black pepper

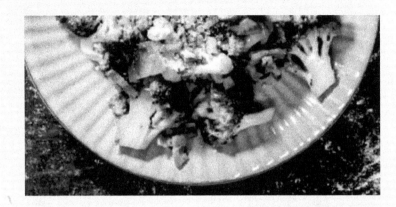

DIRECTIONS
1. Take a medium skillet pan, place it over high heat, add bacon slice and cook for 3 to 5 minutes until crispy.
2. Transfer bacon to a cutting board and then chop it into small pieces.
3. Reduce the heat to medium-low level, add broccoli florets into the pan, stir well into the bacon grease, add butter, then toss until mixed and cook for 5 minutes until tender.
4. Season the broccoli florets with salt, black pepper, and Italian seasoning, add chopped bacon, stir well and cook for 2 minutes until thoroughly heated.
5. Serve.

NUTRITIONAL FACTS: 77 Calories; 5 g Fats; 5 g Protein; 1 g Net Carb; 2 g Fiber;

253. BROCCOLI SALAD WITH BACON

PREPARATION: 5' **COOKING:** 0' **SERVES:** 2

INGREDIENTS
- 1 cup broccoli florets, chopped
- 4 tbsp. whipped topping
- 2 tbsp. shredded cheddar cheese
- 3 slices of turkey bacon, cooked, chopped
- 1/3 tsp garlic powder

Seasoning:
- 1/8 tsp salt
- 1/8 tsp dried parsley

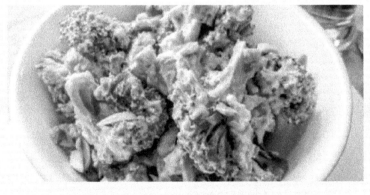

DIRECTIONS
1. Take a medium bowl, place whipped topping in it, whisk in garlic powder and parsley, and then fold in broccoli florets.
2. Top with bacon and cheddar cheese and serve.

NUTRITIONAL FACTS: 119 Calories; 10 g Fats; 3.5 g Protein; 2 g Net Carb; 0.5 g Fiber;

254. ROASTED GREEN BEANS

PREPARATION: 5'   COOKING: 25'   SERVES: 2

INGREDIENTS

- ½ pound green beans
- ½ cup grated parmesan cheese
- 3 tbsp. coconut oil
- ½ tsp garlic powder

Seasoning:
- 1/3 tsp salt
- 1/8 tsp ground black pepper

DIRECTIONS

1. Turn on the oven, then set it to 425 degrees F, and let preheat.
2. Take a baking sheet, line green beans on it, and set aside until required.
3. Prepare the dressing, and for this, place remaining ingredients in a bowl, except for cheese and whisk until combined.
4. Drizzle the dressing over green beans, toss until well coated, and then bake for 20 minutes until green beans are tender-crisp.
5. Then sprinkle cheese on top of beans and continue roasting for 3 to 5 minutes or until cheese melts and nicely golden brown.
6. Serve.

NUTRITIONAL FACTS: 119 Calories; 9 g Fats; 5 g Protein; 4.5 g Net Carb; 3 g Fiber;

255. FRIED CAULIFLOWER AND EGG RICE

PREPARATION: 5'   COOKING: 12'   SERVES: 2

INGREDIENTS

- 14 ounces canned artichoke hearts, drained
- A pinch of salt and black pepper
- 2 cups baby spinach
- 2 tablespoons parsley, chopped
- 1 cup mozzarella, shredded
- Juice of 1 lemon
- 1 and ¾ cup coconut milk
- ½ cup chicken stock
- 2 garlic cloves, minced
- 3 tablespoons ghee, melted
- A pinch of red pepper flakes

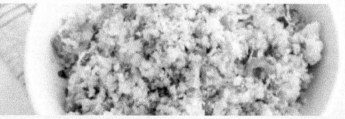

DIRECTIONS

1. Take a large skillet pan, place it over medium-high heat, add coconut oil and riced cauliflower, and cook for 5 minutes until softened.
2. Then add green onions, stir well and cook for 3 minutes until onions are tender.
3. Season with salt, sprinkle garlic over cauliflower, cook for 1 minute until fragrant, then pour in the egg, stir well and cook for 2 minutes until the egg has scrambled to desire level, stirring continuously.
4. Drizzle with soy sauce and sesame oil and Serve.

NUTRITIONAL FACTS: 57 Calories; 4 g Fats; 3 g Protein; 1.7 g Net Carb; 0.5 g Fiber

256. SPINACH ZUCCHINI BOATS

PREPARATION: 5' **COOKING:** 10' **SERVES:** 2

INGREDIENTS

- 1 large zucchini
- ¾ cup spinach
- 1 ½ tbsp. whipped topping
- 3 tbsp. grated parmesan cheese
- ½ tsp garlic powder

Seasoning:
- ½ tsp salt
- ½ tsp ground black pepper

DIRECTIONS

1. Turn on the oven, then set it to 350 degrees F, and let preheat.
2. Take a skillet pan, place it over medium heat, add spinach and cook for 5 to 7 minutes or until spinach leaves have wilted and their moisture has evaporated completely.
3. Sprinkle garlic powder, ¼ tsp each of salt and black pepper over spinach, add whipped topping and 2 tbsp. cheese and stir well until the cheese has melted, remove the pan from heat.
4. Cut off the top and bottom of zucchini, then cut it in half lengthwise and make a well by scooping out pulp along the center, leaving ½-inch shell.
5. Season zucchini with remaining salt and black pepper, place them on a baking sheet and roast for 5 minutes.
6. Then fill zucchini evenly with spinach mixture, top with remaining cheese and broil for 3 minutes until cheese has melted.
7. Serve.

NUTRITIONAL FACTS: 86.5 Calories; 6 g Fats; 4 g Protein; 3.5 g Net Carb; 0.5 g Fiber;

257. GREEN BEANS WITH HERBS

PREPARATION: 5' **COOKING:** 7' **SERVES:** 2

INGREDIENTS

- 3 oz. green beans
- 2 slices of bacon, diced
- 3 tbsp. chopped parsley
- 3 tbsp. chopped cilantro
- 1 tbsp. avocado oil

Seasoning:
- ½ tsp garlic powder
- ¼ tsp salt

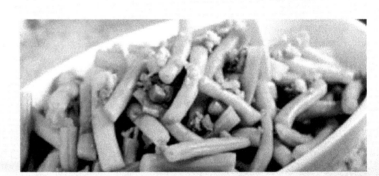

DIRECTIONS

1. Place green beans in a medium heatproof bowl, cover with a plastic wrap, and then microwave for 3 to 4 minutes at high heat setting until tender.
2. Meanwhile, take a medium skillet pan, place it over medium heat and when hot, add bacon and cook for 3 to 4 minutes until crisp.
3. Season bacon with salt, sprinkle with garlic powder and cook for 30 seconds until fragrant, remove the pan from heat.
4. When green beans have steamed, drain them well, rinse under cold water, and then transfer to a bowl.
5. Add bacon and remaining ingredients and toss until well mixed.
6. Serve.

NUTRITIONAL FACTS: 380 Calories; 33.7 g Fats; 15.2 g Protein; 2.4 g Net Carb; 1.4 g Fiber;

258. SALAD SANDWICHES

PREPARATION: 5' COOKING: 0' SERVES: 2

INGREDIENTS

- 1 medium avocado, peeled, pitted, diced
- 2 leaves of iceberg lettuce
- 1-ounce unsalted butter
- 2-ounce cheddar cheese, sliced

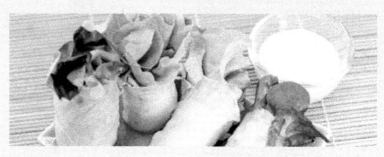

DIRECTIONS

1. Rinse the lettuce leaves, pat dry with a paper towel, and then smear each leaf with butter.
2. Top lettuce with cheese and avocado and serve.

NUTRITIONAL FACTS: 187 Calories; 17 g Fats; 5 g Protein; 4 g Net Carb; 1.5 g Fiber;

259. CELERIAC STUFFED AVOCADO

PREPARATION: 10' COOKING: 0' SERVES: 2

INGREDIENTS

- 1 avocado
- 1 celery root, finely chopped
- 2 tbsp. mayonnaise
- ½ of a lemon, juiced, zested
- 2 tbsp. mayonnaise

Seasoning:
- ¼ tsp salt
-

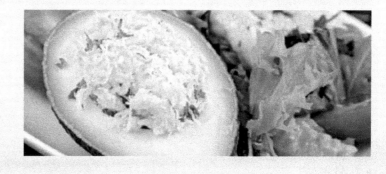

DIRECTIONS

1. Prepare avocado and for this, cut avocado in half and then remove its pit.
2. Place remaining ingredients in a bowl, stir well until combined and evenly stuff this mixture into avocado halves.
3. Serve.

NUTRITIONAL FACTS: 285 Calories; 27 g Fats; 2.8 g Protein; 4.4 g Net Carb; 2.6 g Fiber;

260. COBB SALAD

PREPARATION: 5' COOKING: 10' SERVES: 1

INGREDIENTS

- 1 large egg, hard-boiled, peeled, diced
- 2 oz. chicken thigh
- 2 1/2 slices bacon, cooked, crumbled
- ½ of a medium avocado, diced
- ½ cup chopped lettuce

Seasoning:
- 1 cup of water
- 3 tbsp. apple cider vinegar
- 1 ½ tbsp. coconut oil
- ¼ tsp salt
- 1/8 tsp ground black pepper

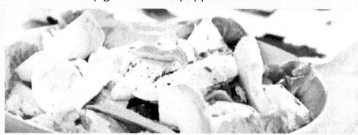

DIRECTIONS

1. Cook chicken thigh and for this, place chicken thighs in an instant pot, pour in 1 cup water, and shut the pot with a lid.
2. Cook the chicken for 5 minutes at high pressure, and when done, let the pressure release naturally.
3. Meanwhile, cook the bacon and for this, take a skillet pan, place it over medium heat and when hot, add bacon slices.
4. Cook the bacon for 3 to 5 minutes until golden brown, then transfer them to a cutting board and chop the bacon, reserve the bacon grease in the pan for the next meal.
5. When chicken thigh has cooked, transfer it to a bowl and shred the chicken with two forks, reserving the chicken broth for later use.
6. Assemble the salad and for this, place lettuce in a salad plate, top with chicken, bacon, diced eggs, avocado, and chicken in horizontal rows.
7. Prepare the dressing and for this, whisk together salt, black pepper, vinegar, and oil until incorporated and then drizzle the dressing generously over the salad.
8. Serve.

NUTRITIONAL FACTS: 206 Calories; 11.8 g Fats; 19.2 g Protein; 6 g Net Carb; 3 g Fiber;

261. CABBAGE HASH BROWNS

PREPARATION: 10' COOKING: 12' SERVES: 2

INGREDIENTS

- 1 ½ cup shredded cabbage
- 2 slices of bacon
- 1/2 tsp garlic powder
- 1 egg

Seasoning:
- 1 tbsp. coconut oil
- ½ tsp salt
- 1/8 tsp ground black pepper

DIRECTIONS

1. Crack the egg in a bowl, add garlic powder, black pepper, and salt, whisk well, then add cabbage, toss until well mixed and shape the mixture into four patties.
2. Take a large skillet pan, place it over medium heat, add oil and when hot, add patties in it and cook for 3 minutes per side until golden brown.
3. Transfer hash browns to a plate, then add bacon into the pan and cook for 5 minutes until crispy.
4. Serve hash browns with bacon.

NUTRITIONAL FACTS: 336 Calories; 29.5 g Fats; 16 g Protein; 0.9 g Net Carb; 0.8 g Fiber;

262. ASPARAGUS, WITH BACON AND EGGS

PREPARATION: 5'   COOKING: 12'   SERVES: 2

INGREDIENTS
- 4 oz. asparagus
- 2 slices of bacon, diced
- 1 egg

Seasoning:
- ¼ tsp salt
- 1/8 tsp ground black pepper

DIRECTIONS
1. Take a skillet pan, place it over medium heat, add bacon, and cook for 4 minutes until crispy.
2. Transfer cooked bacon to a plate, then add asparagus into the pan and cook for 5 minutes until tender-crisp.
3. Crack the egg over the cooked asparagus, season with salt and black pepper, then switch heat to medium-low level and cook for 2 minutes until egg white has set.
4. Chop the cooked bacon slices, sprinkle over egg and asparagus and serve.

NUTRITIONAL FACTS: 179 Calories; 15.3 g Fats; 9 g Protein; 0.7 g Net Carb; 0.6 g Fiber;

263. BELL PEPPER EGGS

PREPARATION: 10'   COOKING: 4'   SERVES: 2

INGREDIENTS
- 1 green bell pepper,
- 2 eggs

Seasoning:
- 1 tsp coconut oil
- ¼ tsp salt
- ¼ tsp ground black pepper

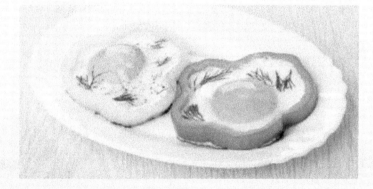

DIRECTIONS
1. Prepare pepper rings, and for this, cut out two slices from the pepper, about ¼-inch, and reserve remaining bell pepper for later use.
2. Take a skillet pan, place it over medium heat, grease it with oil, place pepper rings in it, and then crack an egg into each ring.
3. Season eggs with salt and black pepper, cook for 4 minutes or until eggs have cooked to the desired level.
4. Transfer eggs to a plate and serve.

NUTRITIONAL FACTS: 110.5 Calories; 8 g Fats; 7.2 g Protein; 1.7 g Net Carb; 1.1 g Fiber;

264. OMELET-STUFFED PEPPERS

PREPARATION: 5' COOKING: 20' SERVES: 2

INGREDIENTS

- 1 large green bell pepper, halved, cored
- 2 eggs
- 2 slices of bacon, chopped, cooked
- 2 tbsp. grated parmesan cheese

Seasoning:
- 1/3 tsp salt
- ¼ tsp ground black pepper

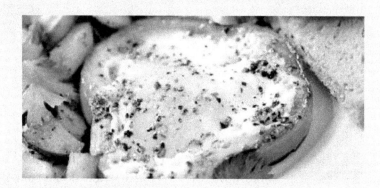

DIRECTIONS

1. Turn on the oven, then set it to 400 degrees F, and let preheat.
2. Then take a baking dish, pour in 1 tbsp. water, place bell pepper halved in it, cut-side up, and bake for 5 minutes.
3. Meanwhile, crack eggs in a bowl, add chopped bacon and cheese, season with salt and black pepper, and whisk until combined.
4. After 5 minutes of baking time, remove baking dish from the oven, evenly fill the peppers with egg mixture and continue baking for 15 to 20 minutes until eggs has set.
5. Serve.

NUTRITIONAL FACTS: 428 Calories; 35.2 g Fats; 23.5 g Protein; 2.8 g Net Carb; 1.5 g Fiber;

265. BACON AVOCADO BOMBS

PREPARATION: 10' COOKING: 10' SERVES: 2

INGREDIENTS

- 1 avocado, halved, pitted
- 4 slices of bacon
- 2 tbsp. grated parmesan cheese

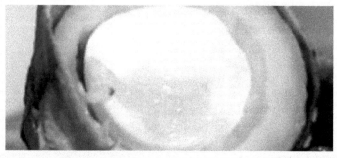

DIRECTIONS

1. Turn on the oven and broiler and let it preheat.
2. Meanwhile, prepare the avocado and for that, cut it in half, then remove its pit, and then peel the skin.
3. Evenly one half of the avocado with cheese, replace with the other half of avocado and then wrap avocado with bacon slices.
4. Take a baking sheet, line it with aluminum foil, place wrapped avocado on it, and broil for 5 minutes per side, flipping carefully with tong halfway.
5. When done, cut each avocado in half crosswise and serve

NUTRITIONAL FACTS: 378 Calories; 33.6 g Fats; 15.1 g Protein; 0.5 g Net Carb; 2.3 g Fiber;

266. EGG IN A HOLE WITH EGGPLANT

PREPARATION: 5' **COOKING:** 15' **SERVES:** 2

INGREDIENTS
- 1 large eggplant
- 2 eggs
- 1 tbsp. coconut oil, melted
- 1 tsp unsalted butter
- 2 tbsp. chopped green onions
- ¾ tsp salt

Seasoning:
- ¾ tsp ground black pepper

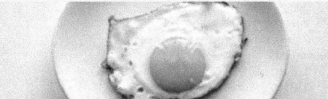

DIRECTIONS
1. Set the grill and let it preheat at the high setting.
2. Meanwhile, prepare the eggplant, and for this, cut two slices from eggplant, about 1-inch thick, and reserve the remaining eggplant for later use.
3. Brush slices of eggplant with oil, season with salt on both sides, then place the slices on grill and cook for 3 to 4 minutes per side.
4. Transfer grilled eggplant to a cutting board, let it cool for 5 minutes and then make a home in the center of each slice by using a cookie cutter.
5. Take a frying pan, place it over medium heat, add butter and when it melts, add eggplant slices in it and crack an egg into its each hole.
6. Let the eggs cook for 3 to 4 minutes, then carefully flip the eggplant slice and continue cooking for 3 minutes until the egg has thoroughly cooked.
7. Season egg with salt and black pepper, transfer them to a plate, then garnish with green onions and serve.

NUTRITIONAL FACTS: 184 Calories; 14.1 g Fats; 7.8 g Protein; 3 g Net Carb; 3.5 g Fiber;

267. FRITTATA WITH SPINACH AND MEAT

PREPARATION: 10' **COOKING:** 20' **SERVES:** 2

INGREDIENTS
- 4 oz. ground turkey
- 3 oz. of spinach leaves
- 1/3 tsp minced garlic
- 1/3 tsp coconut oil
- 2 eggs

Seasoning:
- 1/3 tsp salt
- ¼ tsp ground black pepper

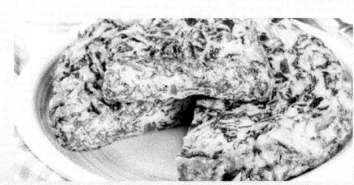

DIRECTIONS
1. Turn on the oven, then set it to 400 degrees F, and let it preheat.
2. Meanwhile, take a skillet pan, place it over medium heat, and add spinach and cook for 3 to 5 minutes until spinach leaves have wilted, remove the pan from heat.
3. Take a small heatproof skillet pan, place it over medium heat, add ground turkey and cook for 5 minutes until thoroughly cooked.
4. Then add spinach, season with salt and black pepper, stir well, then remove the pan from heat and spread the mixture evenly in the pan.
5. Crack eggs in a bowl, season with salt and black pepper, then pour this mixture over spinach mixture in the pan and bake for 10 to 15 minutes until frittata has thoroughly cooked and the top is golden brown.
6. When done, let frittata rest in the pan for 5 minutes, then cut it into slices and serve.

NUTRITIONAL FACTS: 166 Calories; 13 g Fats; 10 g Protein; 0.5 g Net Carb; 0.5 g Fiber;

268. AVOCADO EGG BOAT WITH CHEDDAR

PREPARATION: 5'   COOKING: 15'   SERVES: 2

INGREDIENTS
- 1 avocado, halved, pitted
- 2 eggs
- 2 tbsp. chopped bacon
- 2 tbsp. shredded cheddar cheese

Seasoning:
- 1/8 tsp salt
- 1/8 tsp ground black pepper

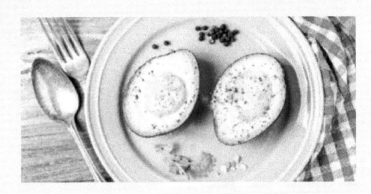

DIRECTIONS
1. Turn on the oven, then set it to 400 degrees F and let it preheat.
2. Meanwhile, prepare avocado and for this, cut it into half lengthwise and then remove the pit.
3. Scoop out some of the flesh from the center, crack an egg into each half, and then sprinkle with bacon and season with salt and black pepper.
4. Sprinkle cheese over egg and avocado and then bake for 10 to 15 minutes or until the yolk has cooked to desired level.
5. Serve.

NUTRITIONAL FACTS: 263.5 Calories; 21.4 g Fats; 12 g Protein; 1.3 g Net Carb; 4.6 g Fiber

CHAPTER 14.
POULTRY

269. PANCAKES

PREPARATION: 5' COOKING: 6' SERVES: 2

INGREDIENTS

- ¼ cup almond flour
- 1 ½ tbsp. unsalted butter
- 2 oz. cream cheese, softened
- 2 eggs

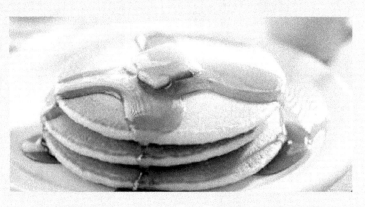

DIRECTIONS

1. Take a bowl, crack eggs in it, whisk well until fluffy, and then whisk in flour and cream cheese until well combined.
2. Take a skillet pan, place it over medium heat, add butter and when it melts, drop pancake batter in four sections, spread it evenly, and cook for 2 minutes per side until brown.
3. Serve.

NUTRITIONAL FACTS: 166.8 Calories; 15 g Fats; 5.8 g Protein; 1.8 g Net Carb; 0.8 g Fiber;

270. CHEESE ROLL-UPS

PREPARATION: 5' COOKING: 0' SERVES: 2

INGREDIENTS

- 2 oz. mozzarella cheese, sliced, full-fat
- 1-ounce butter, unsalted

DIRECTIONS

1. Cut cheese into slices and then cut butter into thin slices.
2. Top each cheese slice with a slice of butter, roll it and then serve.

NUTRITIONAL FACTS: 166 Calories; 15 g Fats; 6.5 g Protein; 2 g Net Carb; 0 g Fiber;

271. SCRAMBLED EGGS WITH SPINACH AND CHEESE

PREPARATION: 5'   COOKING: 5'   SERVES: 2

INGREDIENTS
- 2 oz. spinach
- 2 eggs
- 1 tbsp. coconut oil
- 2 tbsp. grated mozzarella cheese, full-fat

Seasoning:
- ¼ tsp salt
- 1/8 tsp ground black pepper
- 1/8 tsp red pepper flakes

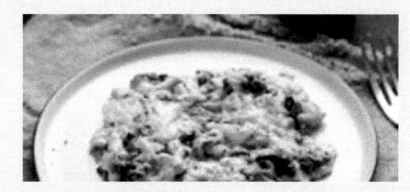

DIRECTIONS
1. Take a medium bowl, crack eggs in it, add salt and black pepper and whisk until combined.
2. Take a medium skillet pan, place it over medium heat, add oil and when hot, add spinach and cook for 1 minute until leaves wilt.
3. Pour eggs over spinach, stir and cook for 1 minute until just set.
4. Stir in cheese, then remove the pan from heat and sprinkle red pepper flakes on top.
5. Serve.

NUTRITIONAL FACTS: 171 Calories; 14 g Fats; 9.2 g Protein; 1.1 g Net Carb; 1.7 g Fiber;

272. EGG WRAPS

PREPARATION: 5'   COOKING: 5'   SERVES: 2

INGREDIENTS
- 2 eggs
- 1 tbsp. coconut oil

Seasoning:
- ¼ tsp salt
- 1/8 tsp ground black pepper

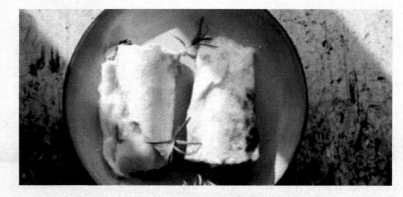

DIRECTIONS
1. Take a medium bowl, crack eggs in it, add salt and black pepper, and then whisk until blended.
2. Take a frying pan, place it over medium-low heat, add coconut oil and when it melts, pour in half of the egg, spread it evenly into a thin layer by rotating the pan and cook for 2 minutes.
3. Then flip the pan, cook for 1 minute, and transfer to a plate.
4. Repeat with the remaining egg to make another wrap, then roll each egg wrap and serve.

NUTRITIONAL FACTS: 68 Calories; 4.7 g Fats; 5.5 g Protein; 0.5 g Net Carb; 0 g Fiber;

273. CHAFFLES WITH POACHED EGGS

PREPARATION: 5' COOKING: 10' SERVES: 2

INGREDIENTS

- 2 tsp coconut flour
- ½ cup shredded cheddar cheese, full-fat
- 3 eggs

Seasoning:
- ¼ tsp salt
- 1/8 tsp ground black pepper

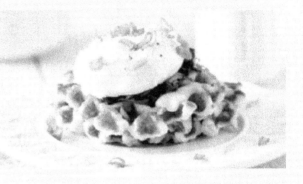

DIRECTIONS

1. Switch on a mini waffle maker and let it preheat for 5 minutes.
2. Meanwhile, take a medium bowl, place all the ingredients in it, reserving 2 eggs and then mix by using an immersion blender until smooth.
3. Ladle the batter evenly into the waffle maker, shut with lid, and let it cook for 3 to 4 minutes until firm and golden brown.
4. Meanwhile, prepare poached eggs, and for this, take a medium bowl half full with water, place it over medium heat and bring it to a boil.
5. Then crack an egg in a ramekin, carefully pour it into the boiling water and cook for 3 minutes.
6. Transfer egg to a plate lined with paper towels by using a slotted spoon and repeat with the other egg.
7. Top chaffles with poached eggs, season with salt and black pepper, and then serve.

NUTRITIONAL FACTS: 265 Calories; 18.5 g Fats; 17.6 g Protein; 3.4 g Net Carb; 6 g Fiber;

274. CHAFFLE WITH SCRAMBLED EGGS

PREPARATION: 5' COOKING: 10' SERVES: 2

INGREDIENTS

- 2 tsp coconut flour
- ½ cup shredded cheddar cheese, full-fat
- 3 eggs
- 1-ounce butter, unsalted

Seasoning:
- ¼ tsp salt
- 1/8 tsp ground black pepper
- 1/8 tsp dried oregano

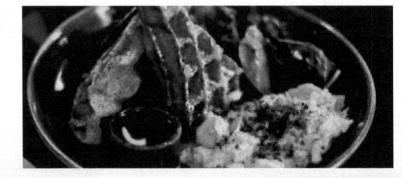

DIRECTIONS

1. Switch on a mini waffle maker and let it preheat for 5 minutes.
2. Meanwhile, take a medium bowl, place all the ingredients in it, reserving 2 eggs and then mix by using an immersion blender until smooth.
3. Ladle the batter evenly into the waffle maker, shut with lid, and let it cook for 3 to 4 minutes until firm and golden brown.
4. Meanwhile, prepare scrambled eggs and for this, take a medium bowl, crack the eggs in it and whisk them with a fork until frothy, and then season with salt and black pepper.
5. Take a medium skillet pan, place it over medium heat, add butter and when it melts, pour in eggs and cook for 2 minutes until creamy, stirring continuously.
6. Top chaffles with scrambled eggs, sprinkle with oregano, and then serve.

NUTRITIONAL FACTS: 265 Calories; 18.5 g Fats; 17.6 g Protein; 3.4 g Net Carb; 6 g Fiber;

275. SHEET PAN EGGS WITH MUSHROOMS AND SPINACH

PREPARATION: 5'   COOKING: 12'   SERVES: 2

INGREDIENTS
- 2 eggs
- 1 tsp chopped jalapeno pepper
- 1 tbsp. chopped mushrooms
- 1 tbsp. chopped spinach
- 1 tbsp. chopped chard

Seasoning:
- 1/3 tsp salt
- 1/4 tsp ground black pepper

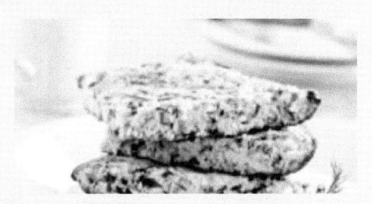

DIRECTIONS
1. Turn on the oven, then set it to 350 degrees F and let it preheat.
2. Take a medium bowl, crack eggs in it, add salt and black pepper, then add all the vegetables and stir until combined.
3. Take a medium sheet ball or rimmed baking sheet, grease it with oil, pour prepared egg batter on it, and then bake for 10 to 12 minutes until done.
4. Cut egg into two squares and then serve.

NUTRITIONAL FACTS: 165 Calories; 10.7 g Fats; 14 g Protein; 1.5 g Net Carb; 0.5 g Fiber;

276. NO BREAD BREAKFAST SANDWICH

PREPARATION: 10'   COOKING: 15'   SERVES: 2

INGREDIENTS
- 2 slices of ham
- 4 eggs
- 1 tsp tabasco sauce
- 3 tbsp. butter, unsalted
- 2 tsp grated mozzarella cheese

Seasoning:
- ¼ tsp salt
- 1/8 tsp ground black pepper

DIRECTIONS
1. Take a frying pan, place it over medium heat, add butter and when it melt, crack an egg in it and fry for 2 to 3 minutes until cooked to desired level.
2. Transfer fried egg to a plate, fry remaining eggs in the same manner and when done, season eggs with salt and black pepper.
3. Prepare the sandwich and for this, use a fried egg as a base for sandwich, then top with a ham slice, sprinkle with a tsp of ham and cover with another fried egg.
4. Place egg into the pan, return it over low heat and let it cook until cheese melts.
5. Prepare another sandwich in the same manner and then serve.

NUTRITIONAL FACTS: 180 Calories; 15 g Fats; 10 g Protein; 1 g Net Carb; 0 g Fiber;

277. SCRAMBLED EGGS WITH BASIL AND BUTTER

PREPARATION: 5'   COOKING: 5'   SERVES: 2

INGREDIENTS

- 1 tbsp. chopped basil leaves
- 2 tbsp. butter, unsalted
- 2 tbsp. grated cheddar cheese
- 2 eggs
- 2 tbsp. whipping cream

Seasoning:
- 1/8 tsp salt
- 1/8 tsp ground black pepper

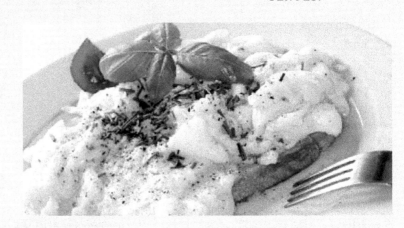

DIRECTIONS

1. Take a medium bowl, crack eggs in it, add salt, black pepper, cheese and cream and whisk until combined.
2. Take a medium pan, place it over low heat, add butter and when it melts, pour in the egg mixture and cook for 2 to 3 minutes until eggs have scrambled to the desired level.
3. When done, distribute scrambled eggs between two plates, top with basil leaves and then serve.

NUTRITIONAL FACTS: 320 Calories; 29 g Fats; 13 g Protein; 1.5 g Net Carb; 0 g Fiber;

278. BACON, AND EGGS

PREPARATION: 5'   COOKING: 10'   SERVES: 2

INGREDIENTS

- 2 eggs
- 4 slices of turkey bacon
- ¼ tsp salt
- ¼ tsp ground black pepper

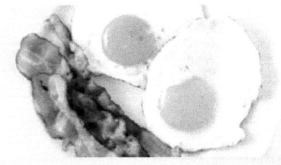

DIRECTIONS

1. Take a skillet pan, place it over medium heat, add bacon slices in it and cook for 5 minutes until crispy.
2. Transfer bacon slices to a plate and set aside until required, reserving the fat in the pan.
3. Cook the egg in the pan one at a time, and for this, crack an egg in the pan and cook for 2 to 3 minutes or more until the egg has cooked to desire level.
4. Transfer egg to a plate and cook the other egg in the same manner.
5. Season eggs with salt and black pepper and then serve with cooked bacon.

NUTRITIONAL FACTS: 136 Calories; 11 g Fats; 7.5 g Protein; 1 g Net Carb; 0 g Fiber

279. BOILED EGGS

PREPARATION: 5' **COOKING:** 10' **SERVES:** 2

INGREDIENTS

- 2 eggs
- ½ of a medium avocado

Seasoning:
- ¼ tsp salt
- ¼ tsp ground black pepper

DIRECTIONS

1. Place a medium pot over medium heat, fill it half full with water and bring it to boil.
2. Then carefully place the eggs in the boiling water and boil the eggs for 5 minutes until soft-boiled, 8 minutes for medium-boiled, and 10 minutes for hard-boiled.
3. When eggs have boiled, transfer them to a bowl containing chilled water and let them rest for 5 minutes.
4. Then crack the eggs with a spoon and peel them.
5. Cut each egg into slices, season with salt and black pepper, and serve with diced avocado.

NUTRITIONAL FACTS: 112 Calories; 9.5 g Fats; 5.5 g Protein; 1 g Net Carb; 0 g Fiber;

280. SPICY CHEESE CHICKEN SOUP

PREPARATION: 15' **COOKING:** 40' **SERVES:** 4

INGREDIENTS

- ½ cup salsa enchilada verde
- 2 cups chicken, cooked and shredded
- 2 cups chicken or bone broth
- 1 cup cheddar cheese, shredded
- 4 ounces cream cheese
- ½ tsp chili powder
- ½ tsp cumin, ground
- ½ tsp fresh cilantro, chopped
- Salt and black pepper to taste

DIRECTIONS

1. Combine the cream cheese, salsa verde, and broth in a food processor.
2. Pulse until smooth. Transfer the mixture to a pot and place over medium heat.
3. Cook until hot, but do not bring to a boil.
4. Add chicken, chili powder, and cumin, and cook for about 3-5 minutes, or until it is heated through. Stir in Cheddar cheese. Season with salt and pepper to taste.
5. Serve hot in individual bowls sprinkled with fresh cilantro.

NUTRITIONAL FACTS: Calories 346, Net Carbs 3g, Fat 23g, Protein 25g

281. CHEESE & SPINACH STUFFED CHICKEN

PREPARATION: 50' COOKING: 40' SERVES: 4

INGREDIENTS

- 4 chicken breasts, boneless and skinless
- ½ cup mozzarella cheese
- 1 ½ cups Parmesan cheese, shredded
- 6 ounces cream cheese
- 2 cups spinach, chopped
- A pinch of nutmeg
- ½ tsp garlic, minced

Breading
- 2 eggs, beaten
- 1/3 cup almond flour
- 2 tbsp. olive oil
- ½ tsp parsley
- 1/3 cup Parmesan cheese
- A pinch of onion powder

DIRECTIONS

1. Pound the chicken until it doubles in size. Mix cream cheese, spinach, mozzarella cheese, nutmeg, and salt, pepper, and Parmesan cheese in a bowl. Divide the mixture between the chicken breasts and spread it out evenly. Wrap the chicken in a plastic wrap. Refrigerate for 15 minutes.
2. Preheat the oven to 370 F.
3. Beat the eggs and set aside. Combine all of the other breading ingredients in a bowl. Dip the chicken in eggs first, then in the breading mixture.
4. Warm the olive oil in a pan over medium heat. Cook the chicken in the pan until browned, about 5-6 minutes. Place on a lined baking sheet, and bake for 20 minutes. Serve.

NUTRITIONAL FACTS: Calories 491, Net Carbs 3.5g, Fat 36g, Protein 38g

282. CHICKEN & SPINACH GRATIN

PREPARATION: 45' COOKING: 40' SERVES: 6

INGREDIENTS

- 6 chicken breasts, skinless and boneless
- 1 tsp mixed spice seasoning
- Pink salt and black pepper to season
- 2 loose cups baby spinach
- 3 tsp olive oil
- 4 oz. cream cheese, cubed
- 1 ¼ cups mozzarella cheese, shredded
- 4 tbsp. water

DIRECTIONS

1. Preheat oven to 375 F.
2. Season chicken with spice mix, salt, and black pepper. Pat with your hands to have the seasoning stick on the chicken.
3. Put in the casserole dish and layer spinach over the chicken.
4. Mix the oil with cream cheese, mozzarella, salt, and black pepper and stir in water a tablespoon at a time.
5. Pour the mixture over the chicken and cover the pot with aluminum foil.
6. Bake for 20 minutes, remove foil and continue cooking for 15 minutes until a beautiful golden brown color is formed on top.
7. Take out and allow sitting for 5 minutes. Serve warm with braised asparagus.

NUTRITIONAL FACTS: Calories 340, Net Carbs 1g, Fat 30.2g, Protein 15g

283. WEEKEND CHICKEN WITH GRAPEFRUIT & LEMON

PREPARATION: 30'   COOKING: 40'   SERVES: 4

INGREDIENTS

- 1 cup omission IPA
- A pinch of garlic powder
- 1 tsp grapefruit zest
- 3 tbsp. lemon juice
- ½ tsp coriander, ground
- 1 tbsp. fish sauce
- 2 tbsp. butter
- ¼ tsp xanthan gum
- 3 tbsp. swerve sweetener
- 20 chicken wing pieces
- Salt and black pepper to taste

DIRECTIONS

1. Combine lemon juice and zest, fish sauce, coriander, omission IPA, sweetener, and garlic powder in a saucepan.
2. Bring to a boil, cover, lower the heat, and let simmer for 10 minutes.
3. Stir in the butter and xanthan gum. Set aside. Season the wings with some salt and pepper.
4. Preheat the grill and cook for 5 minutes per side.
5. Serve topped with the sauce.

NUTRITIONAL FACTS: Calories 365, Net Carbs 4g, Fat 25g, Protein 21g

284. BACON-WRAPPED CHICKEN WITH GRILLED ASPARAGUS

PREPARATION: 50'   COOKING: 40'   SERVES: 4

INGREDIENTS

- 2 tbsp. fresh lemon juice
- 6 chicken breasts
- 8 bacon slices
- 1 tbsp. olive oil
- 1 lb. asparagus spears
- 3 tbsp. olive oil
- Salt and black pepper to taste
- Manchego cheese for topping

DIRECTIONS

1. Preheat the oven to 400 F.
2. Season chicken breasts with salt and black pepper, and wrap 2 bacon slices around each chicken breast. Arrange on a baking sheet that is lined with parchment paper, drizzle with oil, and bake for 25-30 minutes until bacon is brown and crispy.
3. Preheat the grill.
4. Brush the asparagus spears with olive oil and season with salt. Grill turning frequently until slightly charred, 5-10 minutes.
5. Remove to a plate and drizzle with lemon juice. Grate over Manchego cheese so that it melts a little on contact with the hot asparagus and forms a cheesy dressing.

NUTRITIONAL FACTS: Calories 468, Net Carbs 2g, Fat 38g, Protein 26g

285. BOK CHOY CAESAR SALAD WITH CHICKEN

PREPARATION: 1H 20' **COOKING:** 40' **SERVES:** 4

INGREDIENTS

Chicken
- 4 chicken thighs, boneless and skinless
- ¼ cup lemon juice
- 2 garlic cloves, minced
- 2 tbsp. olive oil

Salad
- ½ cup caesar salad dressing, sugar-free
- 2 tbsp. olive oil
- 12 bok choy leaves
- 3 Parmesan cheese crisps
- Parmesan cheese, grated or garnishing

DIRECTIONS

1. Combine the chicken ingredients in a Ziploc bag. Seal the bag, shake to combine, and refrigerate for 1 hour.
2. Preheat the grill to medium heat, and grill the chicken about 4 minutes per side.
3. Cut bok choy leaves lengthwise, and brush it with oil. Grill for about 3 minutes. Place on a serving platter. Top with the chicken, and drizzle the dressing over. Sprinkle with Parmesan cheese and finish with Parmesan crisps to serve.

NUTRITIONAL FACTS: Calories 529, Net Carbs 5g, Fat 39g, Protein 33g

286. TURKEY PATTIES WITH CUCUMBER SALSA

PREPARATION: 30' **COOKING:** 40' **SERVES:** 4

INGREDIENTS

- 2 spring onions, thinly sliced
- 1 pound turkey, ground
- 1 egg
- 2 garlic cloves, minced
- 1 tbsp. herbs, chopped
- 1 small chili pepper, deseeded and diced
- 2 tbsp. ghee

Cucumber Salsa:
- 1 tbsp. apple cider vinegar
- 1 tbsp. dill, chopped
- 1 garlic clove, minced
- 2 cucumbers, grated
- 1 cup sour cream
- 1 jalapeño pepper, minced
- 2 tbsp. olive oil

DIRECTIONS

1. Place all of the turkey ingredients, except the ghee, in a bowl. Mix to combine. Make patties out of the mixture.
2. Melt ghee in a skillet over medium heat. Cook the patties for 3 minutes per side.
3. Place all of the salsa ingredients in a bowl and mix to combine. Serve the patties topped with salsa.

NUTRITIONAL FACTS: Calories 475, Net Carbs 5g, Fat 38g, Protein 26g

287. CHILI CHICKEN KABOBS WITH TAHINI DRESSING

PREPARATION: 20' + 2H REFRIGERATION **COOKING:** 10' **SERVES:** 6

INGREDIENTS

- 3 tbsp. soy sauce
- 1 tbsp. ginger-garlic paste
- 2 tbsp. swerve brown sugar
- 2 tbsp. olive oil
- 3 chicken breasts, cut into bite-sized cubes
- ½ cup tahini
- ½ tsp garlic powder
- Salt and chili pepper to taste

DIRECTIONS

1. In a bowl, whisk soy sauce, ginger-garlic paste, swerve brown sugar, chili pepper, and olive oil. Put the chicken in a zipper bag, pour the marinade over, seal, and shake for an even coat. Marinate in the fridge for 2 hours.
2. Preheat a grill to 400 F and thread the chicken on skewers. Cook for 10 minutes in total with three to four turnings to be golden brown. Plate them.
3. Mix the tahini, garlic powder, salt, and ¼ cup of warm water in a bowl. Serve the chicken skewers and tahini dressing with cauliflower fried rice.

NUTRITIONAL FACTS: Calories 225, Net Carbs 2g, Fat 17.4g, Protein 15g

288. ASIAN CHICKEN WITH FRESH LIME-PEANUT SAUCE

PREPARATION: 1H 30' **COOKING:** 40' **SERVES:** 6

INGREDIENTS

- 1 tbsp. wheat-free soy sauce
- 1 tbsp. sugar-free fish sauce
- 1 tbsp. lime juice
- 1 tsp coriander
- 1 tsp garlic, minced
- 1 tsp ginger, minced
- 1 tbsp. olive oil
- 1 tbsp. rice wine vinegar
- 1 tsp cayenne pepper
- 1 tbsp. erythritol
- 6 chicken thighs

Sauce:
- ½ cup peanut butter
- 1 tsp garlic, minced
- 1 tbsp. lime juice
- 2 tbsp. water
- 1 tsp ginger, minced
- 1 tbsp. jalapeño, chopped
- 2 tbsp. rice wine vinegar
- 2 tbsp. erythritol
- 1 tbsp. fish sauce

DIRECTIONS

1. Combine all of the chicken ingredients in a large Ziploc bag.
2. Seal the bag and shake to combine.
3. Refrigerate for about 1 hour.
4. Remove from the fridge about 15 minutes before cooking.
5. Preheat the grill to medium, and grill the chicken for about 7 minutes per side.
6. Meanwhile, whisk together all of the sauce ingredients in a mixing bowl.
7. Serve the chicken drizzled with peanut sauce.

NUTRITIONAL FACTS: Calories 492, Net Carbs 3g, Fat 36g, Protein 35g

289. CHICKEN WITH EGGPLANT & TOMATOES

PREPARATION: 25' **COOKING:** 10' **SERVES:** 4

INGREDIENTS

- 2 tbsp. ghee
- 1 lb. chicken thighs
- Salt and black pepper to taste
- 2 cloves garlic, minced
- 1 (14 oz.) can whole tomatoes
- 1 eggplant, diced
- 10 fresh basil leaves, chopped + extra to garnish

DIRECTIONS

1. Melt ghee in a saucepan over medium heat, season the chicken with salt and black pepper, and fry for 4 minutes on each side until golden brown. Remove the chicken onto a plate.
2. Sauté the garlic in the ghee for 2 minutes, pour in the tomatoes, and cook covered for 8 minutes. Include the eggplant and basil. Cook for 4 minutes.
3. Season the sauce with salt and black pepper, stir and add the chicken. Coat with sauce and simmer for 3 minutes.
4. Serve chicken with sauce on a bed of squash pasta garnished with basil.

NUTRITIONAL FACTS: Calories 468, Net Carbs 2g, Fat 39.5g, Protein 26g

290. ROSEMARY CHICKEN WITH AVOCADO SAUCE

PREPARATION: 22' **COOKING:** 30' **SERVES:** 4

INGREDIENTS

- 1 avocado pitted
- ½ cup mayonnaise
- 3 tbsp. ghee
- 4 chicken breasts
- Salt and black pepper to taste
- 1 cup rosemary, chopped
- ½ cup chicken broth

DIRECTIONS

1. Spoon avocado, mayonnaise, and salt into a food processor and puree until a smooth sauce is derived. Adjust the taste with salt. Pour sauce into a jar and refrigerate.
2. Melt ghee in a large skillet, season chicken with salt and black pepper, and fry for 4 minutes on each side to a golden brown. Remove chicken to a plate.
3. Pour the broth in the same skillet and add the cilantro. Bring to simmer covered for 3 minutes and add the chicken. Cover, and cook on low heat for 5 minutes until the liquid has reduced and chicken is fragrant.
4. Dish chicken only into serving plates and spoon the mayo-avocado sauce over.
5. Serve warm with buttered green beans and baby carrots.

NUTRITIONAL FACTS: Calories 398, Net Carbs 4g, Fat 32g, Protein 24g

291. TASTY CHICKEN WITH BRUSSEL SPROUTS

PREPARATION: 120' COOKING: 40' SERVES: 8

INGREDIENTS

- 5 pounds whole chicken
- 1 bunch oregano
- 1 bunch thyme
- 1 tbsp. marjoram
- 1 tbsp. parsley
- 1 tbsp. olive oil
- 2 pounds Brussel sprouts
- 1 lemon
- 4 tbsp. butter

DIRECTIONS

1. Preheat your oven to 450 F.
2. Stuff the chicken with oregano, thyme, and lemon.
3. Make sure the wings are tucked over and behind.
4. Roast for 15 minutes. Reduce the heat to 325 F, and cook for 40 minutes.
5. Spread the butter over the chicken and sprinkle parsley and marjoram.
6. Add the Brussel sprouts. Return to oven and bake for 40 more minutes.
7. Let sit for 10 minutes before carving.

NUTRITIONAL FACTS: Calories 430, Net Carbs 5g, Fat 32g, Protein 30g

CHAPTER 15. BEEF

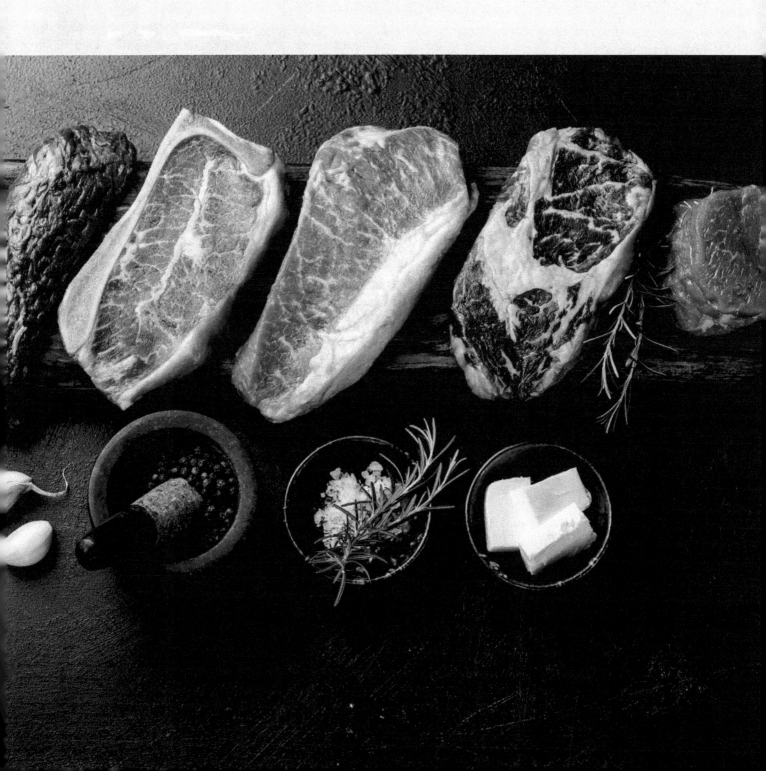

292. BEEF AND BROCCOLI

PREPARATION: 5'   **COOKING:** 10'   **SERVES:** 2

INGREDIENTS

- 6 slices of beef roast, cut into strips
- 1 scallion, chopped
- 3 oz. broccoli florets, chopped
- 1 tbsp. avocado oil
- 1 tbsp. butter, unsalted

Seasoning:
- ¼ tsp salt
- 1/8 tsp ground black pepper
- 1 ½ tbsp. soy sauce
- 3 tbsp. chicken broth

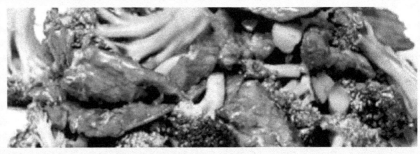

DIRECTIONS

1. Take a medium skillet pan, place it over medium heat, add oil and when hot, add beef strips and cook for 2 minutes until hot.
2. Transfer beef to a plate, add scallion to the pan, then add butter and cook for 3 minutes until tender.
3. Add remaining ingredients, stir until mixed, switch heat to the low level and simmer for 3 to 4 minutes until broccoli is tender.
4. Return beef to the pan, stir until well combined and cook for 1 minute.
5. Serve.

NUTRITIONAL FACTS: 245 Calories; 15.7 g Fats; 21.6 g Protein; 1.7 g Net Carb; 1.3 g Fiber;

293. BEEF WITH CABBAGE NOODLES

PREPARATION: 5'   **COOKING:** 18'   **SERVES:** 2

INGREDIENTS

- 4 oz. ground beef
- 1 cup chopped cabbage
- 4 oz. tomato sauce
- ½ tsp minced garlic
- ½ cup of water

Seasoning:
- ½ tbsp. coconut oil
- ½ tsp salt
- ¼ tsp Italian seasoning
- 1/8 tsp dried basil

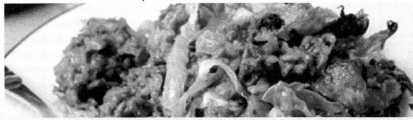

DIRECTIONS

1. Take a skillet pan, place it over medium heat, add oil and when hot, add beef and cook for 5 minutes until nicely browned.
2. Meanwhile, prepare the cabbage and for it, slice the cabbage into thin shred.
3. When the beef has cooked, add garlic, season with salt, basil, and Italian seasoning, stir well and continue cooking for 3 minutes until beef has thoroughly cooked.
4. Pour in tomato sauce and water, stir well and bring the mixture to boil.
5. Then reduce heat to medium-low level, add cabbage, stir well until well mixed and simmer for 3 to 5 minutes until cabbage is softened, covering the pan.
6. Uncover the pan and continue simmering the beef until most of the cooking liquid has evaporated.
7. Serve.

NUTRITIONAL FACTS: 188.5 Calories; 12.5 g Fats; 15.5 g Protein; 2.5 g Net Carb; 1 g Fiber;

294. GARLIC HERB BEEF ROAST

PREPARATION: 5' COOKING: 10' SERVES: 2

INGREDIENTS
- 6 slices of beef roast
- ½ tsp garlic powder
- 1/3 tsp dried thyme
- ¼ tsp dried rosemary
- 2 tbsp. butter, unsalted

Seasoning:
- 1/3 tsp salt
- 1/4 tsp ground black pepper

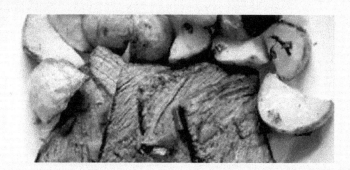

DIRECTIONS
1. Prepare the spice mix and for this, take a small bowl, place garlic powder, thyme, rosemary, salt, and black pepper and then stir until mixed.
2. Sprinkle spice mix on the beef roast.
3. Take a medium skillet pan, place it over medium heat, add butter and when it melts, add beef roast and then cook for 5 to 8 minutes until golden brown and cooked.
4. Serve.

NUTRITIONAL FACTS: 140 Calories; 12.7 g Fats; 5.5 g Protein; 0.1 g Net Carb; 0.2 g Fiber;

295. GARLICKY STEAKS WITH ROSEMARY

PREPARATION: 25' COOKING: 12' SERVES: 2

INGREDIENTS
- 2 beef steaks
- 1/4 of a lime, juiced
- 1 ½ tsp garlic powder
- ¾ tsp dried rosemary
- 2 ½ tbsp. avocado oil

Seasoning:
- ½ tsp salt
- ¼ tsp ground black pepper

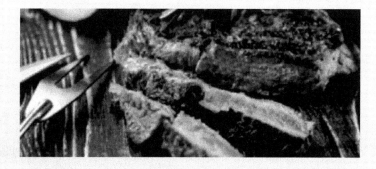

DIRECTIONS
1. Prepare steaks, and for this, sprinkle garlic powder on all sides of steak.
2. Take a shallow dish, place 1 ½ tbsp. oil and lime juice in it, whisk until combined, add steaks, turn to coat and let it marinate for 20 minutes at room temperature.
3. Then take a griddle pan, place it over medium-high heat and grease it with remaining oil.
4. Season marinated steaks with salt and black pepper, add to the griddle pan and cook for 7 to 12 minutes until cooked to the desired level.
5. When done, wrap steaks in foil for 5 minutes, then cut into slices across the grain.
6. Sprinkle rosemary over steaks slices and then serve.

NUTRITIONAL FACTS: 213 Calories; 13 g Fats; 22 g Protein; 1 g Net Carb; 0 g Fiber;

296. ROAST BEEF AND MOZZARELLA PLATE

PREPARATION: 5'   COOKING: 0'   SERVES: 2

INGREDIENTS

- 4 slices of roast beef
- ½ ounce chopped lettuce
- 1 avocado, pitted
- 2 oz. mozzarella cheese, cubed
- ½ cup mayonnaise

Seasoning:
- ¼ tsp salt
- 1/8 tsp ground black pepper
- 2 tbsp. avocado oil

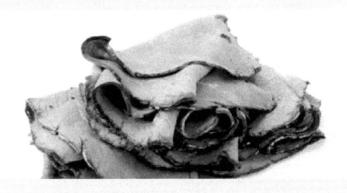

DIRECTIONS

1. Scoop out flesh from avocado and divide it evenly between two plates.
2. Add slices of roast beef, lettuce, and cheese and then sprinkle with salt and black pepper.
3. Serve with avocado oil and mayonnaise.

NUTRITIONAL FACTS: 267.7 Calories; 24.5 g Fats; 9.5 g Protein; 1.5 g Net Carb; 2 g Fiber;

297. SPROUTS STIR-FRY WITH KALE, BROCCOLI, AND BEEF

PREPARATION: 5'   COOKING: 8'   SERVES: 2

INGREDIENTS

- 3 slices of beef roast, chopped
- 2 oz. Brussels sprouts, halved
- 4 oz. broccoli florets
- 3 oz. kale
- 1 ½ tbsp. butter, unsalted
- 1/8 tsp red pepper flakes

Seasoning:
- ¼ tsp garlic powder
- ¼ tsp salt
- 1/8 tsp ground black pepper

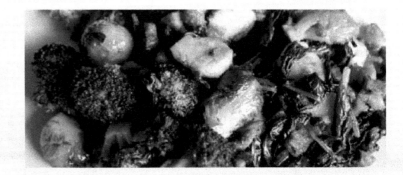

DIRECTIONS

1. Take a medium skillet pan, place it over medium heat, add ¾ tbsp. butter and when it melts, add broccoli florets and sprouts, sprinkle with garlic powder, and cook for 2 minutes.
2. Season vegetables with salt and red pepper flakes, add chopped beef, stir until mixed and continue cooking for 3 minutes until browned on one side.
3. Then add kale along with remaining butter, flip the vegetables and cook for 2 minutes until kale leaves wilts.
4. Serve.

NUTRITIONAL FACTS: 125 Calories; 9.4 g Fats; 4.8 g Protein; 1.7 g Net Carb; 2.6 g Fiber;

298. BEEF AND VEGETABLE SKILLET

PREPARATION: 5' COOKING: 15' SERVES: 2

INGREDIENTS

- 3 oz. spinach, chopped
- ½ pound ground beef
- 2 slices of bacon, diced
- 2 oz. chopped asparagus

Seasoning:
- 3 tbsp. coconut oil
- 2 tsp dried thyme
- 2/3 tsp salt
- ½ tsp ground black pepper

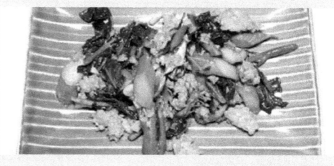

DIRECTIONS

1. Take a skillet pan, place it over medium heat, add oil and when hot, add beef and bacon and cook for 5 to 7 minutes until slightly browned.
2. Then add asparagus and spinach, sprinkle with thyme, stir well and cook for 7 to 10 minutes until thoroughly cooked.
3. Season skillet with salt and black pepper and serve.

NUTRITIONAL FACTS: 332.5 Calories; 26 g Fats; 23.5 g Protein; 1.5 g Net Carb; 1 g Fiber;

299. BEEF, PEPPER AND GREEN BEANS STIR-FRY

PREPARATION: 5' COOKING: 18' SERVES: 2

INGREDIENTS

- 6 oz. ground beef
- 2 oz. chopped green bell pepper
- 4 oz. green beans
- 3 tbsp. grated cheddar cheese

Seasoning:
- ½ tsp salt
- ¼ tsp ground black pepper
- ¼ tsp paprika

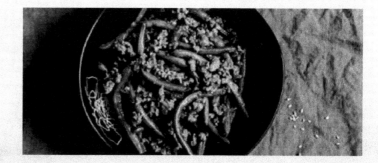

DIRECTIONS

1. Take a skillet pan, place it over medium heat, add ground beef and cook for 4 minutes until slightly browned.
2. Then add bell pepper and green beans, season with salt, paprika, and black pepper, stir well and continue cooking for 7 to 10 minutes until beef and vegetables have cooked through.
3. Sprinkle cheddar cheese on top, then transfer pan under the broiler and cook for 2 minutes until cheese has melted and the top is golden brown.
4. Serve.

NUTRITIONAL FACTS: 282.5 Calories; 17.6 g Fats; 26.1 g Protein; 2.9 g Net Carb; 2.1 g Fiber;

300. ROAST BEEF AND VEGETABLE PLATE

PREPARATION: 10' **COOKING:** 10' **SERVES:** 2

INGREDIENTS

- 2 scallions, chopped in large pieces
- 1 ½ tbsp. coconut oil
- 4 thin slices of roast beef
- 4 oz. cauliflower and broccoli mix
- 1 tbsp. butter, unsalted
- 1 tsp dried parsley

Seasoning:
- 1/2 tsp salt
- 1/3 tsp ground black pepper

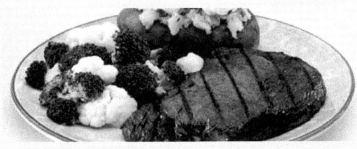

DIRECTIONS

1. Turn on the oven, then set it to 400 degrees F, and let it preheat.
2. Take a baking sheet, grease it with oil, place slices of roast beef on one side, and top with butter.
3. Take a separate bowl, add cauliflower and broccoli mix, add scallions, drizzle with oil, season with remaining salt and black pepper, toss until coated and then spread vegetables on the empty side of the baking sheet.
4. Bake for 5 to 7 minutes until beef is nicely browned and vegetables are tender-crisp, tossing halfway.
5. Distribute beef and vegetables between two plates and then serve.

NUTRITIONAL FACTS: 313 Calories; 26 g Fats; 15.6 g Protein; 2.8 g Net Carb; 1.9 g Fiber;

301. CHEESY MEATLOAF

PREPARATION: 5' **COOKING:** 4' **SERVES:** 2

INGREDIENTS

- 4 oz. ground turkey
- 1 egg
- 1 tbsp. grated mozzarella cheese
- ¼ tsp Italian seasoning
- ½ tbsp. soy sauce

Seasoning:
- ¼ tsp salt
- 1/8 tsp ground black pepper

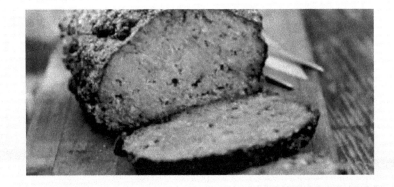

DIRECTIONS

1. Take a bowl, place all the ingredients in it, and stir until mixed.
2. Take a heatproof mug, spoon in prepared mixture and microwave for 3 minutes at high heat setting until cooked.
3. When done, let meatloaf rest in the mug for 1 minute, then take it out, cut it into two slices and serve.

NUTRITIONAL FACTS: 196.5 Calories; 13.5 g Fats; 18.7 g Protein; 18.7 g Net Carb; 0 g Fiber;

302. STEAK AND CHEESE PLATE

PREPARATION: 5'   COOKING: 10'   SERVES: 2

INGREDIENTS

- 1 green onion, chopped
- 2 oz. chopped lettuce
- 2 beef steaks
- 2 oz. of cheddar cheese, sliced
- ½ cup mayonnaise

Seasoning:
- ¼ tsp salt
- 1/8 tsp ground black pepper
- 3 tbsp. avocado oil

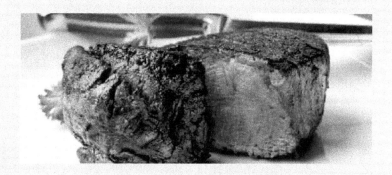

DIRECTIONS

1. Prepare the steak, and for this, season it with salt and black pepper.
2. Take a medium skillet pan, place it over medium heat, add oil and when hot, add seasoned steaks, and cook for 7 to 10 minutes until cooked to the desired level.
3. When done, distribute steaks between two plates, add scallion, lettuce, and cheese slices.
4. Drizzle with remaining oil and then serve with mayonnaise.

NUTRITIONAL FACTS: 714 Calories; 65.3 g Fats; 25.3 g Protein; 4 g Net Carb; 5.3 g Fiber;

303. BEEF CLOD VINDALOO

PREPARATION: 15'   COOKING: 15'   SERVES: 3

INGREDIENTS

- ½ Serrano pepper, chopped
- ¼ teaspoon cumin seeds
- ¼ teaspoon minced ginger
- ¼ teaspoon cayenne pepper
- ¼ teaspoon salt
- ¼ teaspoon ground paprika
- 1 cup water
- 9 ounces (255 g) beef clod, chopped

DIRECTIONS

1. Put Serrano pepper, cumin seeds, minced ginger, cayenne pepper, salt, ground paprika, and water in a food processor. Blend the mixture until smooth.
2. Transfer the mixture in a bowl and add the chopped beef clod. Toss to coat well.
3. Transfer the beef clod and the mixture in the Instant Pot and close the lid.
4. Select Manual mode and set cooking time for 15 minutes on High Pressure.
5. When timer beeps, use a natural pressure release for 10 minutes, then release any remaining pressure. Open the lid.
6. Serve immediately.

NUTRITIONAL FACTS: Calories: 376 Fat: 27.4g Protein: 29.9g Carbs: 0.7g Net carbs: 0.4g Fiber: 0.3g

304. BEEF MASALA CURRY

PREPARATION: 10' **COOKING:** 20' **SERVES:** 4

INGREDIENTS

- 2 tomatoes, quartered
- 1 small onion, quartered
- 4 garlic cloves, chopped
- ½ cup fresh cilantro leaves
- 1 teaspoon garam masala
- ½ teaspoon ground coriander
- 1 teaspoon ground cumin
- ½ teaspoon cayenne
- 1 teaspoon salt
- 1 pound (454 g) beef chuck roast, cut into 1-inch cubes

DIRECTIONS

1. In a blender, combine the tomatoes, onion, garlic, and cilantro.
2. Process until the vegetables are puréed. Add the garam masala, coriander, cumin, cayenne, and salt. Process for several more seconds.
3. To the Instant Pot, add the beef and pour the vegetable purée on top.
4. Lock the lid. Select Manual mode and set cooking time for 20 minutes on High Pressure.
5. When timer beeps, let the pressure release naturally for 10 minutes, then release any remaining pressure. Unlock the lid.
6. Stir and serve immediately.

NUTRITIONAL FACTS: Calories: 309 Fat: 21.0g Protein: 24.0g Carbs: 6.0g Net carbs: 4.0g Fiber: 2.0g

305. BEEF RIBS WITH RADISHES

PREPARATION: 20' **COOKING:** 56' **SERVES:** 4

INGREDIENTS

- ¼ teaspoon ground coriander
- ¼ teaspoon ground cumin
- 1 teaspoon kosher salt, plus more to taste
- ½ teaspoon smoked paprika
- Pinch of ground allspice (optional)
- 4 (8-ounce / 227-g) bone-in beef short ribs
- 2 tablespoons avocado oil
- 1 cup water
- 2 radishes, ends trimmed, leaves rinsed and roughly chopped
- Freshly ground black pepper, to taste

DIRECTIONS

1. In a small bowl, mix together the coriander, cumin, salt, paprika, and allspice. Rub the spice mixture all over the short ribs.
2. Set the Instant Pot to Sauté mode and add the oil to heat. Add the short ribs, bone side up. Brown for 4 minutes on each side.
3. Pour the water into the Instant Pot. Secure the lid. Press the Manual button and set cooking time for 45 minutes on High Pressure.
4. When timer beeps, allow the pressure to release naturally for 10 minutes, then release any remaining pressure. Open the lid.
5. Remove the short ribs to a serving plate.
6. Add the radishes to the sauce in the pot. Place a metal steaming basket directly on top of the radishes and place the radish leaves in the basket.
7. Secure the lid. Press the Manual button and set cooking time for 3 minutes on High Pressure.
8. When timer beeps, quick release the pressure. Open the lid. Transfer the leaves to a serving bowl. Sprinkle with salt and pepper.
9. Remove the radishes and place on top of the leaves. Serve hot with the short ribs.

NUTRITIONAL FACTS: Calories: 450 Fat: 24.8g Protein: 45.4g Carbs: 12.3g Net carbs: 9.4g Fiber: 2.9g

306. BEEF SHAMI KABOB

PREPARATION: 15' **COOKING:** 35' **SERVES:** 4

INGREDIENTS

- 1 pound (454 g) beef chunks, chopped
- 1 teaspoon ginger paste
- ½ teaspoon ground cumin
- 2 cups water
- ¼ cup almond flour
- 1 egg, beaten
- 1 tablespoon coconut oil

DIRECTIONS

1. Put the beef chunks, ginger paste, ground cumin, and water in the Instant Pot.
2. Select Manual mode and set cooking time for 30 minutes on High Pressure.
3. When timer beeps, make a quick pressure release. Open the lid.
4. Drain the water from the meat. Transfer the beef in the blender. Add the almond flour and beaten egg. Blend until smooth. Shape the mixture into small meatballs.
5. Heat the coconut oil on Sauté mode and put the meatballs inside.
6. Cook for 2 minutes on each side or until golden brown.
7. Serve immediately.

NUTRITIONAL FACTS: Calories: 179 Fat: 9.5g Protein: 20.1g Carbs: 2.9g Net carbs: 2.6g Fiber: 0.3g

307. BEEF SHAWARMA AND VEGGIE SALAD BOWLS

PREPARATION: 10' **COOKING:** 19' **SERVES:** 4

INGREDIENTS

- 2 teaspoons olive oil
- 1½ pounds (680 g) beef flank steak, thinly sliced
- Sea salt and freshly ground black pepper, to taste
- 1 teaspoon cayenne pepper
- ½ teaspoon ground bay leaf
- ½ teaspoon ground allspice
- ½ teaspoon cumin, divided
- ½ cup Greek yogurt
- 2 tablespoons sesame oil
- 1 tablespoon fresh lime juice
- 2 English cucumbers, chopped
- 1 cup cherry tomatoes, halved
- 1 red onion, thinly sliced
- ½ head romaine lettuce, chopped

DIRECTIONS

1. Press the Sauté button to heat up the Instant Pot. Then, heat the olive oil and cook the beef for about 4 minutes.
2. Add all seasonings, 1½ cups of water, and secure the lid.
3. Choose Manual mode. Set the cook time for 15 minutes on High Pressure.
4. Once cooking is complete, use a natural pressure release. Carefully remove the lid.
5. Allow the beef to cool completely.
6. To make the dressing, whisk Greek yogurt, sesame oil, and lime juice in a mixing bowl.
7. Then, divide cucumbers, tomatoes, red onion, and romaine lettuce among four serving bowls. Dress the salad and top with the reserved beef flank steak. Serve warm.

NUTRITIONAL FACTS: Calories: 367 Fat: 19.1g Protein: 39.5g Carbs: 8.4g Net carbs: 5.0g Fiber: 3.4g

308. BEEF SHOULDER ROAST

PREPARATION: 15'   **COOKING:** 46'   **SERVES:** 6

INGREDIENTS

- 2 tablespoons peanut oil
- 2 pounds (907 g) shoulder roast
- ¼ cup coconut aminos
- 1 teaspoon porcini powder
- 1 teaspoon garlic powder
- 1 cup beef broth
- 2 cloves garlic, minced
- 2 tablespoons champagne vinegar
- ½ teaspoon hot sauce
- 1 teaspoon celery seeds
- 1 cup purple onions, cut into wedges
- 1 tablespoon flaxseed meal, plus 2 tablespoons water

DIRECTIONS

1. Press the Sauté button to heat up the Instant Pot. Then, heat the peanut oil and cook the beef shoulder roast for 3 minutes on each side.
2. In a mixing dish, combine coconut aminos, porcini powder, garlic powder, broth, garlic, vinegar, hot sauce, and celery seeds.
3. Pour the broth mixture into the Instant Pot. Add the onions to the top.
4. Secure the lid. Choose Meat/Stew mode and set cooking time for 40 minutes on High Pressure.
5. Once cooking is complete, use a natural pressure release for 15 minutes, then release any remaining pressure. Carefully remove the lid.
6. Make the slurry by mixing flaxseed meal with 2 tablespoons of water. Add the slurry to the Instant Pot.
7. Press the Sauté button and allow it to cook until the cooking liquid is reduced and thickened slightly. Serve warm.

NUTRITIONAL FACTS: Calories: 313 Fat: 16.1g Protein: 33.5g Carbs: 6.5g Net carbs: 3.1g Fiber: 3.4g

309. BEEF STUFFED KALE ROLLS

PREPARATION: 15'   **COOKING:** 30'   **SERVES:** 4

INGREDIENTS

- 8 ounces (227 g) ground beef
- 1 teaspoon chives
- ¼ teaspoon cayenne pepper
- 4 kale leaves
- 1 tablespoon cream cheese
- ¼ cup heavy cream
- ½ cup chicken broth

DIRECTIONS

1. In the mixing bowl, combine the ground beef, chives, and cayenne pepper.
2. Then fill and roll the kale leaves with ground beef mixture.
3. Place the kale rolls in the Instant Pot.
4. Add cream cheese, heavy cream, and chicken broth. Close the lid.
5. Select Manual mode and set cooking time for 30 minutes on High Pressure
6. When timer beeps, make a quick pressure release. Open the lid.
7. Serve warm.

NUTRITIONAL FACTS: Calories: 153 Fat: 7.4g Protein: 18.7g Carbs: 2.2g Net carbs: 1.9g Fiber: 0.3g

310. BEEF, BACON AND CAULIFLOWER RICE CASSEROLE

PREPARATION: 15' **COOKING:** 26' **SERVES:** 5

INGREDIENTS

- 2 cups fresh cauliflower florets
- 1 pound (454 g) ground beef
- 5 slices uncooked bacon, chopped
- 8 ounces (227 g) unsweetened tomato puree
- 1 cup shredded Cheddar cheese, divided
- 1 teaspoon garlic powder
- ½ teaspoon paprika
- ½ teaspoon sea salt
- ¼ teaspoon ground black pepper
- ¼ teaspoon celery seed
- 1 cup water
- 1 medium Roma tomato, sliced

DIRECTIONS

1. Spray a round soufflé dish with coconut oil cooking spray. Set aside.
2. Add the cauliflower florets to a food processor and pulse until a riced. Set aside.
3. Select Sauté mode. Once the pot is hot, crumble the ground beef into the pot and add the bacon. Sauté for 6 minutes or until the ground beef is browned and the bacon is cooked through.
4. Transfer the beef, bacon, and rendered fat to a large bowl.
5. Add the cauliflower rice, tomato puree ½ cup Cheddar cheese, garlic powder, paprika, sea salt, black pepper, and celery seed to the bowl with the beef and bacon. Mix well to combine.
6. Add the mixture to the prepared dish and use a spoon to press and smooth the mixture into an even layer.
7. Place the trivet in the Instant Pot and add the water to the bottom of the pot. Place the dish on top of the trivet.
8. Lock the lid. Select Manual mode and set cooking time for 20 minutes on High Pressure.
9. When cooking is complete, quick release the pressure.
10. Open the lid. Arrange the tomato slices in a single layer on top of the casserole and sprinkle the remaining cheese over top.
11. Secure the lid and let the residual heat melt the cheese for 5 minutes.
12. Open the lid, remove the dish from the pot.
13. Transfer the casserole to a serving plate and slice into 5 equal-sized wedges. Serve warm.

NUTRITIONAL FACTS: Calories: 350 Fat: 22.7g Protein: 30.0g Carbs: 8.0g Net carbs: 6.0g Fiber: 2.0g

CHAPTER 16.
PORK RECIPES

311. CILANTRO GARLIC PORK CHOPS

PREPARATION: 10' **COOKING:** 15' **SERVES:** 4

INGREDIENTS

- 1 pound boneless center-cut pork chops, pounded to ¼ inch thick
- Sea salt, for seasoning
- Freshly ground black pepper, for seasoning
- ¼ cup good-quality olive oil, divided
- ¼ cup finely chopped fresh cilantro
- 1 tablespoon minced garlic
- Juice of 1 lime

DIRECTIONS

1. Marinate the pork. Pat the pork chops dry and season them lightly with salt and pepper. Place them in a large bowl, add 2 tablespoons of the olive oil, and the cilantro, garlic, and lime juice. Toss to coat the chops. Cover the bowl and marinate the chops at room temperature for 30 minutes.
2. Cook the pork. In a large skillet over medium-high heat, warm the remaining 2 tablespoons of olive oil. Add the pork chops in a single layer and fry them, turning them once, until they're just cooked through and still juicy, 6 to 7 minutes per side.
3. Serve. Divide the chops between four plates and serve them immediately.

NUTRITIONAL FACTS: Calories: 249 Total fat: 16g Total carbs: 2g Fiber: 0g ;Net carbs: 2g Sodium: 261mg Protein: 25g

312. SPINACH FETA STUFFED PORK

PREPARATION: 15' **COOKING:** 30' **SERVES:** 4

INGREDIENTS

- 4 ounces crumbled feta cheese
- ¾ cup chopped frozen spinach, thawed and liquid squeezed out
- 3 tablespoons chopped Kalamata olives
- 4 (4-ounce) center pork chops, 2 inches thick
- Sea salt, for seasoning
- Freshly ground black pepper, for seasoning
- 3 tablespoons good-quality olive oil

DIRECTIONS

1. Preheat the oven. Set the oven temperature to 400°F.
2. Make the filling. In a small bowl, mix together the feta, spinach, and olives until everything is well combined.
3. Stuff the pork chops. Make a horizontal slit in the side of each chop to create a pocket, making sure you don't cut all the way through. Stuff the filling equally between the chops and secure the slits with toothpicks. Lightly season the stuffed chops with salt and pepper.
4. Brown the chops. In a large oven-safe skillet over medium-high heat, warm the olive oil.
5. Add the chops and sear them until they're browned all over, about 10 minutes in total.
6. Roast the chops. Place the skillet in the oven and roast the chops for 20 minutes or until they're cooked through.
7. Serve. Let the meat rest for 10 minutes and then remove the toothpicks. Divide the pork chops between four plates and serve them immediately.

NUTRITIONAL FACTS: Calories: 342 Total fat: 24g Total carbs: 3g Fiber: 1g ;Net carbs: 2g Sodium: 572mg Protein: 28g

313. COCONUT MILK GINGER MARINATED PORK TENDERLOIN

PREPARATION: 5' **COOKING:** 25' **SERVES:** 4

INGREDIENTS

- ¼ cup coconut oil, divided
- 1½ pounds boneless pork chops, about ¾ inch thick
- 1 tablespoon grated fresh ginger
- 2 teaspoons minced garlic
- 1 cup coconut milk
- 1 teaspoon chopped fresh basil
- Juice of 1 lime
- ½ cup shredded unsweetened coconut

DIRECTIONS

1. Brown the pork. In a large skillet over medium heat, warm 2 tablespoons of the coconut oil. Add the pork chops to the skillet and brown them all over, turning them several times, about 10 minutes in total.
2. Braise the pork. Move the pork to the side of the skillet and add the remaining 2 tablespoons of coconut oil. Add the ginger and garlic and sauté until they've softened, about 2 minutes. Stir in the coconut milk, basil, and lime juice and move the pork back to the center of the skillet. Cover the skillet and simmer until the pork is just cooked through and very tender, 12 to 15 minutes.
3. Serve. Divide the pork chops between four plates and top them with the shredded coconut.

NUTRITIONAL FACTS: Calories: 479 Total fat: 38g Total carbs: 6g Fiber: 3g; Net carbs: 3g Sodium: 318mg Protein: 32g

314. GRILLED PORK CHOPS WITH GREEK SALSA

PREPARATION: 15' **COOKING:** 15' **SERVES:** 4

INGREDIENTS

- ¼ cup good-quality olive oil, divided
- 1 tablespoon red wine vinegar
- 3 teaspoons chopped fresh oregano, divided
- 1 teaspoon minced garlic
- 4 (4-ounce) boneless center-cut loin pork chops
- ½ cup halved cherry tomatoes
- ½ yellow bell pepper, diced
- ½ English cucumber, chopped
- ¼ red onion, chopped
- 1 tablespoon balsamic vinegar
- Sea salt, for seasoning
- Freshly ground black pepper, for seasoning

DIRECTIONS

1. Marinate the pork. In a medium bowl, stir together 3 tablespoons of the olive oil, the vinegar, 2 teaspoons of the oregano, and the garlic. Add the pork chops to the bowl, turning them to get them coated with the marinade. Cover the bowl and place it in the refrigerator for 30 minutes.
2. Make the salsa. While the pork is marinating, in a medium bowl, stir together the remaining 1 tablespoon of olive oil, the tomatoes, yellow bell pepper, cucumber, red onion, vinegar, and the remaining 1 teaspoon of oregano. Season the salsa with salt and pepper. Set the bowl aside.
3. Grill the pork chops. Heat a grill to medium-high heat. Remove the pork chops from the marinade and grill them until just cooked through, 6 to 8 minutes per side.
4. Serve. Rest the pork for 5 minutes. Divide the pork between four plates and serve them with a generous scoop of the salsa.

NUTRITIONAL FACTS: Calories: 277 Total fat: 19g Total carbs: 4g Fiber: 1g; Net carbs: 3g Sodium: 257mg; Protein: 25g

315. GRILLED HERBED PORK KEBABS

PREPARATION: 10' **COOKING:** 15' **SERVES:** 4

INGREDIENTS

- ¼ cup good-quality olive oil
- 1 tablespoon minced garlic
- 2 teaspoons dried oregano
- 1 teaspoon dried basil
- 1 teaspoon dried parsley
- ½ teaspoon sea salt
- 1/4 teaspoon freshly ground black pepper
- 1 (1-pound) pork tenderloin, cut into 1½-inch pieces

DIRECTIONS

1. Marinate the pork. In a medium bowl, stir together the olive oil, garlic, oregano, basil, parsley, salt, and pepper. Add the pork pieces and toss to coat them in the marinade. Cover the bowl and place it in the refrigerator for 2 to 4 hours.
2. Make the kebabs. Divide the pork pieces between four skewers, making sure to not crowd the meat.
3. Grill the kebabs. Preheat your grill to medium-high heat. Grill the skewers for about 12 minutes, turning to cook all sides of the pork, until the pork is cooked through.
4. Serve. Rest the skewers for 5 minutes. Divide the skewers between four plates and serve them immediately.

NUTRITIONAL FACTS: Calories: 261 Total fat: 18g Total carbs: 1g Fiber: 0g; Net carbs: 1g Sodium: 60mg Protein: 24

316. ITALIAN SAUSAGE BROCCOLI SAUTÉ

PREPARATION: 10' **COOKING:** 20' **SERVES:** 4

INGREDIENTS

- 2 tablespoons good-quality olive oil
- 1 pound Italian sausage meat, hot or mild
- 4 cups small broccoli florets
- 1 tablespoon minced garlic
- Freshly ground black pepper, for seasoning

DIRECTIONS

1. Cook the sausage. In a large skillet over medium heat, warm the olive oil. Add the sausage and sauté it until it's cooked through, 8 to 10 minutes. Transfer the sausage to a plate with a slotted spoon and set the plate aside.
2. Sauté the vegetables. Add the broccoli to the skillet and sauté it until its tender, about 6 minutes. Stir in the garlic and sauté for another 3 minutes.
3. Finish the dish. Return the sausage to the skillet and toss to combine it with the other ingredients. Season the mixture with pepper.
4. Serve. Divide the mixture between four plates and serve it immediately.

NUTRITIONAL FACTS: Calories: 486 Total fat: 43g Total carbs: 7g Fiber: 2g ;Net carbs: 5g Sodium: 513mg Protein: 19g

317. CLASSIC SAUSAGE AND PEPPERS

PREPARATION: 10' COOKING: 35' SERVES: 6

INGREDIENTS

- 1½ pounds sweet Italian sausages (or hot if you prefer)
- 2 tablespoons good-quality olive oil
- 1 red bell pepper, cut into thin strips
- 1 yellow bell pepper, cut into thin strips
- 1 orange bell pepper, cut into thin strips
- 1 red onion, thinly sliced
- 1 tablespoon minced garlic
- ½ cup white wine
- Sea salt, for seasoning
- Freshly ground black pepper, for seasoning

DIRECTIONS

1. Cook the sausage. Preheat a grill to medium-high and grill the sausages, turning them several times, until they're cooked through, about 12 minutes in total. Let the sausages rest for 15 minutes and then cut them into 2-inch pieces.
2. Sauté the vegetables. In a large skillet over medium-high heat, warm the olive oil. Add the red, yellow, and orange bell peppers, and the red onion and garlic and sauté until they're tender, about 10 minutes.
3. Finish the dish. Add the sausage to the skillet along with the white wine and sauté for 10 minutes.
4. Serve. Divide the mixture between four plates, season it with salt and pepper, and serve.

NUTRITIONAL FACTS: Calories: 450 Total fat: 40g Total carbs: 5g Fiber: 1g; Net carbs: 4g Sodium: 554mg Protein: 17g

318. LEMON-INFUSED PORK RIB ROAST

PREPARATION: 10' COOKING: 1H SERVES: 6

INGREDIENTS

- ¼ cup good-quality olive oil
- Zest and juice of 1 lemon
- Zest and juice of 1 orange
- 4 rosemary sprigs, lightly crushed
- 4 thyme sprigs, lightly crushed
- 1 (4-bone) pork rib roast, about 2½ pounds
- 6 garlic cloves, peeled
- Sea salt, for seasoning
- Freshly ground black pepper, for seasoning

DIRECTIONS

1. Make the marinade. In a large bowl, combine the olive oil, lemon zest, lemon juice, orange zest, orange juice, rosemary sprigs, and thyme sprigs.
2. Marinate the roast. Use a small knife to make six 1-inch-deep slits in the fatty side of the roast. Stuff the garlic cloves in the slits. Put the roast in the bowl with the marinade and turn it to coat it well with the marinade. Cover the bowl and refrigerate it overnight, turning the roast in the marinade several times.
3. Preheat the oven. Set the oven temperature to 350°F.
4. Roast the pork. Remove the pork from the marinade and season it with salt and pepper, then put it in a baking dish and let it come to room temperature. Roast the pork until it's cooked through (145°F to 160°F internal temperature), about 1 hour. Throw out any leftover marinade.
5. Serve. Let the pork rest for 10 minutes, then cut it into slices and arrange the slices on a platter. Serve it warm.

NUTRITIONAL FACTS: Calories: 403 Total fat: 30g Total carbs: 1g Fiber: 0g; Net carbs: 1g Sodium: 113mg Protein: 30g

319. PORK MEATBALL PARMESAN

PREPARATION: 15' COOKING: 30' SERVES: 6

INGREDIENTS

For The Meatballs:
- 1¼ Pounds ground pork
- ½ cup almond flour
- ½ cup Parmesan cheese
- 1 egg, lightly beaten
- 1 tablespoon chopped fresh parsley
- 1 teaspoon minced garlic
- 1 teaspoon chopped fresh oregano
- ¼ teaspoon sea salt
- 1/8 teaspoon freshly ground black pepper
- 2 tablespoons good-quality olive oil

FOR THE PARMIGIANA:
- 1 cup sugar-free tomato sauce
- 1 cup shredded mozzarella cheese

DIRECTIONS

1. Make the meatballs. In a large bowl, mix together the ground pork, almond flour, Parmesan, egg, parsley, garlic, oregano, salt, and pepper until everything is well mixed. Roll the pork mixture into 1½-inch meatballs.
2. Cook the meatballs. In a large skillet over medium-high heat, warm the olive oil. Add the meatballs to the skillet and cook them, turning them several times, until they're completely cooked through, about 15 minutes in total.

TO MAKE THE PARMIGIANA:

3. Preheat the oven. Set the oven temperature to 350°F.
4. Assemble the parmigiana. Transfer the meatballs to a 9-by-9-inch baking dish and top them with the tomato sauce. Sprinkle with the mozzarella and bake for 15 minutes or until the cheese is melted and golden.
5. Serve. Divide the meatballs and sauce between six bowls and serve it immediately.

NUTRITIONAL FACTS: Calories: 403 Total fat: 32g Total carbs: 1g Fiber: 0g; Net carbs: 1g Sodium: 351mg Protein: 25g

CHAPTER 17.
LAMB RECIPES

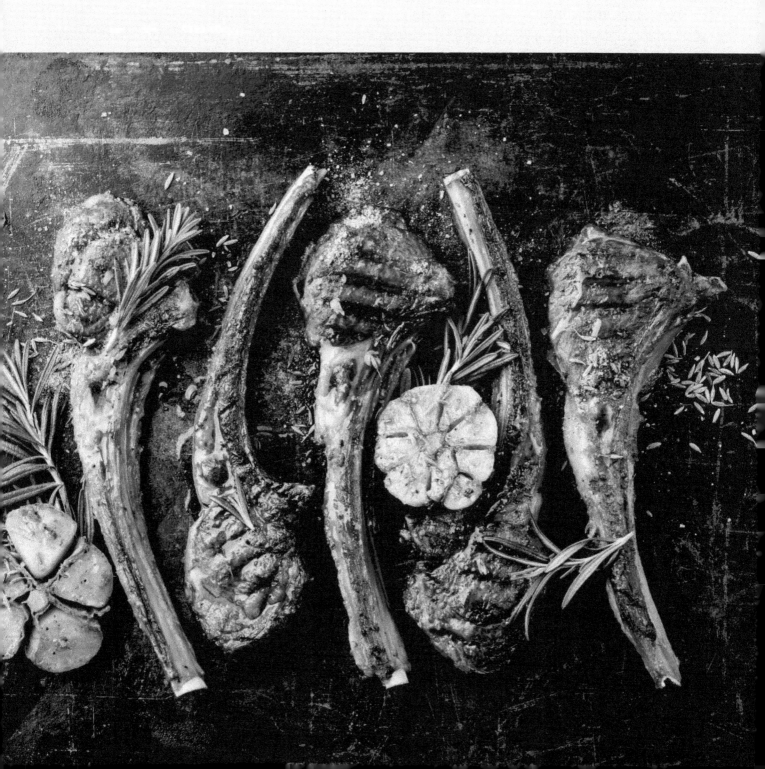

320. CHIPOTLE LAMB RIBS

PREPARATION: 15' COOKING: 20' SERVES: 6

INGREDIENTS

- 2-pound lamb ribs
- 1 tablespoon chipotle pepper, minced
- 2 tablespoons sesame oil
- 1 teaspoon apple cider vinegar

DIRECTIONS

1. Mix lamb ribs with all ingredients and leave to marinate for 10 minutes.
2. Then transfer the lamb ribs and all marinade in the baking tray and cook the meat in the oven at 360F for 40 minutes. Flip the ribs on another side after 20 minutes of cooking.

NUTRITIONAL FACTS: Calories 392 Fat 24.7 Fiber 0 Carbs 0.2 Protein 39.6

321. LAMB AND PECAN SALAD

PREPARATION: 10' COOKING: 10' SERVES: 4

INGREDIENTS

- 2 lamb chops
- 1 tablespoon sesame oil
- 2 pecans, chopped
- 2 cups lettuce, chopped
- 1 teaspoon cayenne pepper
- 1 tablespoon avocado oil

DIRECTIONS

1. Sprinkle the lamb chops with cayenne pepper and put in the hot skillet.
2. Add sesame oil and roast the meat for 4 minutes per side.
3. Then chops the lamb chops and put them in the salad bowl.
4. Add all remaining ingredients and carefully mix the salad.

NUTRITIONAL FACTS: Calories 168 Fat 12.1 Fiber 1 Carbs 2.3 Protein 12.9

322. HOT SAUCE LAMB

PREPARATION: 10' **COOKING:** 35' **SERVES:** 4

INGREDIENTS
- 2 teaspoons paprika
- 1-pound lamb fillet, chopped
- 1 tablespoon coconut oil
- 4 tablespoons keto hot sauce
- ½ cup of water

DIRECTIONS
1. Pour water in the saucepan and bring it to boil.
2. Add lamb and boil it for 20 minutes.
3. After this, preheat the skillet well.
4. Add boiled lamb fillet, coconut oil, and paprika.
5. Roast the ingredients for 6 minutes per side or until the meat is light brown.
6. Then add hot sauce and carefully mix the meal.

NUTRITIONAL FACTS: Calories 245 Fat 11.9 Fiber 0.4 Carbs 0.8 Protein 32.1

323. MUSTARD LAMB CHOPS

PREPARATION: 10' **COOKING:** 40' **SERVES:** 4

INGREDIENTS
- 1 cup spinach
- 3 tablespoons mustard
- 2 tablespoons sesame oil
- ½ teaspoon ground turmeric
- 4 lamb chops

DIRECTIONS
1. Blend the spinach and mix it with mustard, sesame oil, and ground turmeric.
2. Then rub the lamb chops with the mustard mixture and put in the baking pan.
3. Bake the meat at 355F for 40 minutes. Flip the meat after 20 minutes of cooking.

NUTRITIONAL FACTS: Calories 102 Fat 9.3 Fiber 1.5 Carbs 3.4 Protein 2.3

324. GINGER LAMB CHOPS

PREPARATION: 15'   COOKING: 30'   SERVES: 6

INGREDIENTS
- 6 lamb chops
- 1 tablespoon keto tomato paste
- 1 teaspoon minced ginger
- 2 tablespoons avocado oil
- 1 teaspoon plain yogurt

DIRECTIONS
1. Mix plain yogurt with keto tomato paste and minced ginger.
2. Then put the lamb chops in the yogurt mixture and marinate for 10-15 minutes.
3. After this, transfer the mixture in the tray, add avocado oil, and cook the meat at 360F in the oven for 30 minutes.

NUTRITIONAL FACTS: Calories 330 Fat 26.6 Fiber 0.4 Carbs 1 Protein 19.3

325. PARMESAN LAMB

PREPARATION: 10'   COOKING: 20'   SERVES: 4

INGREDIENTS
- 4 lamb chops
- 2 oz. Parmesan, grated
- ½ cup plain yogurt
- 3 scallions, sliced
- 1 tablespoon butter, softened

DIRECTIONS
1. Melt the butter in the saucepan. Add scallions and roast it for 3-4 minutes.
2. Then stir the scallions and add lamb chops.
3. Roast them for 2 minutes per side.
4. Add yogurt and close the lid. Cook the meat for 10 minutes.
5. After this, top the meat with Parmesan and cook it for 2 minutes more.

NUTRITIONAL FACTS: Calories 262 Fat 12.6 Fiber 0.6 Carbs 5.2 Protein 30.5

326. CLOVE LAMB

PREPARATION: 10' **COOKING:** 25' **SERVES:** 4

INGREDIENTS

- 1 teaspoon ground clove
- 2 tablespoons butter
- 1 teaspoon ground paprika
- 1 teaspoon dried rosemary
- ¼ cup of water
- 12 oz. lamb fillet

DIRECTIONS

1. In the shallow bowl, mix ground clove with ground paprika, and dried rosemary.
2. Rub the lamb fillet with spices and grease with butter.
3. Then put the meat in the hot skillet and roast it for 5 minutes per side on the low heat.
4. Add water. Close the lid and cook the lamb on medium heat for 15 minutes.

NUTRITIONAL FACTS: Calories 55 Fat 6 Fiber 0.5 Carbs 0.8 Protein 0.2

327. CARROT LAMB ROAST

PREPARATION: 10' **COOKING:** 40' **SERVES:** 4

INGREDIENTS

- 1-pound lamb loin
- 1 carrot, chopped
- 1 teaspoon dried thyme
- 2 tablespoons coconut oil
- 1 teaspoon salt

DIRECTIONS

1. Put all ingredients in the baking tray, mix well.
2. Bake the mixture in the preheated to 360F oven for 40 minutes.

NUTRITIONAL FACTS: Calories 295 Fat 17.9 Fiber 0.5 Carbs 1.7 Protein 30.3

328. LAMB AND CELERY CASSEROLE

PREPARATION: 10'   **COOKING:** 45'   **SERVES:** 2

INGREDIENTS

- ¼ cup celery stalk, chopped
- 2 lamb chops, chopped
- ½ cup Mozzarella, shredded
- 1 teaspoon butter
- ¼ cup coconut cream
- 1 teaspoon taco seasonings

DIRECTIONS

1. Mix lamb chops with taco seasonings and put in the casserole mold.
2. Add celery stalk, coconut cream, and shredded mozzarella.
3. Then add butter and cook the casserole in the preheated to 360F oven for 45 minutes.

NUTRITIONAL FACTS: Calories 283 Fat 19. 3Fiber 0.9 Carbs 3.3 Protein 24.8

329. LAMB IN ALMOND SAUCE

PREPARATION: 10'   **COOKING:** 30'   **SERVES:** 6

INGREDIENTS

- 14 oz. lamb fillet, cubed
- 1 cup organic almond milk
- 1 teaspoon almond flour
- 1 teaspoon ground nutmeg
- ½ teaspoon ground cardamom
- 1 tablespoon olive oil
- 1 tablespoon lemon juice
- 1 tablespoon butter
- ½ teaspoon minced garlic

DIRECTIONS

1. Preheat the olive oil in the saucepan.
2. Meanwhile, mix lamb, ground nutmeg, ground cardamom, and minced garlic.
3. Put the lamb in the hot olive oil. Roast the meat for 2 minutes per side.
4. Then add butter, lemon juice, and almond milk. Carefully mix the mixture.
5. Cook the meal for 15 minutes on medium heat.
6. Then add almond flour, stir well and simmer the meal for 10 minutes more.

NUTRITIONAL FACTS: Calories 258 Fat 19 Fiber 1.1 Carbs 2.7 Protein 19.7

330. SWEET LEG OF LAMB

PREPARATION: 10'   COOKING: 45'   SERVES: 6

INGREDIENTS

- 2 pounds lamb leg
- 1 tablespoon Erythritol
- 3 tablespoons coconut milk
- 1 teaspoon chili flakes
- 1 teaspoon ground turmeric
- 1 teaspoon cayenne pepper
- 3 tablespoons coconut oil

DIRECTIONS

1. In the shallow bowl, mix cayenne pepper, ground turmeric, chili flakes, and Erythritol.
2. Rub the lamb leg with spices.
3. Melt the coconut oil in the saucepan.
4. Add lamb leg and roast it for 10 minutes per side on low heat.
5. After this, add coconut milk and cook the meal for 30 minutes on low heat. Flip the meat on another side from time to time.

NUTRITIONAL FACTS: Calories 350 Fat 18.8 Fiber 0.3 Carbs 0.8 Protein 42.8

331. COCONUT LAMB SHOULDER

PREPARATION: 10'   COOKING: 75'   SERVES: 5

INGREDIENTS

- 2-pound lamb shoulder
- 1 teaspoon ground cumin
- 2 tablespoons butter
- ¼ cup of coconut milk
- 1 teaspoon coconut shred
- ½ cup kale, chopped

DIRECTIONS

1. Put all ingredients in the saucepan and mix well.
2. Close the lid and cook the meal on low heat for 75 minutes.

NUTRITIONAL FACTS: Calories 414 Fat 21.2 Fiber 0.5 Carbs 1.7 Protein 51.5

332. LAVENDER LAMB

PREPARATION: 10' **COOKING:** 35' **SERVES:** 4

INGREDIENTS

- 4 lamb chops
- 1 teaspoon dried lavender
- 2 tablespoons butter
- 1 teaspoon cumin seeds
- 1 cup of water

DIRECTIONS

1. Toss the butter in the saucepan and melt it.
2. Add lamb chops and roast them for 3 minutes.
3. Then add dried lavender, cumin seeds, and water.
4. Close the lid and cook the meat for 30 minutes on medium-low heat.

NUTRITIONAL FACTS: Calories 211 Fat 12.1 Fiber 0.1 Carbs 0.2 Protein 24

333. DILL LAMB SHANK

PREPARATION: 10' **COOKING:** 40' **SERVES:** 3

INGREDIENTS

- 3 lamb shanks (4 oz. each)
- 1 tablespoon dried dill
- 1 teaspoon peppercorns
- 3 cups of water
- 1 carrot, chopped
- 1 teaspoon salt

DIRECTIONS

1. Bring the water to boil.
2. Add lamb shank, dried dill, peppercorns, carrot, and salt.
3. Close the lid and cook the meat in medium heat for 40 minutes.

NUTRITIONAL FACTS: Calories 224 Fat 84 Fiber 0.8 Carbs 3 Protein 32.3

334. MEXICAN LAMB CHOPS

PREPARATION: 10' **COOKING:** 15' **SERVES:** 4

INGREDIENTS
- 4 lamb chops
- 1 tablespoon Mexican seasonings
- 2 tablespoons sesame oil
- 1 teaspoon butter

DIRECTIONS
1. Rub the lamb chops with Mexican seasonings.
2. Then melt the butter in the skillet. Add sesame oil.
3. Then add lamb chops and roast them for 7 minutes per side on medium heat.

NUTRITIONAL FACTS: Calories 323 Fat 14 Fiber 0 Carbs 1.1 Protein 24.1

335. TENDER LAMB STEW

PREPARATION: 10' **COOKING:** 60' **SERVES:** 4

INGREDIENTS
- 1-pound lamb fillet, chopped
- 3 cups of water
- 1 zucchini, chopped
- ½ cup leek, chopped
- 1 teaspoon ground paprika
- 1 teaspoon cayenne pepper
- 1 teaspoon salt
- 1 teaspoon butter

DIRECTIONS
1. Put all ingredients in the saucepan. Mix the mixture and close the lid.
2. Cook the stew on medium-low heat for 60 minutes.

NUTRITIONAL FACTS: Calories 237 Fat 9.5 Fiber 1.1 Carbs 3.8 Protein 32.7

336. LIME LAMB

PREPARATION: 10'   COOKING: 40'   SERVES: 4

INGREDIENTS

- 2 lamb shanks
- ½ lime
- 1 teaspoon salt
- 1 teaspoon Erythritol
- 3 tablespoons butter

DIRECTIONS

1. Melt the butter in the saucepan.
2. Add lamb shanks in the hot butter and roast them for 5 minutes per side on the medium heat.
3. Then sprinkle the meat with salt and Erythritol.
4. Close the lid and simmer the meat on low heat for 30 minutes.

NUTRITIONAL FACTS: Calories 158 Fat 11.8 Fiber 0.2 Carbs 2.1 Protein 12.1

337. LAMB SAUTE WITH MINT AND LEMON

PREPARATION: 10'   COOKING: 45'   SERVES: 4

INGREDIENTS

- 1-pound lamb fillet
- 1 teaspoon dried mint
- 1 teaspoon lemon zest, grated
- 2 cups of water
- 1 carrot, chopped
- 1 teaspoon keto tomato paste
- 1 teaspoon cayenne pepper

DIRECTIONS

1. Chop the lamb fillet roughly and put it in the saucepan.
2. Roast the meat for 2 minutes per side.
3. Add dried mint, lemon zest, carrot, keto tomato paste, and cayenne pepper.
4. Then add water and carefully stir the ingredients.
5. Close the lid and cook the saute on medium heat for 40 minutes.

NUTRITIONAL FACTS: Calories 220 Fat 8.4 Fiber 0.6 Carbs 2.1 Protein 32.1

338. PANCETTA LAMB

PREPARATION: 10' **COOKING:** 35' **SERVES:** 5

INGREDIENTS

- 1-pound lamb fillet
- 2 oz. pancetta, sliced
- 1 teaspoon chili powder
- 1 teaspoon ground turmeric
- 1 tablespoon coconut oil

DIRECTIONS

1. Cut the lamb fillet into 5 servings.
2. Then mix meat with chili powder and ground turmeric.
3. After this, wrap every lamb fillet with pancetta.
4. Preheat the coconut oil in the skillet.
5. Add meat and roast it for 3 minutes.
6. After this, transfer the meat in the preheated to 360F oven and cook for 30 minutes.

NUTRITIONAL FACTS: Calories 257 Fat 14.2 Fiber 0.3 Carbs 0.7 Protein 29.8

339. SWEET LAMB WITH OREGANO

PREPARATION: 10' **COOKING:** 25' **SERVES:** 4

INGREDIENTS

- 1-pound lamb fillet, sliced
- 1 teaspoon dried oregano
- 1 teaspoon Erythritol
- 3 tablespoons butter
- 1 tablespoon apple cider vinegar

DIRECTIONS

1. Melt butter in the saucepan.
2. Add dried oregano, Erythritol, and apple cider vinegar. Bring the liquid to boil.
3. Add sliced lamb fillet and roast it for 20 minutes. Stir the meat from time to time.

NUTRITIONAL FACTS: Calories 289 Fat 17 Fiber 0.2 Carbs 1.5 Protein 32

340. VEAL AND CABBAGE SALAD

PREPARATION: 10' **COOKING:** 0' **SERVES:** 4

INGREDIENTS
- 1-pound veal, boiled, chopped
- 1 cup white cabbage, shredded
- 1 tablespoon olive oil
- 1 teaspoon apple cider vinegar
- 1 teaspoon dried dill
- 1 teaspoon salt

DIRECTIONS
1. Put all ingredients in the salad bowl.
2. Carefully mix the salad.

NUTRITIONAL FACTS: Calories 230 Fat 12.1 Fiber 0.5 Carbs 1.2 Protein 27.9

341. NUTMEG LAMB

PREPARATION: 15' **COOKING:** 25' **SERVES:** 4

INGREDIENTS
- 13 oz. rack of lamb
- 1 teaspoon ground nutmeg
- 1 tablespoon coconut oil
- ½ teaspoon ground black pepper

DIRECTIONS
1. Rub the lamb with ground nutmeg and ground black pepper.
2. Then melt the coconut oil in the skillet.
3. Add rack of lamb and roast it on medium heat for 10 minutes per side.

NUTRITIONAL FACTS: Calories 188 Fat 11.8 Fiber 0.2 Carbs 0.4 Protein 18.8

342. OIL AND HERBS LAMB

PREPARATION: 10' **COOKING:** 65' **SERVES:** 4

INGREDIENTS

- 11 oz. rack of lamb, trimmed
- 3 tablespoons olive oil
- 1 tablespoon Italian seasonings

DIRECTIONS

1. Mix the Italian seasonings with olive oil.
2. Then sprinkle the rack of lamb with oily mixture and bake in the oven at 360F for 65 minutes.
3. Slice the cooked lamb.

NUTRITIONAL FACTS: Calories 232 Fat 18.4 Fiber 0 Carbs 0.4 Protein 15.9

343. TOMATO LAMB RIBS

PREPARATION: 10' **COOKING:** 30' **SERVES:** 4

INGREDIENTS

- 11 oz. lamb ribs, roughly chopped
- 2 teaspoons keto tomato paste
- 2 tablespoons sesame oil
- 1 teaspoon cayenne pepper
- 1 tablespoon apple cider vinegar
- A pinch of red pepper flakes

DIRECTIONS

1. Roast lamb ribs in the sesame oil for 4 minutes per side.
2. Then add keto tomato paste, cayenne pepper, apple cider vinegar, and keto tomato paste.
3. Carefully stir the lamb ribs and close the lid.
4. Cook the lamb ribs on medium heat for 20 minutes.

NUTRITIONAL FACTS: Calories 222 Fat 14.5 Fiber 0.2 Carbs 0.8 Protein 20.9

CHAPTER 18.
SEAFOODS

344. SALMON WITH GREEN BEANS

PREPARATION: 10' COOKING: 20' SERVES: 2

INGREDIENTS
- 6 oz. green beans
- 3 oz. unsalted butter
- 2 salmon fillets

Seasoning:
- ½ tsp garlic powder
- ½ tsp salt
- ½ tsp cracked black pepper

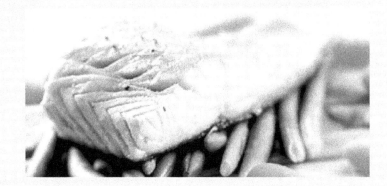

DIRECTIONS
1. Take a frying pan, place butter in it and when it starts to melts, add beans and salmon in fillets in it, season with garlic powder, salt, and black pepper, and cook for 8 minutes until salmon is cooked, turning halfway through and stirring the beans frequently.
2. When done, evenly divide salmon and green beans between two plates and serve.

NUTRITIONAL FACTS: 352 Calories; 29 g Fats; 19 g Protein; 3.5 g Net Carb; 1.5 g Fiber;

345. SALMON SHEET PAN

PREPARATION: 10' COOKING: 20' SERVES: 2

INGREDIENTS
- 2 salmon fillets
- 2 oz. cauliflower florets
- 2 oz. broccoli florets
- 1 tsp minced garlic
- 1 tbsp. chopped cilantro

Seasoning:
- 2 tbsp. coconut oil
- 2/3 tsp salt
- ¼ tsp ground black pepper

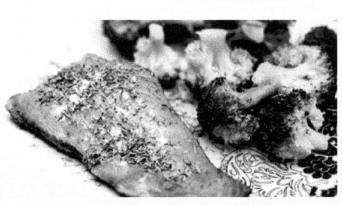

DIRECTIONS
1. Turn on the oven, then set it to 400 degrees F, and let it preheat.
2. Place oil in a small bowl, add garlic and cilantro, stir well, and microwave for 1 minute or until the oil has melted.
3. Take a rimmed baking sheet, place cauliflower and broccoli florets in it, drizzle with 1 tbsp. of coconut oil mixture, season with 1/3 tsp salt, 1/8 tsp black pepper and bake for 10 minutes.
4. Then push the vegetables to a side, place salmon fillets in the pan, drizzle with remaining coconut oil mixture, season with remaining salt and black pepper on both sides and bake for 10 minutes until salmon is fork-tender.
5. Serve.

NUTRITIONAL FACTS: 450 Calories; 23.8 g Fats; 36.9 g Protein; 5.9 g Net Carb; 2.4 g Fiber;

346. FISH WITH KALE AND OLIVES

PREPARATION: 5' COOKING: 12' SERVES: 2

INGREDIENTS

- 2 pacific whitening fillets
- 2 oz. chopped kale
- 3 tbsp. coconut oil
- 2 scallion, chopped
- 6 green olives

Seasoning:
- 1/2 tsp salt
- 1/3 tsp ground black pepper
- 3 drops of liquid stevia

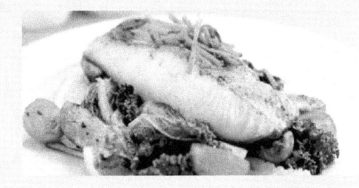

DIRECTIONS

1. Take a large skillet pan, place it over medium-high heat, add 4 tbsp. water, then add kale, toss and cook for 2 minutes until leaves are wilted but green.
2. When done, transfer kale to a strainer placed on a bowl and set aside until required.
3. Wipe clean the pan, add 2 tbsp. oil, and wait until it melts.
4. Season fillets with 1/3 tsp salt and ¼ tsp black pepper, place them into the pan skin-side up and cook for 4 minutes per side until fork tender.
5. Transfer fillets to a plate, add remaining oil to the pan, then add scallion and olives and cook for 1 minute.
6. Return kale into the pan, stir until mixed, cook for 1 minute until hot and then season with remaining salt and black pepper.
7. Divide kale mixture between two plates, top with cooked fillets, and then serve.

NUTRITIONAL FACTS: 454 Calories; 35.8 g Fats; 16 g Protein; 13.5 g Net Carb; 3.5 g Fiber;

347. CARDAMOM SALMON

PREPARATION: 5' COOKING: 20' SERVES: 2

INGREDIENTS

- 2 salmon fillets
- ¾ tsp salt
- 2/3 tbsp. ground cardamom
- 1 tbsp. liquid stevia
- 1 ½ tbsp. avocado oil

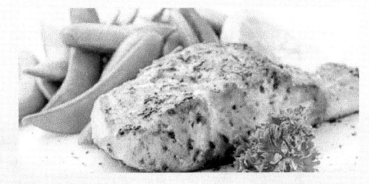

DIRECTIONS

1. Turn on the oven, then set it to 275 degrees F and let it preheat.
2. Meanwhile, prepare the sauce and for this, place oil in a small bowl, and whisk in cardamom and stevia until combined.
3. Take a baking dish, place salmon in it, brush with prepared sauce on all sides, and let it marinate for 20 minutes at room temperature.
4. Then season salmon with salt and bake for 15 to 20 minutes until thoroughly cooked.
5. When done, flake salmon with two forks and then serve.

NUTRITIONAL FACTS: 143.3 Calories; 10.7 g Fats; 11.8 g Protein; 0 g Net Carb; 0 g Fiber;

348. GARLIC BUTTER SALMON

PREPARATION: 10'   COOKING: 15'   SERVES: 2

INGREDIENTS

- 2 salmon fillets, skinless
- 1 tsp minced garlic
- 1 tbsp. chopped cilantro
- 1 tbsp. unsalted butter
- 2 tbsp. grated cheddar cheese

Seasoning:
- ½ tsp salt
- ¼ tsp ground black pepper

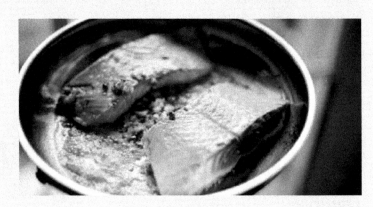

DIRECTIONS

1. Turn on the oven, then set it to 350 degrees F, and let it preheat.
2. Meanwhile, taking a rimmed baking sheet, grease it with oil, place salmon fillets on it, season with salt and black pepper on both sides.
3. Stir together butter, cilantro, and cheese until combined, then coat the mixture on both sides of salmon in an even layer and bake for 15 minutes until thoroughly cooked.
4. Then Turn on the broiler and continue baking the salmon for 2 minutes until the top is golden brown.
5. Serve.

NUTRITIONAL FACTS: 128 Calories; 4.5 g Fats; 41 g Protein; 1 g Net Carb; 0 g Fiber;

349. STIR-FRY TUNA WITH VEGETABLES

PREPARATION: 5'   COOKING: 15'   SERVES: 2

INGREDIENTS

- 4 oz. tuna, packed in water
- 2 oz. broccoli florets
- ½ of red bell pepper, cored, sliced
- ½ tsp minced garlic
- ½ tsp sesame seeds

Seasoning:
- 1 tbsp. avocado oil
- 2/3 tsp soy sauce
- 2/3 tsp apple cider vinegar
- 3 tbsp. water

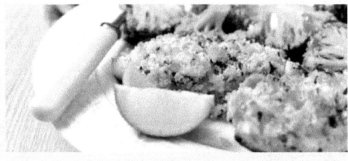

DIRECTIONS

1. Take a skillet pan, add ½ tbsp. oil and when hot, add bell pepper and cook for 3 minutes until tender-crisp.
2. Then add broccoli floret, drizzle with water and continue cooking for 3 minutes until steamed, covering the pan.
3. Uncover the pan, cook for 2 minutes until all the liquid has evaporated, and then push bell pepper to one side of the pan.
4. Add remaining oil to the other side of the pan, add tuna and cook for 3 minutes until seared on all sides.
5. Then drizzle with soy sauce and vinegar, toss all the ingredients in the pan until mixed and sprinkle with sesame seeds.
6. Serve.

NUTRITIONAL FACTS: 99.7 Calories; 5.1 g Fats; 11 g Protein; 1.6 g Net Carb; 1 g Fiber;

350. BAKED FISH WITH FETA AND TOMATO

PREPARATION: 5'   COOKING: 15'   SERVES: 2

INGREDIENTS

- 2 pacific whitening fillets
- 1 scallion, chopped
- 1 Roma tomato, chopped
- 1 tsp fresh oregano
- 1-ounce feta cheese, crumbled

Seasoning:
- 2 tbsp. avocado oil
- 1/3 tsp salt
- 1/4 tsp ground black pepper
- ¼ crushed red pepper

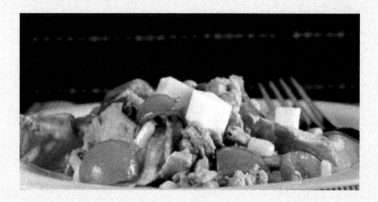

DIRECTIONS

1. Turn on the oven, then set it to 400 degrees F and let it preheat.
2. Take a medium skillet pan, place it over medium heat, add oil and when hot, add scallion and cook for 3 minutes.
3. Add tomatoes, stir in ½ tsp oregano, 1/8 tsp salt, black pepper, red pepper, pour in ¼ cup water and bring it to simmer.
4. Sprinkle remaining salt over fillets, add to the pan, drizzle with remaining oil, and then bake for 10 to 12 minutes until fillets are fork-tender.
5. When done, top fish with remaining oregano and cheese and then serve.

NUTRITIONAL FACTS: 427.5 Calories; 29.5 g Fats; 26.7 g Protein; 8 g Net Carb; 4 g Fiber;

351. CHILI-GLAZED SALMON

PREPARATION: 5'   COOKING: 10'   SERVES: 2

INGREDIENTS

- 2 salmon fillets
- 2 tbsp. sweet chili sauce
- 2 tsp chopped chives
- ½ tsp sesame seeds

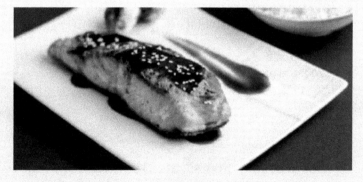

DIRECTIONS

1. Turn on the oven, then set it to 400 degrees F and let it preheat.
2. Meanwhile, place salmon in a shallow dish, add chili sauce and chives and toss until mixed.
3. Transfer prepared salmon onto a baking sheet lined with parchment sheet, drizzle with remaining sauce and bake for 10 minutes until thoroughly cooked.
4. Garnish with sesame seeds and Serve.

NUTRITIONAL FACTS: 112.5 Calories; 5.6 g Fats; 12 g Protein; 3.4 g Net Carb; 0 g Fiber;

352. CREAMY TUNA, SPINACH, AND EGGS PLATES

PREPARATION: 5' **COOKING:** 0' **SERVES:** 2

INGREDIENTS

- 2 oz. of spinach leaves
- 2 oz. tuna, packed in water
- 2 eggs, boiled
- 4 tbsp. cream cheese, full-fat

Seasoning:
- ¼ tsp salt
- 1/8 tsp ground black pepper

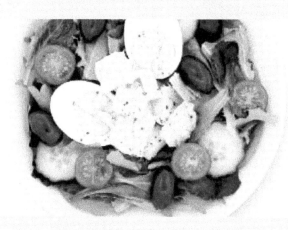

DIRECTIONS

1. Take two plates and evenly distribute spinach and tuna between them.
2. Peel the eggs, cut them into half, and divide them between the plates and then season with salt and black pepper.
3. Serve with cream cheese.

NUTRITIONAL FACTS: 212 Calories; 14.1 g Fats; 18 g Protein; 1.9 g Net Carb; 1.3 g Fiber;

353. TUNA AND AVOCADO

PREPARATION: 5' **COOKING:** 0' **SERVES:** 2

INGREDIENTS

- 2 oz. tuna, packed in water
- 1 avocado, pitted
- 8 green olives
- ½ cup mayonnaise, full-fat

Seasoning:
- 1/3 tsp salt
- 1/4 tsp ground black pepper

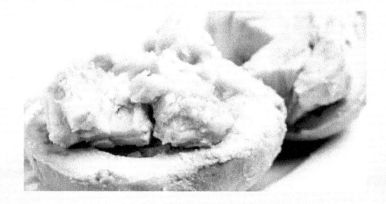

DIRECTIONS

1. Cut avocado into half, then remove the pit, scoop out the flesh and distribute between two plates.
2. Add tuna and green olives and then season with salt and black pepper.
3. Serve with mayonnaise.

NUTRITIONAL FACTS: 680 Calories; 65.6 g Fats; 10.2 g Protein; 2.2 g Net Carb; 9.7 g Fiber;

354. GARLIC OREGANO FISH

PREPARATION: 5' COOKING: 12' SERVES: 2

INGREDIENTS

- 2 pacific whitening fillets
- 1 tsp minced garlic
- 1 tbsp. butter, unsalted
- 2 tsp dried oregano

Seasoning:
- 1/3 tsp salt
- 1/4 tsp ground black pepper

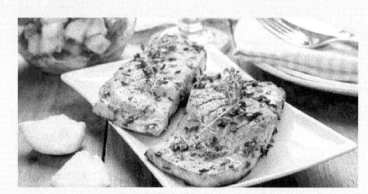

DIRECTIONS

1. Turn on the oven, then set it to 400 degrees F and let it preheat.
2. Meanwhile, take a small saucepan, place it over low heat, add butter and when it melts, stir in garlic and cook for 1 minute, remove the pan from heat.
3. Season fillets with salt and black pepper, and place them on a baking dish greased with oil.
4. Pour butter mixture over fillets, then sprinkle with oregano and bake for 10 to 12 minutes until thoroughly cooked.
5. Serve.

NUTRITIONAL FACTS: 199.5 Calories; 7 g Fats; 33.5 g Protein; 0.9 g Net Carb; 0.1 g Fiber;

355. BACON WRAPPED SALMON

PREPARATION: 5' COOKING: 10' SERVES: 2

INGREDIENTS

- 2 salmon fillets, cut into four pieces
- 4 slices of bacon
- 2 tsp avocado oil
- 2 tbsp. mayonnaise

Seasoning:
- ½ tsp salt
- ½ tsp ground black pepper

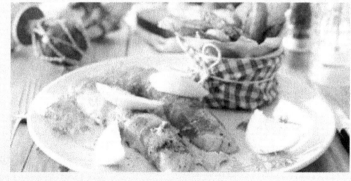

DIRECTIONS

1. Turn on the oven, then set it to 375 degrees F and let it preheat.
2. Meanwhile, place a skillet pan, place it over medium-high heat, add oil and let it heat.
3. Season salmon fillets with salt and black pepper, wrap each salmon fillet with a bacon slice, then add to the pan and cook for 4 minutes, turning halfway through.
4. Then transfer skillet pan containing salmon into the oven and cook salmon for 5 minutes until thoroughly cooked.
5. Serve salmon with mayonnaise

NUTRITIONAL FACTS: 190.7 Calories; 16.5 g Fats; 10.5 g Protein; 0 g Net Carb; 0 g Fiber;

356. FISH AND SPINACH PLATE

PREPARATION: 10' COOKING: 10' SERVES: 2

INGREDIENTS

- 2 pacific whitening fillets
- 2 oz. spinach
- ½ cup mayonnaise
- 1 tbsp. avocado oil
- 1 tbsp. unsalted butter

Seasoning:
- 1/2 tsp salt
- 1/3 tsp ground black pepper

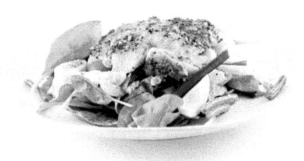

DIRECTIONS

1. Take a frying pan, place it over medium heat, add butter and wait until it melts.
2. Season fillets with 1/3 tsp salt and ¼ tsp black pepper, add to the pan, and cook for 5 minutes per side until golden brown and thoroughly cooked.
3. Transfer fillets to two plates, then distribute spinach among them, drizzle with oil and season with remaining salt and black pepper.
4. Serve with mayonnaise.

NUTRITIONAL FACTS: 389 Calories; 34 g Fats; 7.7 g Protein; 10.6 g Net Carb; 2 g Fiber

357. FISH AND EGG PLATE

PREPARATION: 5' COOKING: 10' SERVES: 2

INGREDIENTS

- 2 eggs
- 1 tbsp. butter, unsalted
- 2 pacific whitening fillets
- ½ oz. chopped lettuce
- 1 scallion, chopped

Seasoning:
- 3 tbsp. avocado oil
- 1/3 tsp salt
- 1/3 tsp ground black pepper

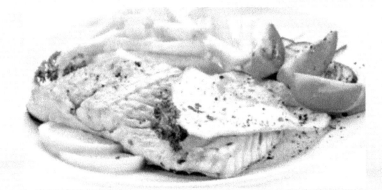

DIRECTIONS

1. Cook the eggs and for this, take a frying pan, place it over medium heat, add butter and when it melts, crack the egg in the pan and cook for 2 to 3 minutes until fried to desired liking.
2. Transfer fried egg to a plate and then cook the remaining egg in the same manner.
3. Meanwhile, season fish fillets with ¼ tsp each of salt and black pepper.
4. When eggs have fried, sprinkle salt and black pepper on them, then add 1 tbsp. oil into the frying pan, add fillets and cook for 4 minutes per side until thoroughly cooked.
5. When done, distribute fillets to the plate, add lettuce and scallion, drizzle with remaining oil, and then serve. vv

358. HERB CRUSTED TILAPIA

PREPARATION: 5' COOKING: 10' SERVES: 2

INGREDIENTS

- 2 fillets of tilapia
- ½ tsp garlic powder
- ½ tsp Italian seasoning
- ½ tsp dried parsley
- 1/3 tsp salt

Seasoning:
- 2 tbsp. melted butter, unsalted
- 1 tbsp. avocado oil

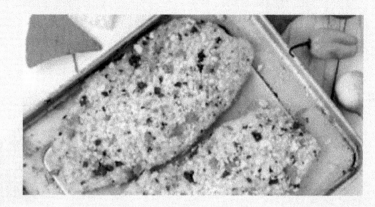

DIRECTIONS

1. Turn on the broiler and then let it preheat.
2. Meanwhile, take a small bowl, place melted butter in it, stir in oil and garlic powder until mixed, and then brush this mixture over tilapia fillets.
3. Stir together remaining spices and then sprinkle them generously on tilapia until well coated.
4. Place seasoned tilapia in a baking pan, place the pan under the broiler and then bake for 10 minutes until tender and golden, brushing with garlic-butter every 2 minutes.
5. Serve.

NUTRITIONAL FACTS: 520 Calories; 35 g Fats; 36.2 g Protein; 13.6 g Net Carb; 0.6 g Fiber;

359. SMOKED SALMON FAT BOMBS

PREPARATION: 5' COOKING: 0' SERVES: 2

INGREDIENTS

- 2 tbsp. cream cheese, softened
- 1 ounce smoked salmon
- 2 tsp bagel seasoning

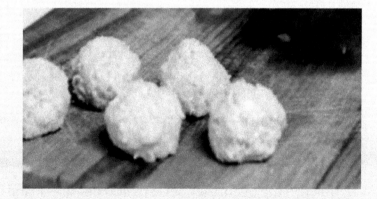

DIRECTIONS

1. Take a medium bowl, place cream cheese and salmon in it, and stir until well combined.
2. Shape the mixture into bowls, roll them into bagel seasoning and then serve.

NUTRITIONAL FACTS: 65 Calories; 4.8 g Fats; 4 g Protein; 0.5 g Net Carb; 0 g Fiber;

360. SHRIMP DEVILED EGGS

PREPARATION: 5' COOKING: 0' SERVES: 2

INGREDIENTS
- 2 eggs, boiled
- 2 oz. shrimps, cooked, chopped
- ½ tsp tabasco sauce
- ½ tsp mustard paste
- 2 tbsp. mayonnaise

Seasoning:
- 1/8 tsp salt
- 1/8 tsp ground black pepper

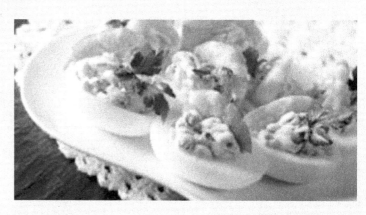

DIRECTIONS
1. Peel the boiled eggs, then slice in half lengthwise and transfer egg yolks to a medium bowl by using a spoon.
2. Mash the egg yolk, add remaining ingredients and stir until well combined.
3. Spoon the egg yolk mixture into egg whites, and then serve.

NUTRITIONAL FACTS: 210 Calories; 16.4 g Fats; 14 g Protein; 1 g Net Carb; 0.1 g Fiber;

361. TUNA MELT JALAPENO PEPPERS

PREPARATION: 5' COOKING: 0' SERVES: 2

INGREDIENTS
- 4 jalapeno peppers
- 1-ounce tuna, packed in water
- 1-ounce cream cheese softened
- 1 tbsp. grated parmesan cheese
- 1 tbsp. grated mozzarella cheese

Seasoning:
- 1 tsp chopped dill pickles
- 1 green onion, green part sliced only

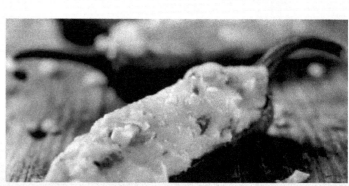

DIRECTIONS
1. Turn on the oven, then set it to 400 degrees F and let it preheat.
2. Prepare the peppers and for this, cut each pepper in half lengthwise and remove seeds and stem.
3. Take a small bowl, place tuna in it, add remaining ingredients except for cheeses, and then stir until combined.
4. Spoon tuna mixture into peppers, sprinkle cheeses on top, and then bake for 7 to 10 minutes until cheese has turned golden brown.
5. Serve.

NUTRITIONAL FACTS: 104 Calories; 6.2 g Fats; 7 g Protein; 2.1 g Net Carb; 1.1 g Fiber;

362. SALMON CUCUMBER ROLLS

PREPARATION: 15' COOKING: 0' SERVES: 2

INGREDIENTS

- 1 large cucumber
- 2 oz. smoked salmon
- 4 tbsp. mayonnaise
- 1 tsp sesame seeds
- **Seasoning:**
- ¼ tsp salt
- ¼ tsp ground black pepper

DIRECTIONS

1. Trim the ends of the cucumber, cut it into slices by using a vegetable peeler, and then place half of the cucumber slices in a dish.
2. Cover with paper towels, layer with remaining cucumber slices, top with paper towels, and let them refrigerate for 5 minutes.
3. Meanwhile, take a medium bowl, place salmon in it, add mayonnaise, season with salt and black pepper, and then stir until well combined.
4. Remove cucumber slices from the refrigerator, place salmon on one side of each cucumber slice, and then roll tightly.
5. Repeat with remaining cucumber, sprinkle with sesame seeds and then serve.

NUTRITIONAL FACTS: 269 Calories; 24 g Fats; 6.7 g Protein; 4 g Net Carb; 2 g Fiber;

363. SESAME TUNA SALAD

PREPARATION: 35' COOKING: 0' SERVES: 2

INGREDIENTS

- 6 oz. of tuna in water
- ½ tbsp. chili-garlic paste
- ½ tbsp. black sesame seeds, toasted
- 2 tbsp. mayonnaise
- 1 tbsp. sesame oil
- **Seasoning:**
- 1/8 tsp red pepper flakes

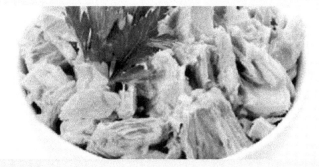

DIRECTIONS

1. Take a medium bowl, all the ingredients for the salad in it except for tuna, and then stir until well combined.
2. Fold in tuna until mixed and then refrigerator for 30 minutes.
3. Serve.

NUTRITIONAL FACTS: 322 Calories; 25.4 g Fats; 17.7 g Protein; 2.6 g Net Carb; 3 g Fiber;

364. BACON WRAPPED MAHI-MAHI

PREPARATION: 10' **COOKING:** 12' **SERVES:** 2

INGREDIENTS

- 2 fillets of mahi-mahi
- 2 strips of bacon
- ½ of lime, zested
- 4 basil leaves
- ½ tsp salt
- **Seasoning:**
- ½ tsp ground black pepper
- 1 tbsp. avocado oil

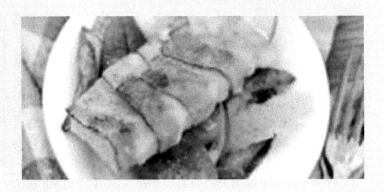

DIRECTIONS

1. Turn on the oven, then set it to 375 degrees F and let them preheat.
2. Meanwhile, season fillets with salt and black pepper, top each fillet with 2 basil leaves, sprinkle with lime zest, wrap with a bacon strip and secure with a toothpick if needed.
3. Take a medium skillet pan, place it over medium-high heat, add oil and when hot, place prepared fillets in it and cook for 2 minutes per side.
4. Transfer pan into the oven and bake the fish for 5 to 7 minutes until thoroughly cooked.
5. Serve.

NUTRITIONAL FACTS: 217 Calories; 11.3 g Fats; 27.1 g Protein; 1.2 g Net Carb; 0.5 g Fiber;

365. TUNA STUFFED AVOCADO

PREPARATION: 5' **COOKING:** 0' **SERVES:** 2

INGREDIENTS

- 1 medium avocado
- ¼ of a lemon, juiced
- 5-ounce tuna, packed in water
- 1 green onion, chopped
- 2 slices of turkey bacon, cooked, crumbled
- **Seasoning:**
- ¼ tsp salt
- ¼ tsp ground black pepper

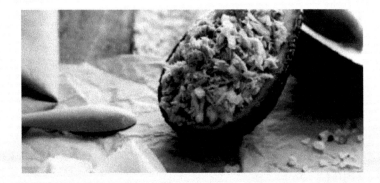

DIRECTIONS

1. Drain tuna, place it in a bowl, and then broke it into pieces with a form.
2. Add remaining ingredients, except for avocado and bacon, and stir until well combined.
3. Cut avocado into half, remove its pit and then stuff its cavity evenly with the tuna mixture.
4. Top stuffed avocados with bacon and Serve.

NUTRITIONAL FACTS: 108.5 Calories; 8 g Fats; 6 g Protein; 0.8 g Net Carb; 2.3 g Fiber;

366. CHEESY GARLIC BREAD WITH SMOKED SALMON

PREPARATION: 10' COOKING: 1' SERVES: 2

INGREDIENTS

- 4 tbsp. almond flour
- ½ tsp baking powder
- 2 tbsp. grated cheddar cheese
- 1 egg
- 2 oz. salmon, cut into thin sliced
- **Seasoning:**
- 1 tbsp. butter, unsalted
- ¼ tsp garlic powder
- 1/8 tsp salt
- ¼ tsp Italian seasoning

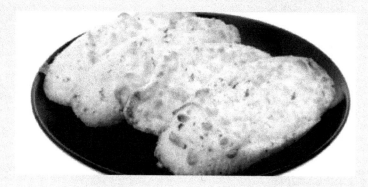

DIRECTIONS

1. Take a heatproof bowl, place all the ingredients in it except for cheese and then stir by using a fork until well combined.
2. Fold in cheese until just mixed and then microwave for 1 minute at high heat setting until thoroughly cooked, else continue cooking for another 15 to 30 seconds.
3. When done, lift out the bread, cool it for 5 minutes and then cut it into slices.
4. Top each slice with salmon and then serve straight away

NUTRITIONAL FACTS: 233 Calories; 18 g Fats; 13.8 g Protein; 1.9 g Net Carb; 1.5 g Fiber;

367. TUNA SALAD PICKLE BOATS

PREPARATION: 10' COOKING: 0' SERVES: 2

INGREDIENTS

- 4 dill pickles
- 4 oz. of tuna, packed in water, drained
- ¼ of lime, juiced
- 4 tbsp. mayonnaise

Seasoning:
- ¼ tsp salt
- 1/8 tsp ground black pepper
- ¼ tsp paprika
- 1 tbsp. mustard paste

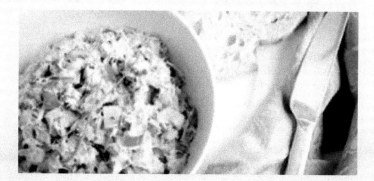

DIRECTIONS

1. Prepare tuna salad and for this, take a medium bowl, place tuna in it, add lime juice, mayonnaise, salt, black pepper, paprika, and mustard and stir until mixed.
2. Cut each pickle into half lengthwise, scoop out seeds, and then fill with tuna salad.
3. Serve.

NUTRITIONAL FACTS: 308.5 Calories; 23.7 g Fats; 17 g Protein; 3.8 g Net Carb; 3.1 g Fiber;

368. KETO TUNA SANDWICH

PREPARATION: 10' **COOKING:** 10' **SERVES:** 2

INGREDIENTS

- 2 oz. tuna, packed in water
- 2 2/3 tbsp. coconut flour
- 1 tsp baking powder
- 2 eggs
- 2 tbsp. mayonnaise

Seasoning:
- 1/4 tsp salt
- 1/4 tsp ground black pepper

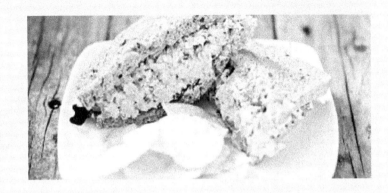

DIRECTIONS

1. Turn on the oven, then set it to 375 degrees F and let it preheat.
2. Meanwhile, prepare the batter for this, add all the ingredients in a bowl, reserving mayonnaise, 1 egg, and 1/8 tsp salt, and then whisk until well combined.
3. Take a 4 by 4 inches heatproof baking pan, grease it with oil, pour in the prepared batter and bake 10 minutes until bread is firm.
4. Meanwhile, prepare tuna and for this, place tuna in a medium bowl, add mayonnaise, season with remaining salt and black pepper, and then stir until combined.
5. When done, let the bread cool in the pan for 5 minutes, then transfer it to a wire rack and cool for 20 minutes.
6. Slice the bread, prepare sandwiches with prepared tuna mixture, and then serve.

NUTRITIONAL FACTS: 255 Calories; 17.8 g Fats; 16.3 g Protein; 3.7 g Net Carb; 3.3 g Fiber;

369. SMOKED SALMON PASTA SALAD

PREPARATION: 10' **COOKING:** 0' **SERVES:** 2

INGREDIENTS

- 1 zucchini, spiralized into noodles
- 4 oz. smoked salmon, break into pieces
- 2 oz. cream cheese
- 2 oz. mayonnaise
- 2 oz. sour cream

Seasoning:
- 1/3 tsp salt
- ¼ tsp ground black pepper
- ¼ tsp hot sauce

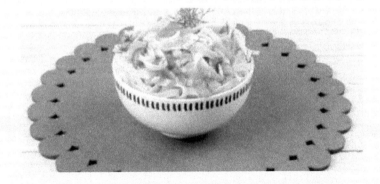

DIRECTIONS

1. Take a medium bowl, place cream cheese in it, add mayonnaise, sour cream, salt, black pepper and hot sauce and stir until well combined.
2. Add zucchini noodles, toss until well coated and then fold in salmon until just mixed.
3. Serve.

NUTRITIONAL FACTS: 458 Calories; 38.7 g Fats; 15.4 g Protein; 6.1 g Net Carb; 1.7 g Fiber;

370. TUNA, DILL AND SPINACH CURRY BOWL

PREPARATION: 5' **COOKING:** 0' **SERVES:** 2

INGREDIENTS

- 3 oz. tuna, packed in water
- 1 green onion, sliced
- 1 tbsp. diced dill pickle
- 1/3 of avocado, sliced
- 1 ounce chopped spinach

Seasoning:
- 1 ½ tsp curry powder
- ¼ tsp of sea salt
- 5 tbsp. mayonnaise

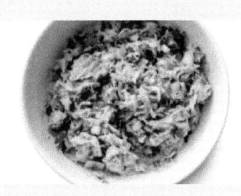

DIRECTIONS

1. Take a medium bowl, place mayonnaise in it, and then stir in curry powder and salt.
2. Add tuna, onion, dill pickle and spinach, toss until well coated, and then top with avocado.
3. Serve.

NUTRITIONAL FACTS: 310 Calories; 28 g Fats; 12.2 g Protein; 1 g Net Carb; 0.5 g Fiber;

371. MAHI-MAHI WITH CHILI LIME BUTTER

PREPARATION: 5' **COOKING:** 10' **SERVES:** 2

INGREDIENTS

- 3 tbsp. coconut oil, divided
- ½ tsp red chili powder
- 2 mahi-mahi fillets
- 1 lime, zested

Seasoning:
- 1/3 tsp salt
- ¼ tsp ground black pepper

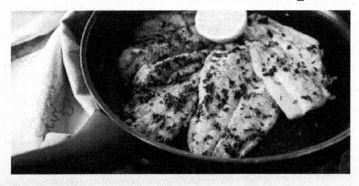

DIRECTIONS

1. Prepare the chili-lime butter and for this, take a small bowl, add 2 tbsp. coconut oil in it and then stir in red chili powder and lime zest until combined, set aside until required.
2. Take a medium skillet pan, place it over medium-high heat, add remaining oil and wait until it melts.
3. Season fillets with salt and black pepper, add to the pan and cook for 5 minutes per side until thoroughly cooked and golden brown.
4. When done, transfer fillets to the plates, top generously with prepared chili-lime butter, and then serve.

NUTRITIONAL FACTS: 298 Calories; 18.2 g Fats; 31.5 g Protein; 0.1 g Net Carb; 0.2 g Fiber;

372. GINGER SESAME GLAZED SALMON

PREPARATION: 10' **COOKING:** 15' **SERVES:** 2

INGREDIENTS

- 2 salmon fillets
- 1 tbsp. soy sauce
- 1 tsp sesame oil
- 2 tsp fish sauce
- 1 tbsp. avocado oil

Seasoning:
- 1 tsp garlic powder
- 1 tsp ginger powder
- ½ tbsp. apple cider vinegar

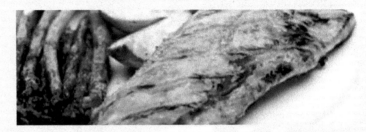

DIRECTIONS

1. Prepare the marinade and for this, take a small bowl, place soy sauce in it and stir in sesame oil, fish sauce, sesame oil, avocado oil, vinegar, ginger powder and garlic powder and stir until mixed.
2. Place salmon fillets in a shallow dish, pour prepared marinate on it, toss until coated, and let it marinate for 10 minutes.
3. When ready to cook, take a griddle pan, place it over medium heat, grease it with oil, and when hot, place marinated salmon fillets on it and then grill for 5 to 7 minutes per side until done.
4. Serve.

NUTRITIONAL FACTS: 370 Calories; 23.5 g Fats; 33 g Protein; 2.5 g Net Carb; 0 g Fiber

373. GARLIC PARMESAN MAHI-MAHI

PREPARATION: 10' **COOKING:** 10' **SERVES:** 2

INGREDIENTS

- 2 fillets of mahi-mahi
- 1 tsp minced garlic
- 1/3 tsp dried thyme
- 1 tbsp. avocado oil
- 1 tbsp. grated parmesan cheese

Seasoning:
- 1/3 tsp salt
- 1/4 tsp ground black pepper

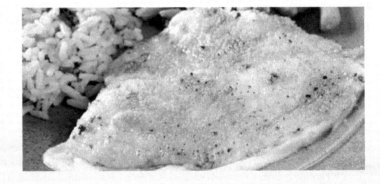

DIRECTIONS

1. Turn on the oven, set it to 425 degrees F and let it preheat.
2. Meanwhile, take a small bowl, place oil in it, add garlic, thyme, cheese and oil and stir until mixed.
3. Season fillets with salt and black pepper, then coat with prepared cheese mixture, place fillets in a baking sheet and then cook for 7 to 10 minutes until thoroughly cooked.
4. Serve.

NUTRITIONAL FACTS: 170 Calories; 7.8 g Fats; 22.3 g Protein; 0.8 g Net Carb; 0 g Fiber;

374. SALMON WITH LIME BUTTER SAUCE

PREPARATION: 20'   **COOKING:** 10'   **SERVES:** 2

INGREDIENTS

- 2 salmon fillets
- 1 lime, juiced, divided
- ½ tbsp. minced garlic
- 3 tbsp. butter, unsalted
- 1 tbsp. avocado oil

Seasoning:
- 1/4 tsp salt
- 1/4 tsp ground black pepper

DIRECTIONS

1. Prepare the fillets and for this, season fillets with salt and black pepper, place them on a shallow dish, drizzle with half of the lime juice and then it marinate for 15 minutes.
2. Meanwhile, prepare the lime butter sauce and for this, take a small saucepan, place it over medium-low heat, add butter, garlic, and half of the lime juice, stir until mixed, and then bring it to a low boil, set aside until required.
3. Then take a medium skillet pan, place it over medium-high heat, add oil and when hot, place marinated salmon in it, cook for 3 minutes per side and then transfer to a plate.
4. Top each salmon with prepared lime butter sauce and then serve.

NUTRITIONAL FACTS: 192 Calories; 18 g Fats; 6 g Protein; 4 g Net Carb; 0 g Fiber;

375. MUSHROOM WITH SALMON

PREPARATION: 5'   **COOKING:** 15'   **SERVES:** 2

INGREDIENTS

- 2 salmon fillets
- 2 oz. sliced mushrooms
- 1 tbsp. avocado oil
- 3 tbsp. butter, unsalted
- ¼ cup of water
- ¼ tsp paprika

Seasoning:
- 3/4 tsp salt
- 1/2 tsp ground black pepper

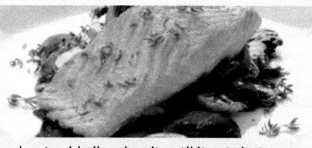

DIRECTIONS

1. Take a medium skillet pan, place it over medium heat, add oil and wait until it gets hot.
2. Season salmon with ½ tsp salt and ¼ tsp black pepper, add them to the pan and cook for 3 minutes per side until brown, set aside until done.
3. Add 2 tbsp. butter into the pan and when it melts, add mushrooms, season with paprika and remaining salt and black pepper, and cook for 3 minutes until sauté.
4. Pour in water, stir well, then add remaining butter and when it melts, return pork chops into the pan and simmer for 3 minutes until cooked.
5. Serve.

NUTRITIONAL FACTS: 420 Calories; 34.2 g Fats; 25 g Protein; 1.8 g Net Carb; 0.3 g Fiber;

376. BLACKENED FISH WITH ZUCCHINI NOODLES

PREPARATION: 10' **COOKING:** 12' **SERVES:** 2

INGREDIENTS

- 1 large zucchini
- 2 fillets of mahi-mahi
- 1 tsp Cajun seasoning
- 2 tbsp. butter, unsalted
- 1 tbsp. avocado oil

Seasoning:
- ½ tsp garlic powder
- 2/3 tsp salt
- ½ tsp ground black pepper

DIRECTIONS

1. Spiralized zucchini into noodles, place them into a colander, sprinkle with 1/3 tsp salt, toss until mixed and set aside until required.
2. Meanwhile, prepare fish and for this, season fillets with remaining salt and ¾ tsp Cajun seasoning.
3. Take a medium skillet pan, place it over medium heat, add butter and when it melts, add prepared fillets, switch heat to medium-high level and cook for 3 to 4 minutes per side until cooked and nicely browned.
4. Transfer fillets to a plate and then reserve the pan for zucchini noodles.
5. Squeeze moisture from the noodles, add them to the skillet pan, add oil, toss until mixed, season with remaining Cajun seasoning and cook for 2 to 3 minutes until noodles have turned soft.
6. Sprinkle with garlic powder, remove the pan from heat and distribute noodles between two plates.
7. Top noodles with a fillet and then serve.

NUTRITIONAL FACTS: 350 Calories; 25 g Fats; 27.1 g Protein; 2.8 g Net Carb; 1.6 g Fiber;

377. ZUCCHINI NOODLES IN CREAMY SALMON SAUCE

PREPARATION: 5' **COOKING:** 7' **SERVES:** 2

INGREDIENTS

- 3 oz. smoked salmon
- 1 zucchini, spiralized into noodles
- 1 tbsp. chopped basil
- 2 oz. whipping cream
- 2 oz. cream cheese, softened

Seasoning:
- 1/3 tsp salt
- 1/3 tsp ground black pepper
- 1 tbsp. avocado oil

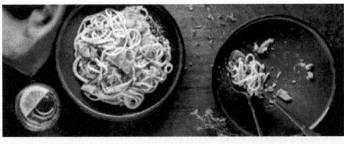

DIRECTIONS

1. Cut zucchini into noodles, place them into a colander, sprinkle with some salt, toss until well coated and set aside for 10 minutes.
2. Meanwhile, take a small saucepan, place it over medium-low heat, add whipped cream in it, add cream cheese, stir until mixed, bring it to a simmer, and cook for 2 minutes or more until smooth.
3. Then switch heat to low heat, add basil into the pan, cut salmon into thin slices, add to the pan, season with ¼ tsp of each salt and black pepper and cook for 1 minute until hot, set aside until required.
4. Take a medium skillet pan, place it over medium-high heat, add oil and when hot, add zucchini noodles and cook for 1 to 2 minutes until fried.
5. Season zucchini with remaining salt and black pepper and then distribute zucchini between two plates.
6. Top zucchini noodles with salmon sauce and then serve.

NUTRITIONAL FACTS: 271 Calories; 22 g Fats; 13.5 g Protein; 4.5 g Net Carb; 1.5 g Fiber;

378. TUNA SALAD CUCUMBER BOATS

PREPARATION: 10' COOKING: 0' SERVES: 2

INGREDIENTS
- 1 cucumber
- 2 oz. tuna, packed in water
- 1 green onion, sliced
- 2 1/2 tbsp. mayonnaise
- 1 tsp mustard paste

Seasoning:
- ¼ tsp salt
- 1/8 tsp ground black pepper

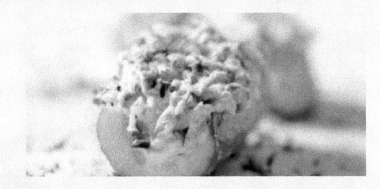

DIRECTIONS
1. Prepare salad and for this, place tuna in a bowl, add onion, mayonnaise and mustard, then add salt and black pepper and stir until combined.
2. Cut cucumber from the middle lengthwise, then scrape out the inside by using a spoon and fill the space with tuna salad.
3. Serve.

NUTRITIONAL FACTS: 190 Calories; 14.2 g Fats; 8.8 g Protein; 3.6 g Net Carb; 2 g Fiber;

379. SALMON WITH ROASTED VEGGIES

PREPARATION: 10' COOKING: 15' SERVES: 2

INGREDIENTS
- 2 fillets of salmon
- 4 oz. asparagus spears cut
- 2 oz. sliced mushrooms
- 2 oz. grape tomatoes
- 2 oz. basil pesto

Seasoning:
- 2/3 tsp salt
- ½ tsp ground black pepper
- 1 tbsp. mayonnaise
- oz. grated mozzarella cheese
- 2 tbsp. avocado oil

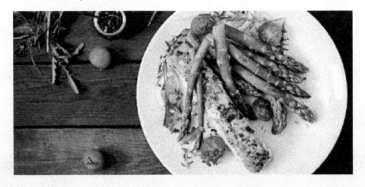

DIRECTIONS
1. Turn on the oven, then set it to 425 degrees F and let it preheat.
2. Take a medium baking sheet lined with parchment paper, place salmon fillets on it and then season with 1/3 tsp salt and ¼ tsp ground black pepper.
3. Take a small bowl, mix together mayonnaise and pesto in it until combined, spread this mixture over seasoned salmon and then top evenly with cheese.
4. Take a medium bowl, place all the vegetables in it, season with remaining salt and black pepper, drizzle with oil and toss until coated.
5. Spread vegetables around prepared fillets and then bake for 12 to 15 minutes until fillets have thoroughly cooked.
6. Serve.

NUTRITIONAL FACTS: 571 Calories; 45.4 g Fats; 34.1 g Protein; 3.5 g Net Carb; 2.2 g Fiber;

380. CHEESY BAKED MAHI-MAHI

PREPARATION: 10' COOKING: 25' SERVES: 2

INGREDIENTS

- 2 fillets of mahi-mahi
- ½ tsp minced garlic
- 2 tbsp. mayonnaise
- 1 tbsp. grated parmesan cheese
- 1 tbsp. grated mozzarella cheese

Seasoning:
- ½ tsp salt
- ¼ tsp ground black pepper
- 1 tbsp. mustard paste
- ¼ of lime, juiced

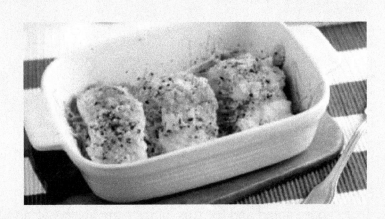

DIRECTIONS

1. Turn on the oven, then set it to 400 degrees F and let it preheat.
2. Meanwhile, take a baking sheet, line it with foil, place fillets on it and then season with salt and black pepper.
3. Take a small bowl, add mayonnaise, stir in garlic, lime juice and mustard until well mixed and then spread this mixture evenly on fillets.
4. Stir together parmesan cheese and mozzarella cheese, sprinkle it over fillets and then bake for 15 to 20 minutes until thoroughly cooked.
5. Then Turn on the broiler and continue cooking the fillets for 2 to 3 minutes until the top is nicely golden brown.
6. Serve.

NUTRITIONAL FACTS: 241 Calories; 13.6 g Fats; 25 g Protein; 1.1 g Net Carb; 0 g Fiber;

CHAPTER 19.
SOUP AND STEW

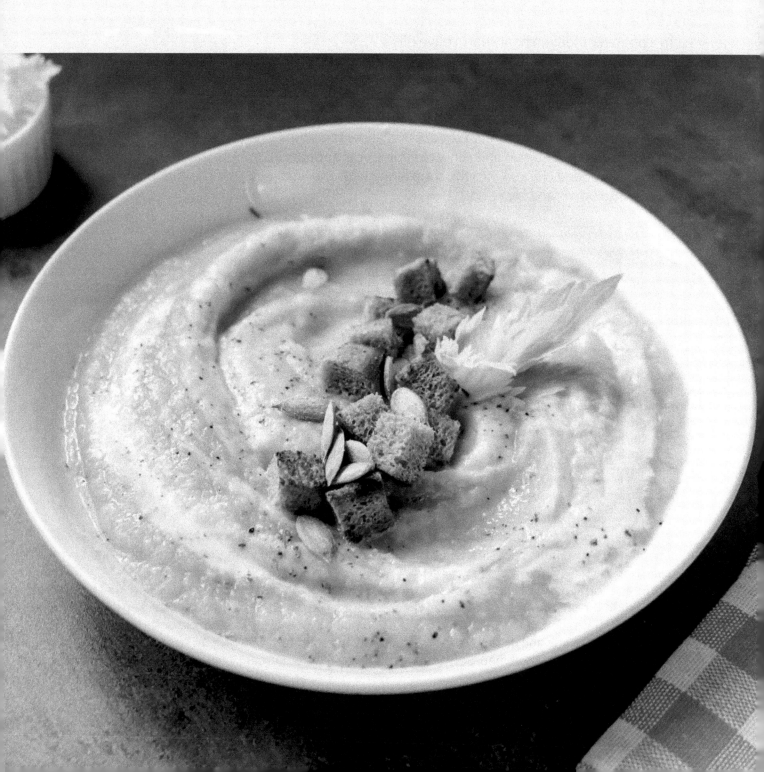

381. CHICKEN ENCHILADA SOUP

PREPARATION: 10' **COOKING:** 45' **SERVES:** 4

INGREDIENTS

- ½ c. fresh cilantro, chopped
- 1 ¼ tsp. chili powder
- 1 c. fresh tomatoes, diced
- 1 med. yellow onion, diced
- 1 sm. red bell pepper, diced
- 1 tbsp. cumin, ground
- 1 tbsp. extra virgin olive oil
- 1 tbsp. lime juice, fresh
- 1 tsp. dried oregano
- 2 cloves garlic, minced
- 2 lg. stalks celery, diced
- 4 c. chicken broth
- 8 oz. chicken thighs, boneless & skinless, shredded
- 8 oz. cream cheese, softened

DIRECTIONS

1. In a pot over medium heat, warm olive oil.
2. Once hot, add celery, red pepper, onion, and garlic. Cook for about 3 minutes or until shiny.
3. Stir the tomatoes into the pot and let cook for another 2 minutes.
4. Add seasonings to the pot, stir in chicken broth and bring to a boil.
5. Once boiling, drop the heat down to low and allow to simmer for 20 minutes.
6. Once simmered, add the cream cheese and allow the soup to return to a boil. *
7. Drop the heat once again and allow to simmer for another 20 minutes.
8. Stir the shredded chicken into the soup along with the lime juice and the cilantro.
9. Spoon into bowls and serve hot!

NUTRITIONAL FACTS: Calories: 420 Carbohydrates: 9 grams Fat: 29.5 grams Protein: 27 grams

382. BUFFALO CHICKEN SOUP

PREPARATION: 20' **COOKING:** 20' **SERVES:** 4

INGREDIENTS

- 4 med. stalks celery, diced
- 2 med. carrots, diced
- 4 chicken breasts, boneless & skinless
- 6 tbsp. butter
- 1 qt. chicken broth
- 2 oz. cream cheese
- ½ c. heavy cream
- ½ c. buffalo sauce 1 tsp. sea salt
- ½ tsp. thyme, dried

For garnish:
- Sour cream
- Green onions, thinly sliced
- Bleu cheese crumbles

DIRECTIONS

1. Set a large pot to warm over medium heat with the olive oil in it.
2. Cook celery and carrot until shiny and tender. Add chicken breasts to the pot and cover. Allow to cook about five to six minutes per side. Once the chicken has cooked and formed some caramelization on each side, remove it from the pot.
3. Shred the chicken breasts and set aside. Pour the chicken broth into the pot with the carrots and celery, then stir in the cream, butter, and cream cheese. * Bring the pot to a boil, then add chicken back to the pot. Stir buffalo sauce into the mix and combine completely. Feel free to increase or decrease as desired.
4. Add seasonings, stir, and drop the heat to low. Allow the soup to simmer for 15 to 20 minutes, or until all the flavors have fully combined. Serve hot with a garnish of sour cream, bleu cheese crumbles, and sliced green onion!

NUTRITIONAL FACTS: Calories: 563 Carbohydrates: 4 grams Fat: 32.5 grams Protein: 57 grams

383. THE SALSA

PREPARATION: 20' **COOKING:** 40' **SERVES:** 1

INGREDIENTS

- One small tomato
- One Thai chili, thinly sliced.
- One teaspoon of caper, fine cut
- Parsley - 2 teaspoons fine cut
- 1/4 of a lemon's juice

DIRECTIONS

1. Remove the eye from the tomato to make the salsa and slice it finely, ensuring that the fluid remains in as much as possible. Combine chile, capers, lemon juice and parsley. You might mix it all in, but the end product is a little different.
2. Oven to 220 degrees Celsius (425 ° F), in one teaspoon, marinate the chicken breast with a little oil and lemon juice. Leave for five to ten minutes.
3. Then add the marinated chicken and cook on either side for about a minute, until pale golden, transfer to the oven (on a baking tray, if your pan is not ovenproof), 8 to 10 minutes or until cooked. Remove from the oven, cover with tape, and wait until eaten for five minutes.
4. Cook the kale for 5 minutes in a steamer in the meantime, add a little butter, fry the red onions and the ginger and then mix in the fluffy but not browned mix.
5. Cook the buckwheat with the remaining teaspoon of turmeric according to the package instructions. Eat rice, tomatoes and salsa. Eat together.

NUTRITIONAL FACTS: Calories: 104, Sodium: 33 mg, Dietary Fibre: 1.6 g, Total Fat: 4.3 g, Total Carbs: 15.3 g, Protein: 1.3 g.

384. RAS-EL-HANOUT HOT SAUCE

PREPARATION: 10' **COOKING:** 10' **SERVES:** 2

INGREDIENTS

- Olive oil
- Lemon slices (juice)
- Teaspoon honey
- 1½ teaspoons Ras el Hanout
- 1/2 red peppers, prepare:

DIRECTIONS

1. Remove the seeds from the pepper.
2. Chopped peppers.
3. Put pepper in a bowl filled with lemon juice, honey and Ras-ElHanout and mix.
4. Then add olive oil drop by drop while continuing to mix. Sweet and Sour Pot:

NUTRITIONAL FACTS: Calories: 1495, Sodium: 33 mg, Dietary Fibre: 1.6 g, Total Fat: 3.1 g, Total Carbs: 16.5 g, Protein: 1.3 g.

385. TERIYAKI SAUCE

PREPARATION: 10' **COOKING:** 30' **SERVES:** 1

INGREDIENTS
- 7fl oz. soy sauce
- 7fl oz. pineapple juice
- 1 teaspoon red wine vinegar
- 1-inch chunk of fresh ginger root, peeled and chopped
- 2 cloves of garlic

DIRECTIONS
1. Place the ingredients into a saucepan, bring them to the boil, reduce the heat and simmer for 10 minutes. Let it cool then remove the garlic and ginger. Store it in a container in the fridge until ready to use. Use as a marinade for meat, fish and tofu dishes.

NUTRITIONAL FACTS: Calories: 267, Sodium: 33 mg, Dietary Fibre: 1.2 g, Total Fat: 4.3 g, Total Carbs: 16.2 g, Protein: 1.3 g.

386. GARLIC VINAIGRETTE

PREPARATION: 10' **COOKING:** 30' **SERVES:** 1

INGREDIENTS
- 1 clove garlic, crushed
- 4 tablespoons olive oil
- 1 tablespoon lemon juice
- Freshly ground black pepper

DIRECTIONS
1. Simply mix all of the ingredients together. It can either be stored or used straight away.

NUTRITIONAL FACTS: Calories: 104, Sodium: 35 mg, Dietary Fibre: 1.3 g, Total Fat: 3.1 g, Total Carbs: 16.2 g, Protein: 1.3 g.

387. LEMON CAPER PESTO

PREPARATION: 10'   **COOKING:** 10'   **SERVES:** 1

INGREDIENTS
- 6 tablespoons fresh parsley leaves
- 3 cloves of garlic
- 2 tablespoons capers
- 2oz cashew nuts
- 2 tablespoons olive oil
- 1 tablespoon lemon juice

DIRECTIONS
1. Place all of the ingredients into a food processor and blitz until smooth. Add a little extra oil if necessary. Serve with pasta, vegetables or meat dishes.

NUTRITIONAL FACTS: Calories: 250, Sodium: 32 mg, Dietary Fibre: 1.6 g, Total Fat: 4.1 g, Total Carbs: 16.4 g, Protein: 1.5 g.

388. PARSLEY PESTO

PREPARATION: 10'   **COOKING:** 10'   **SERVES:** 1

INGREDIENTS
- 3oz Parmesan cheese, finely grated
- 2oz pine nuts
- 6 tablespoons fresh parsley leaves, chopped
- 2 cloves of garlic
- 2 tablespoons olive oil

DIRECTIONS
1. Put all of the ingredients into a food processor or blend until you have a smooth paste.

NUTRITIONAL FACTS: Calories: 104, Sodium: 32 mg, Dietary Fibre: 1.6 g, Total Fat: 4.3 g, Total Carbs: 16.2 g, Protein: 1.3 g.

389. SLOW COOKER TACO SOUP

PREPARATION: 10' **COOKING:** 2H **SERVES:** 8

INGREDIENTS

- ¼ c. sour cream
- ½ c. cheddar cheese, shredded
- 2 c. diced tomatoes
- 2 lbs. ground beef
- 3 tbsp. taco seasoning*
- 4 c. chicken broth
- 8 oz. cream cheese, cubed**

DIRECTIONS

1. Heat a medium saucepan over medium heat and brown the beef.
2. Drain the fat from the beef and then place it into the slow cooker.
3. Add the cream cheese cubes, taco seasoning, and diced tomatoes into the slow cooker.
4. Add the chicken broth, cover and leave to cook on high for two hours.
5. Once the timer is up, stir all the ingredients and spoon the soup into bowls.
6. Serve hot with sour cream and shredded cheese on top!
7. *Check the label! Make sure that the taco seasoning you buy doesn't contain hidden sugars or starches.
8. **Cream cheese is easier to cut when it's very cold and if you carefully spread a little bit of olive oil on the blade of the knife!

NUTRITIONAL FACTS: Calories: 505 Carbohydrates: 8.5 grams Fat: 31.5 grams Protein: 43.5 grams

390. WALNUT VINAIGRETTE

PREPARATION: 10' **COOKING:** 10' **SERVES:** 1

INGREDIENTS

- 1 clove garlic, finely chopped
- 6 tablespoons olive oil
- 3 tablespoons red wine vinegar
- 1 tablespoon walnut oil
- Sea salt
- Freshly ground black pepper

DIRECTIONS

1. Combine all of the ingredients in a bowl or container and season with salt and pepper. Use immediately or store in the fridge.

NUTRITIONAL FACTS: Calories: 109, Sodium: 33 mg, Dietary Fibre: 1.6 g, Total Fat: 4.3 g, Total Carbs: 16.4 g, Protein: 1.6 g.

391. TURMERIC & LEMON DRESSING

PREPARATION: 10' **COOKING:** 30' **SERVES:** 1

INGREDIENTS

- 1 teaspoon turmeric
- 4 tablespoons olive oil
- Juice of 1 lemon

DIRECTIONS

1. Combine all the ingredients in bowl and serve with salads. Eat straight away.

NUTRITIONAL FACTS: Calories: 125, Sodium: 32 mg, Dietary Fibre: 1.6 g, Total Fat: 3.3 g, Total Carbs: 16.3 g, Protein: 1.5 g.

392. WALNUT & MINT PESTO

PREPARATION: 10' **COOKING:** 10' **SERVES:** 1

INGREDIENTS

- 6 tablespoons fresh mint leaves
- 2oz walnuts
- 2 cloves of garlic
- 3½oz Parmesan cheese
- 1 tablespoon lemon juice

DIRECTIONS

1. Put all the ingredients into a food processor and blend until it becomes a smooth paste.

NUTRITIONAL FACTS: Calories: 99, Sodium: 33 mg, Dietary Fibre: 1.6 g, Total Fat: 4.4 g, Total Carbs: 16.4 g, Protein: 1.6 g.

393. WEDDING SOUP

PREPARATION: 5' **COOKING:** 10' **SERVES:** 4

INGREDIENTS

- ½ c. almond flour
- ½ c. parmesan cheese, grated
- ½ sm. yellow onion, diced
- 1 lb. ground beef
- 1 lg. egg, beaten
- 1 tsp. Italian seasoning
- 1 tsp. oregano, fresh & chopped
- 1 tsp. thyme, fresh & chopped
- 2 c. baby leaf spinach, fresh
- 2 c. cauliflower, riced
- 2 med. stalks celery, diced
- 2 tbsp. extra virgin olive oil
- 3 cloves garlic, minced
- 6 c. chicken broth
- Sea salt & pepper to taste

DIRECTIONS

1. In a large mixing bowl, combine almond flour, parmesan cheese, ground beef, egg, salt, pepper, and Italian seasoning. Mix thoroughly by band
2. Shape the meat mixture into one-inch meatballs, cover, and refrigerate until ready to cook.
3. In a large saucepan over medium heat, warm the olive oil.
4. Once the oil is hot, stir the celery and onion into the pan and season to taste with salt and pepper.
5. Stirring often, bring the onion and celery to a lightly cooked state, about six or seven minutes.
6. Add the garlic to the pan, stir to combine, and allow to cook for one more minute.
7. Stir chicken broth, fresh oregano, and the fresh thyme into the pan and stir to combine.
8. Bring the mixture to a boil.
9. Drop the heat to low and allow to simmer for about ten minutes before adding cauliflower and meatballs to it.
10. Allow to cook for about five minutes or until the meatballs are cooked all the way through.
11. Add the spinach to the soup and stir in for about one to two minutes, or until it's sufficiently wilted.
12. Add seasoning as is needed.
13. Serve hot!

NUTRITIONAL FACTS: Calories: 420 Carbohydrates: 4 grams Fat: 26 grams Protein: 6.5 grams

394. VINAIGRETTE

PREPARATION: 10' **COOKING:** 10' **SERVES:** 2

INGREDIENTS

- A teaspoon of yellow mustard
- A spoon of white wine vinegar
- 1 Teaspoon of honey
- 165 ml of prepared olive oil:

DIRECTIONS

1. Mix mustard, vinegar and honey in a bowl.
2. Add a small amount of olive oil and stir until the vinegar thickens.
3. Season with salt and pepper.

NUTRITIONAL FACTS: Calories: 1495, Sodium: 33 mg, Dietary Fibre: 1.4 g, Total Fat: 4.3 g, Total Carbs: 16.2 g, Protein: 1.5 g.

395. MEXICAN PORK STEW

PREPARATION: 15' **COOKING:** 2H 10' **SERVES:** 1

INGREDIENTS

- 3 tbsp. unsalted butter
- 2½ lb. boneless pork ribs, cut into ¾-inch cubes
- 1 large yellow onion, chopped
- 4 garlic cloves, crushed
- 1½ C. homemade chicken broth
- 2 (10-oz.) cans sugar-free diced tomatoes
- 1 C. canned roasted poblano chiles
- 2 tsp. dried oregano
- 1 tsp. ground cumin
- Salt, to taste
- ¼ C. fresh cilantro, chopped
- 2 tbsp. fresh lime juice

DIRECTIONS

1. In a large pan, melt the butter over medium-high heat and cook the pork, onions and garlic for about 5 minutes or until browned.
2. Add the broth and scrape up the browned bits.
3. Add the tomatoes, poblano chiles, oregano, cumin, and salt and bring to a boil.
4. Reduce the heat to medium-low and simmer, covered for about 2 hours.
5. Stir in the fresh cilantro and lime juice and remove from heat.
6. Serve hot.

NUTRITIONAL FACTS: Calories: 288 Carbohydrates: 8.8g Protein: 39.6g Fat: 10.1g Sugar: 4g Sodium: 283mg Fiber: 2.8g

396. CURRY SOUP

PREPARATION: 25' **COOKING:** 20' **SERVES:** 4

INGREDIENTS

- ¾ tsp. cumin
- ¼ c. pumpkin seeds, raw
- ½ tsp. garlic powder
- ½ tsp. paprika ½ tsp. sea salt
- 1 c. coconut milk, unsweetened
- 1 clove garlic, minced
- 1 med. onion, diced
- 2 c. carrots, chopped
- 2 tbsp. curry powder
- 3 c. cauliflower, riced
- 3 tbsp. extra virgin olive oil, divided
- 4 c. kale, chopped
- 4 c. vegetable broth
- Sea salt & pepper to taste

DIRECTIONS

1. Hear a large saute pan over medium heat with 2 tablespoons of olive oil. Once the oil is hot, add the rice cauliflower to the pan along with the curry powder, cumin, salt, paprika, and garlic powder. Stir thoroughly to combine.
2. While cooking, stir occasionally. Once the cauliflower is warmed through, remove it from the heat.
3. In a large pot over medium heat, add the remainder of your olive oil. Once it's hot, add the onion and allow it to cook for about four minutes. Add the garlic, then cook for about another two minutes.
4. To the large pot, add the broth, kale, carrots, and cauliflower. Stir to thoroughly incorporate.
5. Allow the mixture to come to a boil, drop the heat to low, and allow the soup to simmer for about 15 minutes.
6. Stir the coconut milk into the mixture along with salt and pepper to taste.
7. Garnish with pumpkin seeds and serve hot!

NUTRITIONAL FACTS: Calories: 274 Carbs: 11 grams Fat: 19 grams Protein: 15 grams

397. WINTER COMFORT STEW

PREPARATION: 10' COOKING: 50' SERVES: 6

INGREDIENTS

- 2 tbsp. olive oil
- 1 small yellow onion, chopped
- 2 garlic cloves, chopped
- 2 lb. grass-fed beef chuck, cut into 1-inch cubes
- 1 (14-oz.) can sugar-free crushed tomatoes
- 2 tsp. ground allspice
- 1½ tsp. red pepper flakes
- ½ C. homemade beef broth
- 6 oz. green olives, pitted
- 8 oz. fresh baby spinach
- 2 tbsp. fresh lemon juice
- Salt and freshly ground black pepper, to taste
- ¼ C. fresh cilantro, chopped

DIRECTIONS

1. In a pan, heat the oil in a pan over high heat and sauté the onion and garlic for about 2-3 minutes.
2. Add the beef and cook for about 3-4 minutes or until browned, stirring frequently.
3. Add the tomatoes, spices and broth and bring to a boil.
4. Reduce the heat to low and simmer, covered for about 30-40 minutes or until desired doneness of the beef.
5. Stir in the olives and spinach and simmer for about 2-3 minutes.
6. Stir in the lemon juice, salt and black pepper and remove from the heat.
7. Serve hot with the garnishing of cilantro.

NUTRITIONAL FACTS: Calories: 388 Carbohydrates: 8g Protein: 485g Fat: 17.7g Sugar: 2.6g Sodium: 473mgFiber: 3.1g

398. HUNGARIAN PORK STEW

PREPARATION: 15' COOKING: 2H 20' SERVES: 4

INGREDIENTS

- 3 tbsp. olive oil
- 3½ lb. pork shoulder, cut into 4 portions
- 1 tbsp. butter
- 2 medium onions, chopped
- 16 oz. tomatoes, crushed
- 5 garlic cloves, crushed
- 2 Hungarian wax peppers, chopped
- 3 tbsp. Hungarian Sweet paprika
- 1 tbsp. smoked paprika
- 1 tsp. hot paprika
- ½ tsp. caraway seeds
- 1 bay leaf
- 1 C. homemade chicken broth
- 1 packet unflavored gelatin
- 2 tbsp. fresh lemon juice
- Pinch of xanthan gum
- Salt and freshly ground black pepper, to taste

DIRECTIONS

1. In a heavy-bottomed pan, heat 1 tbsp. of oil over high heat and sear the pork for about 2-3 minutes or until browned.
2. Transfer the pork onto a plate and cut into bite-sized pieces.
3. In the same pan, heat 1 tbsp. of oil and butter over medium-low heat and sauté the onions for about 5-6 minutes.
4. With a slotted spoon transfer the onion into a bowl.
5. In the same pan, add the tomatoes and cook for about 3-4 minutes, without stirring.
6. Meanwhile, in a small frying pan, heat the remaining oil over-low heat and sauté the garlic, wax peppers, all kinds of paprika and caraway seeds for about 20-30 seconds.
7. Remove from the heat and set aside.
8. In a small bowl, mix together the gelatin and broth.
9. In the large pan, add the cooked pork, garlic mixture, gelatin mixture and bay leaf and bring t0 a gentle boil.
10. Reduce the heat to low and simmer, covered for about 2 hours.
11. Stir in the xanthan gum and simmer for about 3-5 minutes.
12. Stir in the lemon juice, salt and black pepper and remove from the heat.
13. Serve hot.

NUTRITIONAL FACTS: Calories: 529 Carbohydrates: 5.8g Protein: 38.9g Fat: 38.5g Sugar: 2.6g Sodium: 216mgFiber: 2.1g

399. WEEKEND DINNER STEW

PREPARATION: 15' **COOKING:** 55' **SERVES:** 6

INGREDIENTS

- 1½ lb. grass-fed beef stew meat, trimmed and cubed into 1-inch size
- Salt and freshly ground black pepper, to taste
- 1 tbsp. olive oil
- 1 C. homemade tomato puree
- 4 C. homemade beef broth
- 2 C. zucchini, chopped
- 2 celery ribs, sliced
- ½ C. carrots, peeled and sliced
- 2 garlic cloves, minced
- ½ tbsp. dried thyme
- 1 tsp. dried parsley
- 1 tsp. dried rosemary
- 1 tbsp. paprika
- 1 tsp. onion powder
- 1 tsp. garlic powder

DIRECTIONS

1. In a large bowl, add the beef cubes, salt and black pepper and toss to coat well.
2. In a large pan, heat the oil over medium-high heat and cook the beef cubes for about 4-5 minutes or until browned.
3. Add the remaining ingredients and stir to combine.
4. Increase the heat to high and bring to a boil.
5. Reduce the heat to low and simmer, covered for about 40-50 minutes.
6. Stir in the salt and black pepper and remove from the heat.
7. Serve hot.

NUTRITIONAL FACTS: Calories: 293 Carbohydrates: 8g Protein: 9.3g Fat: 10.7g Sugar: 4g Sodium: 223mg Fiber: 2.3g

400. YELLOW CHICKEN SOUP

PREPARATION: 15' **COOKING:** 25' **SERVES:** 5

INGREDIENTS

- 2½ tsp. ground turmeric
- 1½ tsp. ground cumin
- 1/8 tsp cayenne pepper
- 2 tbsp. butter, divided
- 1 small yellow onion, chopped
- 2 C. cauliflower, chopped
- 2 C. broccoli, chopped
- 4 C. homemade chicken broth
- 1½ C. water
- 1 tsp. fresh ginger root, grated
- 1 bay leaf
- 2 C. Swiss chard, stemmed and chopped finely
- ½ C. unsweetened coconut milk
- 3 (4-oz.) grass-fed boneless, skinless chicken thighs, cut into bite-size pieces
- 2 tbsp. fresh lime juice

DIRECTIONS

1. In a small bowl, mix together the turmeric, cumin and cayenne pepper and set aside.
2. Ina large pan, melt 1 tbsp. of the butter over medium heat and sauté the onion for about 3-4 minutes.
3. Add the cauliflower, broccoli and half of the spice mixture and cook for another 3-4 minutes.
4. Add the broth, water, ginger and bay leaf and bring to a boil.
5. Reduce the heat to low and simmer for about 8-10 minutes.
6. Stir in the Swiss chard and coconut milk and cook for about 1-2 minutes.
7. Meanwhile, in a large skillet, melt the remaining butter over medium heat and sear the chicken pieces for about 5 minutes.
8. Stir in the remaining spice mix and cook for about 5 minutes, stirring frequently.
9. Transfer the soup into serving bowls and top with the chicken pieces.
10. Drizzle with lime juice and serve.

NUTRITIONAL FACTS: Calories: 258 Carbohydrates: 8.4g Protein: 18.4g Fat: 16.8g Sugar: 3g Sodium: 753mg Fiber: 2.9g

401. IDEAL COLD WEATHER STEW

PREPARATION: 20' **COOKING:** 2H 40' **SERVES:** 6

INGREDIENTS

- 3 tbsp. olive oil, divided
- 8 oz. fresh mushrooms, quartered
- 1¼ lb. grass-fed beef chuck roast, trimmed and cubed into 1-inch size
- 2 tbsp. tomato paste
- ½ tsp. dried thyme
- 1 bay leaf
- 5 C. homemade beef broth
- 6 oz. celery root, peeled and cubed
- 4 oz. yellow onions, chopped roughly
- 3 oz. carrot, peeled and sliced
- 2 garlic cloves, sliced
- Salt and freshly ground black pepper, to taste

DIRECTIONS

1. In a Dutch oven, heat 1 tbsp. of the oil over medium heat and cook the mushrooms for about 2 minutes, without stirring.
2. Stir the mushroom and cook for about 2 minutes more.
3. With a slotted spoon, transfer the mushroom onto a plate.
4. In the same pan, heat the remaining oil over medium-high heat and sear the beef cubes for about 4-5 minutes.
5. Stir in the tomato paste, thyme and bay leaf and cook for about 1 minute.
6. Stir in the broth and bring to a boil.
7. Reduce the heat to low and simmer, covered for about 1½ hours.
8. Stir in the mushrooms, celery, onion, carrot and garlic and simmers for about 40-60 minutes.
9. Stir in the salt and black pepper and remove from the heat.
10. Serve hot.

NUTRITIONAL FACTS: Calories: 447 Carbohydrates: 7.4g Protein: 30.8g Fat: 32.3g Sugar: 8g Sodium: 764mg Fiber: 1.9g

402. DELICIOUS TOMATO BASIL SOUP

PREPARATION: 10' **COOKING:** 40' **SERVES:** 4

INGREDIENTS

- ¼ c. olive oil
- ½ c. heavy cream
- 1 lb. tomatoes, fresh
- 4 c. chicken broth, divided
- 4 cloves garlic, fresh
- Sea salt & pepper to taste

DIRECTIONS

1. Preheat oven to 400° Fahrenheit and line a baking sheet with foil.
2. Remove the cores from your tomatoes and place them on the baking sheet along with the cloves of garlic.
3. Drizzle tomatoes and garlic with olive oil, salt, and pepper.
4. Roast at 400° Fahrenheit for 30 minutes.
5. Pull the tomatoes out of the oven and place into a blender, along with the juices that have dripped onto the pan during roasting.
6. Add two cups of the chicken broth to the blender.
7. Blend until smooth, then strain the mixture into a large saucepan or a pot.
8. While the pan is on the stove, whisk the remaining two cups of broth and the cream into the soup.
9. Simmer for about ten minutes.
10. Season to taste, then serve hot!

NUTRITIONAL FACTS: Calories: 225 Carbohydrates: 5.5 grams Fat: 20 grams Protein: 6.5 grams

CHAPTER 20.
BREAD

403. KETO BREAKFAST BREAD

PREPARATION: 15' **COOKING:** 40' **SERVES:** 16

INGREDIENTS

- ½ tsp. xanthan gum
- ½ tsp. salt
- 2 tbsp. coconut oil
- ½ cup butter, melted
- 1 tsp. baking powder
- 2 cups of almond flour
- 7 eggs

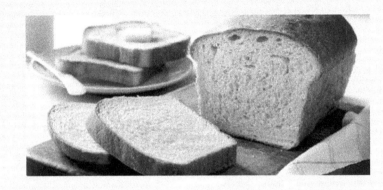

DIRECTIONS

1. Preheat the oven to 355F.
2. Beat eggs in a bowl on high for 2 minutes.
3. Add coconut oil and butter to the eggs and continue to beat.
4. Line a loaf pan with baking paper and pour the beaten eggs.
5. Pour in the rest of the ingredients and mix until it becomes thick.
6. Bake until a toothpick comes out dry, about 40 to 45 minutes.

NUTRITIONAL FACTS: Calories: 234 Fat: 23g Carb: 1g Protein: 7g

404. PUMPKIN BREAD

PREPARATION: 15' **COOKING:** 1H **SERVES:** 8

INGREDIENTS

- 3 tbsp. walnuts, chopped
- 3 tbsp. pumpkin seeds plus extra for topping
- 2 eggs
- ¼ cup no-sugar-added apple sauce
- 2 tbsp. coconut oil
- ¾ cup pumpkin puree
- ½ tbsp. butter
- 1 tbsp. pumpkin pie spice
- ½ tbsp. baking powder
- ½ tsp. salt
- 1 tbsp. psyllium husk powder
- ¼ cup flaxseed
- ½ cup almond flour
- ½ cup coconut flour

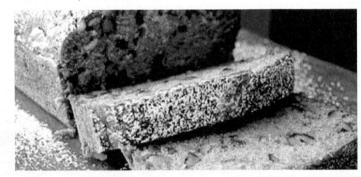

DIRECTIONS

1. Preheat the oven to 400F and grease a baking tray with butter.
2. Combine all the dry ingredients in a bowl except pumpkin seeds.
3. Whisk together apple sauce, eggs, pumpkin puree, and oil in another bowl.
4. Combine the dry mixture with the egg mixture.
5. Transfer the mixture to a baking tray and sprinkle with pumpkin seeds.
6. Place the tray on the lower rack of the oven and bake for 1 hour.
7. Cool, slice, and serve.

NUTRITIONAL FACTS: Calories: 194 Fat: 13.8g Carb: 4.6g Protein: 6.3g

405. GARLIC ALMOND BREAD

PREPARATION: 15' COOKING: 25' SERVES: 8

INGREDIENTS

- 1 cup almond flour
- 3 eggs
- 3 tbsp. butter
- ¼ cup sour cream
- 1 cup cheddar cheese, shredded
- ½ tbsp. baking powder
- ½ tbsp. garlic, minced
- ¼ tsp. salt
- 2 tbsp. parsley, chopped

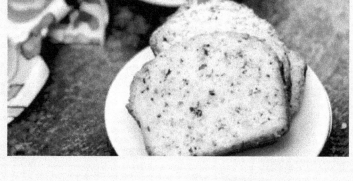

DIRECTIONS

1. Preheat the oven to 350F. Grease a round baking dish.
2. Combine butter, eggs, and sour cream in a bowl and whisk.
3. Combine cheddar cheese, almond flour, baking powder, minced garlic, and salt in another bowl and mix well.
4. Combine flour mixture with egg mixture and let the ingredients integrate.
5. Transfer the batter into the baking dish and sprinkle with parsley.
6. Place in the oven and bake for 25 minutes.
7. Cool, slice, and serve.

NUTRITIONAL FACTS: Calories: 220 Fat: 18.8g Carb: 4.3g Protein: 8.9g

406. KETO CLOUD BREAD

PREPARATION: 10' COOKING: 20' SERVES: 12

INGREDIENTS

- 3 tbsp. cream cheese
- 3 eggs
- ½ tsp. sea salt
- ¼ tsp. baking powder
- ¼ tsp. pepper

DIRECTIONS

1. Preheat oven to 350F.
2. Add egg yolks and cream cheese into a bowl and mix with a hand mixer.
3. In another bowl, add egg whites, pepper, salt and baking powder and mix for 5 minutes or until stiff peaks form.
4. Add the egg yolk mixture and egg white mixture together until mixed well.
5. Transfer mixture into a loaf pan and place into the prepared oven.
6. Bake for 15 to 18 minutes, or until lightly golden.

NUTRITIONAL FACTS: Calories: 28 Fat: 2g Carb: 0 g Protein: 2g

407. ALMOND CINNAMON BREAD

PREPARATION: 10' **COOKING:** 30' **SERVES:** 9

INGREDIENTS

- 2 cups almond flour
- 2 tbsp. coconut flour
- ½ tsp. sea salt
- 1 tsp. baking soda
- ¼ cup flax seed meal.
- 5 eggs plus 1 egg white, whisked
- 1 ½ tsp. juiced lime
- 2 tbsp. no-sugar-added maple syrup
- 3 tbsp. butter, divided and melted
- 1 tbsp. cinnamon plus extra for topping

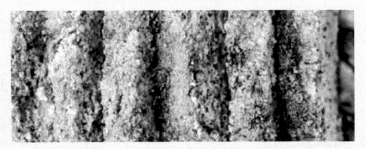

DIRECTIONS

1. Preheat the oven to 350F and line a loaf pan with parchment paper.
2. In a bowl, combine the almond flour, coconut flour, baking soda, salt, ½ tbsp. cinnamon, and flaxseed meal together.
3. In another bowl, add in the egg white and eggs and whisk together. Add in the maple syrup, butter, vinegar, and combine.
4. Pour the flour mixture into the egg mixture then mix to combine.
5. Transfer into the lined loaf pan.
6. Bake at 350F for 30 to 35 minutes. Remove.
7. Combine the remaining cinnamon and melted butter together then use it to rub the baked bread.
8. Cool, slice, and serve.

NUTRITIONAL FACTS: Calories: 221 Fat: 15.4g Carb: 10.7g Protein: 9.3g

408. FLUFFY PALEO BREAD

PREPARATION: 10' **COOKING:** 40' **SERVES:** 15

INGREDIENTS

- 1 ¼ cup almond flour
- 5 eggs
- 1 tsp. lemon juice
- 1/3 cup avocado oil
- 1 dash black pepper
- ½ tsp. sea salt
- 3 to 4 tbsp. tapioca flour
- 1 to 2 tsp. poppy seed
- ¼ cup ground flaxseed
- ½ tsp. baking soda

Top with
- Poppy seeds
- Pumpkin seeds

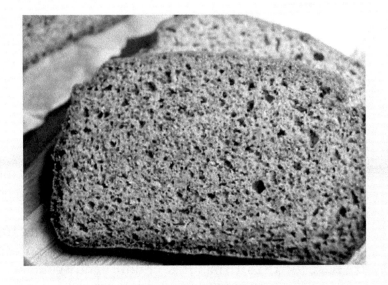

DIRECTIONS

1. Preheat the oven to 350F.
2. Line a baking pan with parchment paper and set aside.
3. In a bowl, add eggs, avocado oil, and lemon juice and whisk until combined.
4. In another bowl, add tapioca flour, almond flour, baking soda, flaxseed, black pepper and poppy seed. Mix.
5. Add the lemon juice mixture into the flour mixture and mix well.
6. Add the batter into the loaf pan. Top with extra pumpkin seeds and poppy seeds.
7. Cover loaf pan and transfer into the prepared oven.
8. Bake for 20 minutes. Remove cover and bake until an inserted knife comes out clean, after about 15 to 20 minutes.
9. Remove from oven and cool.
10. Slice and serve.

NUTRITIONAL FACTS: Calories: 149 Fat: 12.9g Carb: 4.4g Protein: 5g

409. TASTY PSYLLIUM HUSK BREAD

PREPARATION: 5'   **COOKING:** 55'   **SERVES:**

INGREDIENTS

- 6 tbsp. whole psyllium husks (finely ground)
- 1 cup coconut flour
- 8 egg whites
- ¾ tsp. sea salt
- ½ cup avocado oil
- 2 large eggs
- 1 ½ tsp. baking soda
- ¼ cup melted coconut oil
- ¾ cup warm water

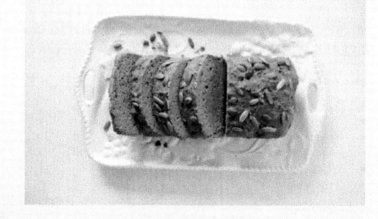

DIRECTIONS

1. Preheat the oven to 350F.
2. Prepare a baking pan with parchment paper.
3. Add every ingredient into a food processor and process until combined.
4. Add batter into the prepared baking pan and spread until even at the top.
5. Transfer baking pan into the preheated oven and bake for 45 to 55 minutes, or until an inserted toothpick comes out clean and bread edges are browned.
6. Remove bread from the oven and cool for 15 minutes.
7. Serve.

NUTRITIONAL FACTS: Calories: 127 Fat: 13.3g Carb: 6g Protein: 3g

410. LOW-CARB HOLIDAY BREAD

PREPARATION: 25' **COOKING:** 1H **SERVES:** 12

INGREDIENTS

- 1 cup almond flour
- ¼ cup coconut flour
- 3 tbsp. sesame seeds
- 3 tbsp. flaxseed
- 2 tbsp. psyllium husk powder
- ½ tbsp. baking powder
- ½ tsp. salt
- 3 eggs
- ½ cup sour cream
- ¼ cup cream cheese
- 1 tbsp. cloves, ground
- ½ tbsp. bitter orange peel, ground
- ½ tbsp. fennel seeds
- 1 tsp. anise seeds
- 1 tsp. cardamom, ground

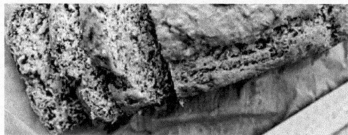

DIRECTIONS

1. Preheat the oven to 400F and lightly grease a loaf pan.
2. Mix all the dry ingredients together in a bowl.
3. Whisk together eggs, sour cream, and cream cheese in another bowl.
4. Combine the dry mixture with the egg mixture and stir well.
5. Transfer the mixture to the loaf pan and place in the oven.
6. Slice and serve.

NUTRITIONAL FACTS: Calories: 85 Fat: 6.6g Carb: 4g Protein: 2.9g

411. SANDWICH BREAD

PREPARATION: 10' **COOKING:** 45' **SERVES:** 8

INGREDIENTS

- ½ cup coconut flour, sifted
- ¼ cup almond flour, sifted
- 6 eggs, whites and yolks separated
- ½ cup coconut oil
- ¼ tsp. salt
- 3 tbsp. water
- 1 tbsp. apple cider vinegar
- ½ tsp. baking powder

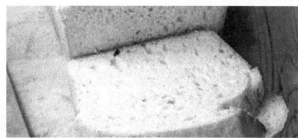

DIRECTIONS

1. Preheat the oven to 350F.
2. Grease an (8 ½ by 4-inch) loaf pan with oil.
3. Place a piece of parchment paper on the bottom of the pan.
4. Cream coconut oil in a food processor and add egg yolks at a time.
5. Pulse to combine coconut oil and yolks.
6. Add sifted coconut and almond flour, baking powder, apple cider vinegar, salt, and water to a food processor and pulse until combined.
7. Take a mixing bowl and beat egg whites.
8. Fold in coconut flour. Mix into egg whites and mix.
9. Pour the batter into prepared loaf pan and bake for 40 to 45 minutes. Cover it with aluminum foil about halfway through.
10. Let it cool and slice.
11. Enjoy.

NUTRITIONAL FACTS: Calories: 146 Fat: 11g Carb: 7g Protein: 5g

412. NO CORN CORNBREAD

PREPARATION: 10' COOKING: 20' SERVES: 8

INGREDIENTS
- ½ cup almond flour
- ¼ cup coconut flour
- ¼ tsp. salt
- ¼ tsp. baking soda
- 3 eggs
- ¼ cup unsalted butter
- 2 tbsp. low-carb sweetener
- ½ cup coconut milk

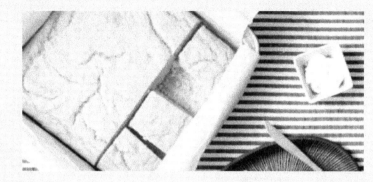

DIRECTIONS
1. Preheat the oven to 325F. Line a baking pan.
2. Mix all the dry ingredients in a bowl.
3. Add all the wet ingredients to the dry ones and blend well.
4. Pour the batter into the baking pan and bake for 20 minutes.
5. Cool, slice, and serve.

NUTRITIONAL FACTS: Calories: 65 Fat: 6g Carb: 2g Protein: 2g

413. DOUBLE CHOCOLATE ZUCCHINI BREAD

PREPARATION: 10' COOKING: 55' SERVES: 12

INGREDIENTS
- ½ cup coconut flour
- ½ cup chocolate chips (sugar free)
- 2 cups zucchini (shredded)
- 1 tsp. vanilla
- 4 large eggs
- ¼ cup coconut oil, melted
- ¼ tsp. salt
- 1 tsp. baking powder
- 1 tsp. baking soda
- ½ tsp. ground cinnamon
- ½ cup low carb sweetener
- ½ cup cocoa powder (unsweetened)

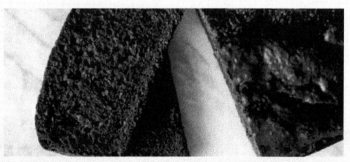

DIRECTIONS
1. In a bowl, combine coconut flour, salt, baking powder, cinnamon, sweetener, baking soda, and cocoa.
2. Blend in the vanilla, coconut oil, and eggs. Mix well.
3. Fold in the chocolate chips and zucchini.
4. Line a loaf pan (9 x 5) with parchment paper and pour the mixture in it.
5. Bake at 350F for 45 to 55 minutes.
6. Remove from the oven and cool.
7. Serve.

NUTRITIONAL FACTS: Calories: 124 Fat: 10g Carb: 7g Protein: 4g

414. KETO BLUEBERRY BREAD

PREPARATION: 15' **COOKING:** 1H 10' **SERVES:** 12

INGREDIENTS

- 10 tbsp. coconut flour
- 1 ½ tsp. baking powder
- ½ tsp. salt
- 2 tbsp. heavy whipping cream
- 1 ½ tsp. vanilla
- 2/3 cup Monkfruit classic
- 2 tbsp. sour cream
- ½ tsp. cinnamon
- ¾ cup fresh blueberries
- 9 tbsp. melted butter
- 6 eggs

For the icing
- ¼ tsp. lemon zest
- 1 tbsp. heavy whipping cream
- dash of vanilla
- 1 tsp. butter (melted)
- 2 tbsp. Monkfruit powdered

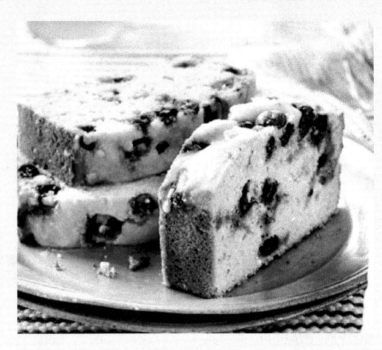

DIRECTIONS

1. Line a regular loaf pan with parchment paper and preheat oven to 350F.
2. Melt butter.
3. Beat eggs, cinnamon, baking powder, salt, vanilla, whipping cream, sour cream, and Monkfruit until combined.
4. Add melted butter and mix well.
5. Add coconut flour and mix well.
6. Add a small amount of batter in the loaf pan and sprinkle with a couple of blueberries. Then spread more batter and sprinkle blueberries on top. Repeat to finish the batter and blueberries.
7. Bake for 65 to 75 minutes. Cool.
8. For the icing, combine all ingredients and whisk.
9. Drizzle over warm bread and serve.

NUTRITIONAL FACTS: Calories: 155 Fat: 13g Carb: 4g Protein: 3g

CHAPTER 21.
PANCAKE AND MUFFINS

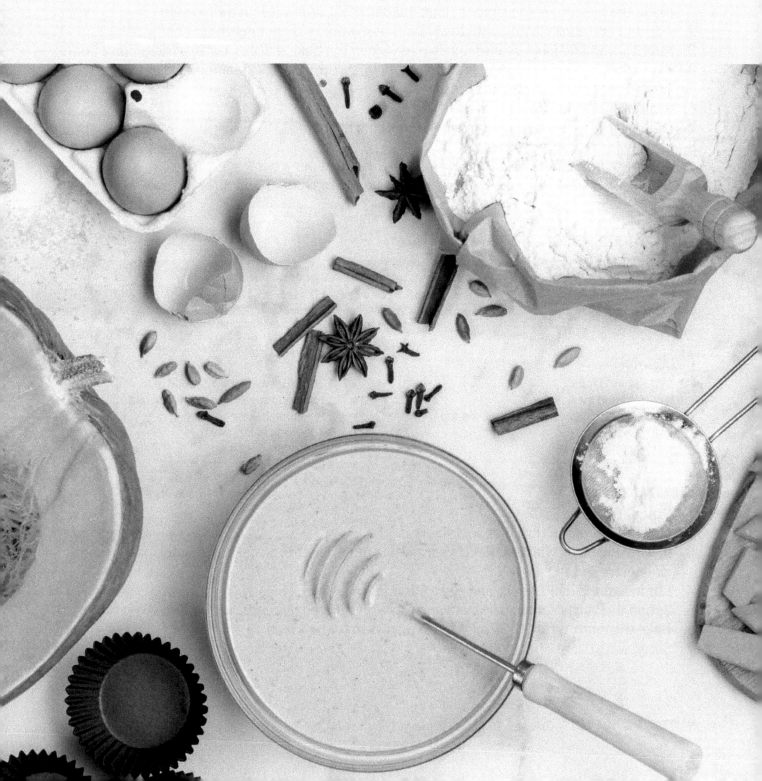

415. ALMOND FRENCH TOAST

PREPARATION: 10' **COOKING:** 20' **SERVES:** 6

INGREDIENTS

- 2 ¼ cups water
- 1 ½ cups almond flour
- ½ cup almond meal
- 1 pinch salt
- 2 large eggs
- 2/3 cup unsweetened coconut milk
- 1 tablespoon sugar-free syrup
- ½ teaspoon sugar-free vanilla extract
- ½ teaspoon cinnamon
- 1 pinch nutmeg

DIRECTIONS

1. Make the base; combine almond flour, almond meal, and water in a saucepot.
2. Add salt and cook stirring until the water has evaporated completely.
3. Pour the almond mixture into 8-inch paper lined the baking dish. Cool in a fridge for 2 hours.
4. Make the custard; combine eggs, coconut milk, syrup, vanilla, cinnamon, and nutmeg.
5. Cut the almond mixture into slices.
6. Dip the slices into the egg mixture.
7. Heat a large non-stick skillet over medium-high heat.
8. Spray with cooking spray.
9. Add the almond bread slice and cook for 2-3 minutes per side.
10. Arrange the slices onto the baking sheet. Bake the toast for 10 minutes.
11. Serve warm.

NUTRITIONAL FACTS: Calories: 9 Fats: 4 Protein: 2

416. HEALTHY MUFFINS

PREPARATION: 10' **COOKING:** 25' **SERVES:** 8

INGREDIENTS

- 1 cup almond flour
- ½ cup almond meal
- 1 tablespoon slivered almonds, for the top
- 2 large eggs
- ¼ cup powdered Erythritol
- Few drops Stevia
- 1/3 cup unsweetened almond milk
- 1 teaspoon sugar-free vanilla extract
- 1 teaspoon baking powder
- ¼ teaspoon baking soda
- ½ teaspoon cinnamon
- 1 pinch salt

DIRECTIONS

1. Preheat oven to 350F.
2. Line 8-hole muffin tin with paper liners.
3. In a mixing bowl, whisk almond flour, almond meal, Erythritol, baking powder, baking soda, cinnamon, and salt.
4. Stir in almond milk, Stevia, and eggs. Stir until smooth.
5. Spoon the batter into paper liners and top with slivered almonds.
6. Bake the muffins for 20-25 minutes or until firm to the touch.
7. Serve warm.

NUTRITIONAL FACTS: Calories: 12 Fats: 6 Protein: 1

417. BISCUITS AND GRAVY

PREPARATION: 10' COOKING: 20' SERVES: 6

INGREDIENTS

- 4 tablespoons melted butter
- 5 medium eggs
- ½ cup coconut flour
- Salt, to taste
- 1 cup grated sharp cheddar
- ¼ teaspoon baking powder

Gravy:
- 1lb. ground pork sausage
- 1 cup chicken stock
- 1 cup heavy cream
- Salt and white pepper, to taste

DIRECTIONS

1. Preheat oven to 400F. Line baking sheet with parchment paper.
2. Combine biscuit ingredients in a bowl, until the dough comes together.
3. Scoop the dough using a scoop onto the baking sheet.
4. Bake the biscuits for 15 minutes.
5. In the meantime, make the gravy; cook the pork sausage in a skillet over medium-high heat until browned. Drain any excess fat.
6. Pour in chicken stock and heavy cream. Simmer until gently thickened.
7. Season to taste with salt and pepper. You can add some thyme, it really improves the flavor.
8. Cut biscuits in half and serve with a generous amount of the gravy.

NUTRITIONAL FACTS: Calories: 12 Fats: 4 Protein: 1

418. BLUEBERRY MUFFINS

PREPARATION: 5' COOKING: 1' SERVES: 2

INGREDIENTS

- 2 tablespoons unsalted butter
- 2 tablespoons softened cream cheese
- 2 small eggs
- 2 tablespoons coconut flour
- 1 teaspoon cinnamon
- 1 teaspoon baking powder
- 15 drops Stevia
- ½ teaspoon sugar-free vanilla
- 1 pinch salt
- 3 tablespoons fresh blueberries
- 2 tablespoons chopped almonds
- 1 tablespoon almond butter, for topping

DIRECTIONS

1. Spray two 6oz. ramekins with cooking spray.
2. Melt butter and cream cheese in a microwave-safe bowl.
3. Whisk in egg with a fork.
4. Add the remaining ingredients and whisk vigorously to prevent from cooking.
5. Spoon the batter into the ramekins.
6. Microwave on high for 60 seconds.
7. Remove the ramekins from the microwave and top with some almond butter.
8. Serve.

NUTRITIONAL FACTS: Calories: 08 Fats: 6 Protein: 1

419. BUTTERMILK PANCAKES

PREPARATION: 10' **COOKING:** 15' **SERVES:** 4

INGREDIENTS

- 2 tablespoons sifted coconut flour
- 3 tablespoons blanched almond flour
- 2 small eggs, room temperature
- ¼ cup unsweetened almond milk
- ½ teaspoon sugar-free vanilla extract
- 1 tablespoon Erythritol
- ½ tablespoon coconut oil
- 1 pinch salt

DIRECTIONS

1. In a large mixing bowl, combine flours, baking powder, sweetener, and salt.
2. In a separate bowl, beat eggs, almond milk, and vanilla.
3. Fold the liquid ingredients into the dry ones.
4. Heat coconut oil in a skillet.
5. Add a ¼ cup of the batter into the heated skillet.
6. Cook for 2 minutes per side.
7. Serve warm.

NUTRITIONAL FACTS: Calories: 10 Fats: 6 Protein: 1

420. CARROT APPLE MUFFINS

PREPARATION: 10' **COOKING:** 30' **SERVES:** 6

INGREDIENTS

- 1 tablespoon coconut oil
- ½ small banana, mashed
- ½ cup grated apple
- 1 small carrot, grated
- 2oz. applesauce
- ¼ cup unsweetened almond milk
- ¾ cup almond flour
- ¼ cup almond meal
- ½ teaspoon allspice
- ¾ teaspoon baking soda
- 1 pinch salt
- 2 tablespoons chopped pecans

DIRECTIONS

1. Preheat oven to 350F.
2. Line 6-hole regular muffin tin with paper liners.
3. Combine coconut oil, banana, apple, applesauce, carrots, egg and milk.
4. Fold in the dry ingredients.
5. Finally, fold in the chopped walnuts.
6. Spoon the mixture into the paper liners and bake for 25-30 minutes.
7. Cool the muffins onto the wire rack for 5 minutes before serving.

NUTRITIONAL FACTS: Calories: 10 Fats: 6 Protein: 1

421. BERRY MUFFINS WITH TOPPING

PREPARATION: 15' **COOKING:** 25' **SERVES:** 6

INGREDIENTS

- ½ cup unsalted butter
- ¼ cup granulated Erythritol
- 2 medium eggs, room temperature
- 2 teaspoons sugar-free vanilla extract
- 1 cup blanched almond flour
- 2 tablespoons sifted coconut flour
- 1 teaspoon baking powder
- 1 pinch salt
- ½ cup fresh mixed berries

Topping:
- 2 tablespoon unsalted butter
- ½ cup blanched almond flour
- 2 tablespoons granulated Erythritol
- 1 tablespoon coconut flour

Icing:
- 2oz. mascarpone cheese
- 1 tablespoon lemon juice
- 2 tablespoons granulated Erythritol
- 10 drops Stevia

DIRECTIONS

1. Preheat oven to 375F. Line 6-hole muffin tin with paper liners.
2. Make the muffins; cream butter and Erythritol in a bowl.
3. Beat in eggs and vanilla. Fold in almond flour, coconut flour, baking powder, and salt. Stir until smooth. Fold in the berries.
4. Spoon the batter into the prepared muffin tin. Place the muffins aside and prepare the topping.
5. Make the topping; place butter in a bowl. Add almond flour, granulated Erythritol, and coconut flour. Rub with clean fingers until a coarse mixture is formed. Sprinkle the muffins with prepared topping.
6. Bake the muffins 20-25 minutes.
7. Make the icing; beat the icing ingredients with an electric whisk until smooth.
8. Remove the muffins from the oven. Allow them to cool before drizzling with prepared icing.
9. Serve.

NUTRITIONAL FACTS: Calories: 10 Fats: 6 Protein: 1

422. CREAMY MONKEY BREAD

PREPARATION: 20' **COOKING:** 1H 10' **SERVES:** 14

INGREDIENTS

- 2 cups almond flour
- ½ cup coconut flour
- ¾ cup psyllium husk
- 4 teaspoons baking powder
- Salt, to taste
- 1 cup granulated Erythritol
- 12 egg whites
- 5 tablespoons cider vinegar
- 2 cups boiling water

Filling:
- 8oz. cream cheese

For topping:
- ½ cup butter
- 1 tablespoon Ceylon cinnamon
- ½ cup powdered Erythritol

DIRECTIONS

1. Preheat oven to 375F.
2. In a large mixing bowl, combine almond flour, coconut flour, psyllium husk, baking powder, salt, and Erythritol.
3. Stir in egg whites and vinegar.
4. Pour in boiling water and mix until combined.
5. Shape the dough into 20 equal balls.
6. Flatten the balls gently and place the cream cheese in the center of each ball. Gently close the cream cheese in a ball of dough, from three sides, leaving the fourth side, open.
7. Place the 10 balls into the greased Bundt pan, open part up. Top with remaining balls, open part down.
8. Place in the oven and bake for 50 minutes.
9. Make the topping; combine the topping ingredients in a bowl. Stir until smooth.
10. Spread the topping over the bread and continue to bake for 15 minutes.
11. Cool the bread on a rack before serving.

NUTRITIONAL FACTS: Calories: 11 Fats: 4 Protein: 1

423. DELICIOUS ROLLS

PREPARATION: 10' **COOKING:** 20' **SERVES:** 6

INGREDIENTS

- 2oz. almond flour
- 2oz. softened cream cheese
- 2 medium eggs, separated
- ½ teaspoon baking powder
- 2 tablespoons olive oil
- ¼ teaspoon cream of tartar
- 1 pinch salt

DIRECTIONS

1. Place cream cheese in a microwave-safe bowl.
2. Microwave the cheese on high for 30 seconds.
3. Whisk in olive oil until smooth.
4. Fold in almond flour, salt, and baking powder.
5. Whisk in egg yolks.
6. Beat egg whites with some salt and cream of tartar until stiff peaks form.
7. Fold the egg whites into the egg yolk mixture, adding gradually.
8. Preheat oven to 375F.
9. Grease a 6-hole muffin tin with some coconut oil.
10. Spoon the batter into the muffin tin. Bake the rolls for 15 minutes.
11. Place on a wire rack to cool before removing from the tin and serving.

NUTRITIONAL FACTS: Calories: 10 Fats: 4 Protein: 1

424. CRAB CAKES WITH VEGGIES

PREPARATION: 10' **COOKING:** 25' **SERVES:** 12

INGREDIENTS

- 1 tablespoon ghee
- ½ cup chopped celery
- ¼ cup chopped green and red bell pepper
- ½ onion, diced
- 1 clove garlic, minced
- 1 small egg
- Salt and pepper, to taste
- 1 tablespoon mayonnaise
- ½ teaspoon chili powder
- ½ teaspoon mustard powder
- 0.5lb. crab meat
- ¼ cup crushed pork rinds
- ¼ cup grated cheddar cheese
- 1 tablespoon avocado oil

DIRECTIONS

1. Heat ghee in a skillet over medium-high heat.
2. Add vegetables and cook stirring for 7-8 minutes. Remove and place aside.
3. In a mixing bowl, combine all the remaining ingredients. Add the cooked vegetables and stir to combine. Let the mixture rest in a fridge for 1 hour.
4. Heat avocado oil in a skillet. Fry the crab cakes until golden.
5. Serve warm.

NUTRITIONAL FACTS: Calories: 10 Fats: 4 Protein: 1

CHAPTER 22.
BASIC CHAFFLES

425. TRADITIONAL CHAFFLE

PREPARATION: 5'   COOKING: 4'   SERVES: 2 MINI WAFFLES

INGREDIENTS

- 1 large egg
- 1/2 cup finely shredded mozzarella

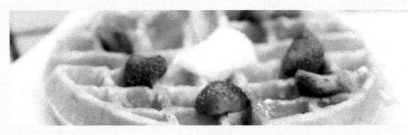

DIRECTIONS

1. Switch on the mini waffle maker according to manufacturer's instructions
2. Spray the waffle iron with non-stick spray
3. Crack egg and combine with cheddar cheese in a small bowl
4. Place half batter on waffle maker and spread evenly.
5. Cook for 4 minutes or until as desired
6. Gently remove from waffle maker and set aside for 2 minutes so it cools down and become crispy
7. Repeat with remaining batter.
8. Serve warm with desired toppings (optional) - butter, strawberries and sugar-free syrup

NUTRITIONAL FACTS: Calories: 363 Protein: 2 Fat: 40 Carbohydrates: 1

426. KETO PLAIN PREPPED CHAFFLES

PREPARATION: 3'   COOKING: 6'   SERVES: 1

INGREDIENTS

- 2 small eggs
- 1/2 cup shredded cheddar cheese

DIRECTIONS

1. Preheat mini waffle maker until hot
2. Whisk egg in a bowl, add cheese, then mix well
3. Stir in the remaining ingredients (except toppings, if any).
4. Grease waffle maker and Scoop 1/2 of the batter onto the waffle maker, spread across evenly
5. Cook until a bit browned and crispy, about 4 minutes.
6. Gently remove from waffle maker and let it cool
7. Repeat with remaining batter.
8. Store in the fridge for 3-5 days.

NUTRITIONAL FACTS: Calories: 363 Protein: 2 Fat: 40 Carbohydrates: 1

427. JALAPENO BACON SWISS CHAFFLE

PREPARATION: 18' **COOKING:** 12' **SERVES:** 2

INGREDIENTS
- Shredded Swiss cheese: ½ cup
- Fresh jalapenos (diced): 1 tablespoon
- Bacon piece: 2 tablespoon
- Egg: 1

DIRECTIONS
1. First, preheat and grease the waffle maker. Using a pan, cook the bacon pieces, put off the heat and shred the cheese and egg. Add in the diced fresh jalapenos and mix evenly. Heat the waffle makers to get the mixture into a crispy form. Repeat the process for the remaining mixture. Serve the dish to enjoy.

NUTRITIONAL FACTS: Calories: 363 Protein: 2 Fat: 40 Carbohydrates: 1

428. CRISPY ZUCCHINI CHAFFLES

PREPARATION: 18' **COOKING:** 12' **SERVES:** 2

INGREDIENTS
- Zucchini: 1 (small – finely grated)
- Egg: 1
- Shredded mozzarella: half cup
- Parmesan: 1 tablespoon
- Pepper: As per your taste
- Basil: 1 teaspoon

DIRECTIONS
1. Preheat and grease the waffle maker. Prepare a mix of all the ingredients in a mixing bowl. Pour the mixture into a large-sized waffle maker and spread evenly. Heat the mixtures to a crunchy form. Repeat the process for the remaining mixture. Serve hot and enjoy the crispy taste.

NUTRITIONAL FACTS: Calories: 363 Protein: 2 Fat: 40 Carbohydrates: 1

429. OKONOMIYAKI CHAFFLE

PREPARATION: 22' **COOKING:** 11' **SERVES:** 2

INGREDIENTS

Okonomiyaki Chaffle
- Mozzarella Cheese: ½ cup
- Baking powder: ½ teaspoon
- Egg: 2
- Cabbage: ¼ cup (shredded)

Sauce
- Soy Sauce: 4 teaspoons
- Swerve/Monk fruit: 2 tablespoons
- Ketchup: 4 tablespoons (sugar-free)
- Worcestershire Sauce: 4 teaspoons

Toppings
- Kewpie Mayo: 2 tablespoons
- Beni Shoga: 2 tablespoons
- Green Onion: 1 stalk
- Bonito Flakes: 4 tablespoons
- Dried Seaweed Powder: 2 tablespoons

DIRECTIONS

1. Prepare a mix of chopped onions and finely cut cabbage and set aside. Using a mixing bowl, prepare another mix for the sauce containing all ingredients for the sauce and also set aside. Quickly, preheat a mini-sized waffle and grease it. In another mixing bowl, prepare a mix of shredded mozzarella cheese with cabbage, beaten eggs and baking powder. Combine the mixture and pour into the lower side of the waffle maker. With the lid closed, cook for 5 minutes to a crunch. Once timed out, take out waffles and serve in a plate. Repeat process for the remaining waffle mixture. Garnish the chaffles with beni shoga, bonito flakes, chopped onions and dried seaweed powder. Pour the prepared sauce with Kewpie mayo. Serve and enjoy.

NUTRITIONAL FACTS: Calories: 363 Protein: 2 Fat: 40 Carbohydrates: 1

430. JALAPENO CHEDDAR CHAFFLE

PREPARATION: 12' **COOKING:** 5' **SERVES:** 2

INGREDIENTS

- Egg: 2
- Deli Jalapeno: 16 slices
- Cheddar cheese: 1½ cup

DIRECTIONS

1. Preheat and grease a waffle maker. Prepare a mixture containing ½ half cheddar with beaten eggs, then mix evenly. Sprinkle some shredded cheese at the base of the waffle maker, then pour the batter on the cheese and top again with more cheese with 4 slices of Jalapeno. With the lid closed, cook for 5 minutes to a crunch. Repeat the process for the remaining mixture. Serve and enjoy.

NUTRITIONAL FACTS: Calories: 363 Protein: 2 Fat: 40 Carbohydrates: 1

KETO WOMEN over 50 276

431. KETO MINTY BASE CHAFFLE

PREPARATION: 30' COOKING: 4' SERVES: 1

INGREDIENTS

- 1 egg
- 1/2 cup cheddar cheese, shredded
- 1 tbsp. mint extract (low carb)

DIRECTIONS

1. Using a mini waffle maker, preheat according to maker's instructions.
2. Combine egg and cheddar cheese in a mixing bowl. Stir thoroughly
3. Add mint extract and place half batter on waffle maker; spread evenly.
4. Cook for 4 minutes or until as desired
5. Gently remove from waffle maker and set aside for 2 minutes so it cools down and become crispy
6. Repeat for remaining batter
7. Garnish with desired toppings

NUTRITIONAL FACTS: 170 calories 2g net carbs 14g fat 10g protein

432. FLUFFY SANDWICH BREAKFAST CHAFFLE

PREPARATION: 5' COOKING: 3' SERVES: 2

INGREDIENTS

- 1/2 tsp Psyllium husk powder (optional)
- 2 tbsp. almond flour
- 1/4 tsp Baking powder (optional)
- 1 large Egg
- 1/2 cup Mozzarella cheese, shredded
- 1 tbsp. vanilla or
- Dash of cinnamon

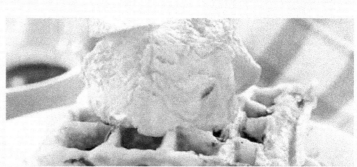

DIRECTIONS

1. Switch on the waffle maker according to manufacturer's instructions
2. Crack egg and combine with cheddar cheese in a small bowl
3. Add remaining ingredients and combine thoroughly.
4. Place half batter on waffle maker and spread evenly.
5. Cook for 4 minutes or until as desired
6. Gently remove from waffle maker and set aside for 2 minutes so it cools down and become crispy
7. Repeat for remaining batter
8. Serve with keto ice cream topping

NUTRITIONAL FACTS: Calories: 363 Protein: 2 Fat: 40 Carbohydrates: 1

433. BACON CHEDDAR CHAFFLE

PREPARATION: 12' COOKING: 6' SERVES: 2

INGREDIENTS

- Egg: 1
- Bacon bite: As per your taste
- Cheddar cheese: 1½ cup

DIRECTIONS

1. First, preheat and grease the waffle maker. Prepare a mix of all ingredients in a bowl, then pour into a waffle maker and heat for 4 minutes in a waffle maker until it turns crispy. Repeat the process for the remaining mixture. Serve the dish to enjoy.

NUTRITIONAL FACTS: Calories: 363 Protein: 2 Fat: 40 Carbohydrates: 1

434. VANILLA KETO CHAFFLE

PREPARATION: 3' COOKING: 4' SERVES: 1

INGREDIENTS

- 1 egg
- 1/2 cup cheddar cheese, shredded
- 1/2 tsp vanilla extract

DIRECTIONS

1. Switch on the waffle maker according to manufacturer's instructions
2. Crack egg and combine with cheddar cheese in a small bowl
3. Add vanilla extract and combine thoroughly.
4. Place half batter on waffle maker and spread evenly.
5. Cook for 4 minutes or until as desired
6. Gently remove from waffle maker and set aside for 2 minutes so it cools down and become crispy
7. Repeat for remaining batter

NUTRITIONAL FACTS: Calories: 163 Protein: 2 Fat: 40 Carbohydrates: 1

435. FLAKY DELIGHT CHAFFLE

PREPARATION: 3' **COOKING:** 4' **SERVES:** 1

INGREDIENTS
- 1 egg
- 1/2 cup cheddar cheese, shredded
- 1/2 cup coconut flakes

DIRECTIONS
1. Switch on the waffle maker according to manufacturer's instructions
2. Crack egg and combine with cheddar cheese in a small bowl
3. Place half batter on waffle maker and spread evenly.
4. Sprinkle coconut flakes and Cook for 4 minutes or until as desired
5. Gently remove from waffle maker and set aside for 2 minutes so it cools down and become crispy
6. Repeat for remaining batter
7. Serve with desired toppings

NUTRITIONAL FACTS: 291 calories 1g net carbs 23g fat 20g protein

436. BASIC KETO CHAFFLE

PREPARATION: 3' **COOKING:** 4' **SERVES:** 1

INGREDIENTS
- 1 egg
- 1/2 cup cheddar cheese, shredded
- 1/2 tbsp. Psyllium husk powder
- 1/2 tbsp. chia seeds

DIRECTIONS
1. Switch on the waffle maker according to manufacturer's instructions
2. Crack egg and combine with cheddar cheese in a small bowl
3. Place half batter on waffle maker and spread evenly.
4. Sprinkle Chia on top, cover and cook for 4 minutes or until as desired
5. Gently remove from waffle maker and set aside for 2 minutes so it cools down and become crispy
6. Repeat for remaining batter
7. Serve with desired toppings

NUTRITIONAL FACTS: Calories: 363 Protein: 2 Fat: 40 Carbohydrates: 1

437. FLUFFY KETO CHAFFLE

PREPARATION: 3'   COOKING: 4'   SERVES: 1

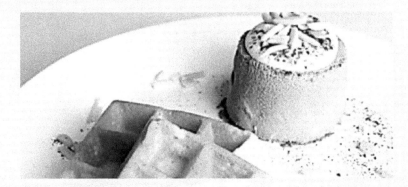

INGREDIENTS
- 1 egg
- 1/2 cup cheddar cheese, shredded

DIRECTIONS
1. Switch on the waffle maker according to manufacturer's instructions
2. Crack egg and combine with cheddar cheese in a small bowl
3. Place half batter on waffle maker and spread evenly.
4. Cook for 4 minutes or until as desired
5. Gently remove from waffle maker and set aside for 2 minutes so it cools down and become crispy
6. Repeat for remaining batter
7. Serve with desired toppings

NUTRITIONAL FACTS: Calories: 363 Protein: 2 Fat: 40 Carbohydrates: 1

438. CRISPY SANDWICH CHAFFLE

PREPARATION: 3'   COOKING: 4'   SERVES: 1

INGREDIENTS
- 1 egg
- 1/2 cup cheddar cheese, shredded
- 1 tbsp. coconut flour

DIRECTIONS
1. Using a mini waffle maker, preheat according to maker's instructions.
2. Combine egg and cheddar cheese in a mixing bowl. Stir thoroughly
3. Add coconut flour for added texture if so desired
4. Place half batter on waffle maker and spread evenly.
5. Cook for 4 minutes or until as desired
6. Gently remove from waffle maker and set aside for 2 minutes so it cools down and become crispy
7. Repeat for remaining batter
8. Stuff 2 chaffles with desired sandwich

NUTRITIONAL FACTS: Calories: 363 Protein: 2 Fat: 40 Carbohydrates: 1

439. KETO SANDWICH CHAFFLE

PREPARATION: 3'   COOKING: 4'   SERVES: 1

INGREDIENTS
- 1 egg
- 1/2 cup cheddar cheese, shredded
- 1 tbsp. almond flour (optional)

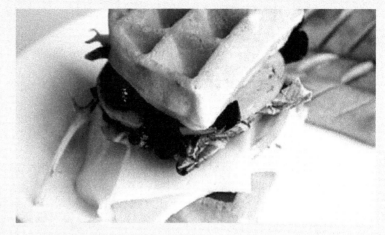

DIRECTIONS
1. Using a mini waffle maker, preheat according to maker's instructions.
2. Combine egg and cheddar cheese in a mixing bowl. Stir thoroughly
3. Add Almond flour for added texture if so desired
4. Place half batter on waffle maker and spread evenly.
5. Cook for 4 minutes or until as desired
6. Gently remove from waffle maker and set aside for 2 minutes so it cools down and become crispy
7. Repeat for remaining batter
8. Stuff 2 chaffles with garnishing to make a sandwich

NUTRITIONAL FACTS: Calories: 363 Protein: 2 Fat: 40 Carbohydrates: 1

440. SIMPLE AND CRISPY CHAFFLE

PREPARATION: 12'   COOKING: 6'   SERVES: 2

INGREDIENTS
- Cheddar cheese: 1/3 cup
- Baking powder: 1/4 teaspoon
- Parmesan cheese (shredded): 1/3 cup
- Egg: 1
- Flaxseed: 1 teaspoon (ground)

DIRECTIONS
1. Prepare a mix containing egg, baking powder, flaxseed, and cheddar seed in a mixing bowl. Preheat and grease the waffle maker. Sprinkle the shredded cheddar cheese at the base of the waffle maker and pour the mixture into the waffle maker, then add some more shredded cheese at the top of the mixture. Heat the mixture to cook to a crispy form. Repeat the process for the remaining mixture. Serve the dish to enjoy.

NUTRITIONAL FACTS: Calories: 363 Protein: 2 Fat: 40 Carbohydrates: 1

441. RICH AND CREAMY MINI CHAFFLE

PREPARATION: 12' **COOKING:** 6' **SERVES:** 2

INGREDIENTS
- Baking powder: ¾ tablespoon
- Eggs: 2
- Cream cheese: 2 tablespoons
- Almond flour: 2 tablespoons
- Water: 2 tablespoon (optional)
- Shredded mozzarella: 1 cup

DIRECTIONS
1. Preheat and grease the waffle maker. Prepare a mix of all the ingredients in a mixing bowl. Pour the mixture into a large-sized waffle maker and spread evenly. Heat the mixtures to a crunchy form for 5 minutes. Repeat the process for the remaining mixture. Serve hot and enjoy the crispy taste.

NUTRITIONAL FACTS: Calories: 363 Protein: 2 Fat: 40 Carbohydrates: 1

CHAPTER 23.
SMOOTHIE AND DRINKS RECIPES

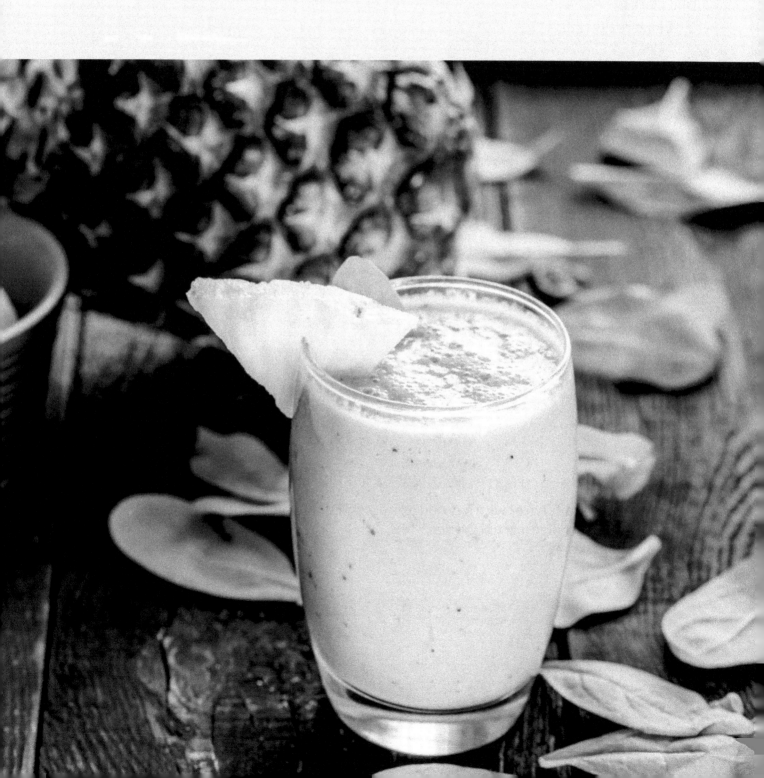

442. KETO TRADITIONAL COFFEE RECIPE

PREPARATION: 2'   **COOKING:** 0'   **SERVES:** 1

INGREDIENTS
- 1 cup black coffee
- 1/2 tsp MCT oil
- 1 Tsp ghee

DIRECTIONS
1. Blend really well.

NUTRITIONAL FACTS: Calories: 143 Fat 17g Carbs 2g Sugar 0.4g Protein 4g

443. VANILLA LATTE MARTINI

PREPARATION: 5'   **COOKING:** 0'   **SERVES:** 2

INGREDIENTS
- 3 ounces vanilla vodka
- 2 ounces homemade coffee liqueur
- 1 tbsp. cream

DIRECTIONS
1. Fill a mixed drink shaker with ice. Add espresso alcohol, vanilla vodka and cream. Shake well and pour into two chilled martini glasses.

NUTRITIONAL FACTS: Calories: 454 Fat 31g Carbs 26g Sugars 4.4g Protein 22g

444. KETO BOOSTED COFFEE RECIPE

PREPARATION: 2' COOKING: 0' SERVES: 16 OUNCES

INGREDIENTS
- 2 cups freshly brewed hot coffee
- 2 tablespoons grass-fed butter
- 1 scoop Perfect Keto Powder
- 1 teaspoon Ceylon cinnamon

DIRECTIONS
1. Add the entirety of the Ingredients: in a blender.
2. Utilizing a submersion blender or frothier, mix on low bringing the accelerate to high for 30 seconds or until foamy.
3. Serve, taste, and serve and enjoy.

NUTRITIONAL FACTS: Calories: 280 Fat 31g Carbs 2.8g Sugar 2.2g Protein: 1g

445. KETO COCONUT COFFEE RECIPE

PREPARATION: 2' COOKING: 0' SERVES: 1

INGREDIENTS
- 1 cup of black coffee
- 1/2 Tsp coconut oil
- 1 Tsp ghee

DIRECTIONS
1. Blend really well.

NUTRITIONAL FACTS: Calories: 179 Fat 21g Carbs 3g Sugar 1.1g Protein 5g

446. KETO FROTHY COFFEE RECIPE

PREPARATION: 2'   COOKING: 0'   SERVES: 1

INGREDIENTS
- 1 cup of black coffee
- 1/2 Tsp coconut oil
- 1 Tsp ghee
- 2 Tsp unsweetened coconut

DIRECTIONS
1. Blend really well.

NUTRITIONAL FACTS: Calories: 190 Fat 22g Carbs 2g Sugar 0.3g Protein 9g

447. KETO COLLAGEN BOOSTED COFFEE

PREPARATION: 2'   COOKING: 0'   SERVES: 1

INGREDIENTS
- 1 cup of black coffee
- 1 Tsp ghee
- 1/2 scoop unflavored hydrolyzed collagen powder

DIRECTIONS
1. Blend really well.

NUTRITIONAL FACTS: Calories 160 Fat 14g Carbs 2g Sugar 3g Protein 5g

448. KETO ICED LEMON COFFEE RECIPE

PREPARATION: 5' **COOKING:** 0' **SERVES:** 1

INGREDIENTS

- 1 cup cold brew coffee
- 1/4 cup ice cubes
- 1/4 cup freshly squeezed lemon juice
- Stevie to taste
- 1 slice of lemon for garnish

DIRECTIONS

1. Add everything into a glass and mix. Toss in a cut of lemon for decoration.

NUTRITIONAL FACTS: Calories: 16 Fat 3g Carbs 4g Sugar 4g Protein 5g

449. LOW CARB BLUEBERRY MOJITOS

PREPARATION: 10' **COOKING:** 0' **SERVES:** 4

INGREDIENTS

- 3/4 cup fresh blueberries
- 3 to 4 tbsp. powdered Swerve Sweetener
- 1/4 cup packed mint leaves
- 1 cup white rum
- 1/3 cup fresh lime juice
- 1/2-liter club soda

DIRECTIONS

1. In a blender, add blueberries and powdered sugar. Mix to a thick puree. Move to a pitcher.
2. Tear mint leaves by way of hand and upload to a tumbler that holds, in any occasion, one liter.
3. Pound with a muddle or the end of a wooden spoon to discharge the oils
4. Add blueberry puree, white rum, lime juice, and dad and blend to join.
5. Fill four highball or basin glasses with squashed ice. Empty mojitos into glasses, embellish with blueberries and mint leaves and serve.

NUTRITIONAL FACTS: Calories 153 Fat 0.1g Carbs 6g Sugar 1g Protein 0.4g

450. APPLE MARTINI

PREPARATION: 5' **COOKING:** 0' **SERVES:** 2

INGREDIENTS
- Apple slice
- 1 teaspoon of low carb sugar syrup
- 2 ounces plain vodka
- 2 ounces of apple-flavored vodka

DIRECTIONS
1. Finely dice the apple cut and put in a mixed drink shaker. Add the sugar syrup and crush them together.
2. Add the two kinds of vodka and ice. Shake well. Strain into a martini glass. The aggregate of 2 grams of carb

NUTRITIONAL FACTS: Calories 300, Fat 19g, Carbs 6g, Sugar 1g, Protein 25g

451. BLUEBERRY MARTINI

PREPARATION: 5' **COOKING:** 0' **SERVES:** 3

INGREDIENTS
- 6-7 good-sized fresh blueberries
- 1 teaspoon of low carb sugar syrup
- 2 ounces plain vodka
- 2 ounces blueberry flavored vodka
-

DIRECTIONS
1. Put the blueberries in a mixed drink shaker. Add the sugar syrup and squash them together.
2. Add the two kinds of vodka and ice. Shake well. Strain into a martini glass. Aggregate of 2 grams of carb

NUTRITIONAL FACTS: Calories 368 Fat 38.85g Carbs 3.7g Sugar 1.28g Protein 1.69g

452. CRANBERRY GINGER MULLED WINE

PREPARATION: 10' COOKING: 30' SERVES: 4

INGREDIENTS
- 1 bottle full-bodied red wine
- 1 cup fresh cranberries
- 1/2 cup granulated erythritol
- juice of half a lemon
- 1 cinnamon stick and 1 inch of ginger root

DIRECTIONS
1. Join all Ingredients: in an enormous pan and bring it to a stew. Stew tenderly over low heat for 30 minutes.
2. Fill mugs and embellishment with cranberries and lemon.

NUTRITIONAL FACTS: Calories 168 Fat 15g Carbs 5g Sugar 2g Protein 4g

453. BLACK BEAUTY – LOW CARB VODKA DRINK

PREPARATION: 5' COOKING: 0' SERVES: 1

INGREDIENTS
- 2 ounces vodka
- 5 fresh blackberries
- ¾ ounce fresh lemon juice
- 2 tsp powdered erythritol
- ¼ tsp black pepper, 5 fresh mint leaves, and Soda water

DIRECTIONS
1. Fill an enormous rocks glass with ice.
2. Join the vodka, blackberries, lemon juice, erythritol, dark pepper, and mint leaves in a mixed drink shaker. Jumble until the foods grown from the ground are squashed and have discharged their juices.
3. Strain the substance of the mixed drink shaker over top of the ice.
4. Top with soft drink water and embellishment with blackberries and a new mint leaf

NUTRITIONAL FACTS: Calories: 180 Fat 0.2g Carbs 5g Sugar 2g Protein 1g

454. LOW CARB STRAWBERRY MARGARITA GUMMY WORMS

PREPARATION: 10' **COOKING:** 5' **SERVES:** 6

INGREDIENTS

- 10 hulled strawberries
- 2 ounces silver tequila
- 3 tsps. gelatin collagen protein
- 2 tablespoons powdered erythritol
- 1 ½ ounces fresh lime juice

DIRECTIONS

1. Put the strawberries and tequila in a blender and heartbeat till clean.
2. Pour the strawberry-and-tequila mixture right into a medium pan and set over low heat.
3. Add the gelatin, erythritol, and lime squeeze and rush to interrupt up the gelatin and be part of the Ingredient. Keep on warming for round 10 minutes, whisking habitually, until the combo is pourable.
4. Move the mixture to a cup or a bowl.
5. Refrigerate for 10 to 15 minutes, till set. Pop the sticky worms out of the shape and serve and enjoy it! Store leftovers inside the icebox for so long as seven days

NUTRITIONAL FACTS: Calories: 50 Fat 0.3g Carbs 2.2g Sugar 0.4g Protein 3.2g

455. DAIRY-FREE BOOSTED KETO COFFEE

PREPARATION: 20' **COOKING:** 15' **SERVES:** 4

INGREDIENTS

- 8 ounces dark roast coffee
- 1 tablespoon butter flavored coconut oil
- 1 scoop Keto Zone French Vanilla
- 1 scoop Collagen Peptides
- 2 teaspoons monk fruit sweetened caramel syrup
- Almond milk

DIRECTIONS

1. Join all Ingredients in a blender or milk frothier. Mix until smooth and rich
2. Serve and enjoy

NUTRITIONAL FACTS: Calories: 440 Fat 48g Carbs 0.2g Sugar 0.4 Protein 4g

456. CACAO COFFEE RECIPE

PREPARATION: 20' **COOKING:** 10' **SERVES:** 2

INGREDIENTS

- 1 cup Cacao nibs
- Boiling water
- 1/2 tsp gelatin
- Coconut oil
- Cinnamon powder

DIRECTIONS

1. Preheat your stove to 350 degrees. Put the cacao nibs in a slim layer on a heating sheet.
2. Put in the stove and let cook for 15 - 18 minutes.
3. Remove from the stove and let cool.
4. To make some Cacao espresso, you will require 1 tsp of Cacao nibs per 1 cup of bubbling water.
5. Put the cacao nibs in your espresso processor and beat multiple times for 2 seconds each. On the off chance that you hold the conservative you will get a powder. Evacuate and put in your French press and add bubbling water.
6. In your cup add your gelatin and some cold water and mix with spoon.
7. Pour in your cacao espresso and add coconut oil and cinnamon.

NUTRITIONAL FACTS: Calories: 335 Fat 19g Carbs 10g Sugar 7g Protein 8g

457. CHOCOLATE-VANILLA ALMOND MILK (SOY, NUTS)

PREPARATION: 5' **COOKING:** 0' **SERVES:** 1

INGREDIENTS

- 2 tbsp. coconut oil
- 1½ cups unsweetened almond milk
- ½ vanilla stick (crushed)
- 1 scoop organic soy protein powder (chocolate flavor)
- 4-6 drops stevia sweetener
- Optional: ½ tsp. cinnamon
- Optional: 1-2 ice cubes

DIRECTIONS

1. Add all the listed ingredients to a blender—except the ice—but including the optional cinnamon if desired.
2. Blend the ingredients for 1 minute; then if desired, add the optional ice cubes and blend for another 30 seconds.
3. Transfer the milk to a large cup or shaker, top with some additional cinnamon, serve, and enjoy!
4. Alternatively, store the smoothie in an airtight container or a mason jar, keep it in the fridge, and consume within 3 days. Store for a maximum of 30 days in the freezer and thaw at room temperature.

NUTRITIONAL FACTS: Calories: 422 kcal Net Carbs: 1.3 g. Fat: 34.8 g. Protein: 25.5 g. Fiber: 2.7 g. Sugar: 0.8 g.

458. NUTTY PROTEIN SHAKE (SOY, PEANUTS, NUTS)

PREPARATION: 5'   **COOKING:** 0'   **SERVES:** 1

INGREDIENTS

- 2 tbsp. coconut oil
- 2 cups unsweetened almond milk
- 2 tbsp. peanut butter (see recipe)
- 1 scoop organic soy protein powder (chocolate flavor)
- 2-4 ice cubes
- 4-6 drops stevia sweetener
- Optional: 1 tsp. vegan creamer
- Optional: 1 tsp. cocoa powder

DIRECTIONS

1. Add all the above listed ingredients—except the optional ingredients—to a blender, and blend for 2 minutes.
2. Transfer the shake to a large cup or shaker. If desired, top the shake with the optional vegan creamer and/or cocoa powder.
3. Stir before serving and enjoy!
4. Alternatively, store the smoothie in an airtight container or a mason jar, keep it in the fridge, and consume within 3 days. Store for a maximum of 30 days in the freezer and thaw at room temperature.

NUTRITIONAL FACTS: Calories: 618 kcal Net Carbs: 4.4 g. Fat: 51.3 g. Protein: 34 g. Fiber: 4.9 g. Sugar: 3 g.

459. CHIA & COCO SHAKE (SOY, PEANUTS)

PREPARATION: 5'   **COOKING:** 0'   **SERVES:** 1

INGREDIENTS

- 1 tbsp. chia seeds
- 6 tbsp. water
- 1 cup coconut milk
- 2 tbsp. peanut butter (see recipe)
- 1 tbsp. MCT oil (or coconut oil)
- 1 scoop organic soy protein powder (chocolate flavor)
- Pinch of Himalayan salt
- 2-4 ice cubes or ½ cup of water

DIRECTIONS

1. Mix the chia seeds and 6 tablespoons of water in a small bowl; let sit for at least 30 minutes.
2. Transfer the soaked chia seeds and all other listed ingredients to a blender and blend for 2 minutes.
3. Transfer the shake to a large cup or shaker, serve, and enjoy!
4. Alternatively, store the smoothie in an airtight container or a mason jar, keep it in the fridge, and consume within 3 days. Store for a maximum of 30 days in the freezer and thaw at room temperature.

NUTRITIONAL FACTS: Calories: 593 kcal Net Carbs: 7.4 g. Fat: 45.6 g. Protein: 36 g. Fiber: 13.9 g. Sugar: 3 g.

460. FAT-RICH PROTEIN ESPRESSO (SOY)

PREPARATION: 5'   **COOKING:** 0'   **SERVES:** 1

INGREDIENTS

- 1 cup espresso (freshly brewed)
- 2 tbsp. coconut butter (or alternatively, use coconut oil)
- 1 scoop organic soy protein (chocolate flavor)
- ½ vanilla stick
- 4 ice cubes or ½ cup boiled water
- Optional: 1 tbsp. cocoa powder
- Optional: ½ tsp. cinnamon
- 2 tbsp. coconut cream

DIRECTIONS

1. Make sure to use fresh, hot espresso.
2. Add all the listed ingredients to a heat-safe blender, including the ice or boiled water and optional ingredients (if desired). Use ice to make iced espresso, or hot water for a warm treat.
3. Blend the ingredients for 1 minute and transfer to a large coffee cup.
4. Top the coffee with the coconut cream, stir, serve and enjoy!
5. Alternatively, store the smoothie in an airtight container or a mason jar, keep it in the fridge, and consume within 3 days. Store for a maximum of 30 days in the freezer and thaw at room temperature.

NUTRITIONAL FACTS: Calories: 441 kca lNet Carbs: 5.6 g. Fat: 34.8 g. Protein: 25.4 g. Fiber: 6.9 g.Sugar: 2.8 g.

461. RASPBERRY PROTEIN SHAKE (SOY)

PREPARATION: 5'   **COOKING:** 0'   **SERVES:** 1

INGREDIENTS

- 1 cup full-fat coconut milk (or alternatively, use almond milk)
- Optional: ¼ cup coconut cream
- 1 scoop organic soy protein (chocolate or vanilla flavor)
- ½ cup raspberries (fresh or frozen)
- 1 tbsp. low-carb maple syrup
- Optional: 2-4 ice cubes

DIRECTIONS

1. Add all the ingredients to a blender, including the optional coconut cream and ice cubes if desired, and blend for 1 minute.
2. Transfer the shake to a large cup or shaker, and enjoy!
3. Alternatively, store the smoothie in an airtight container or a mason jar, keep it in the fridge, and consume within 2 days. Store for a maximum of 30 days in the freezer and thaw at room temperature.

NUTRITIONAL FACTS: Calories: 311 kcal Net Carbs: 6.9 g. Fat: 19.3 g. Protein: 26.8 g. Fiber: 5 g. Sugar: 4.8 g.

462. FOREST FRUIT BLASTER (SOY)

| PREPARATION: 5' | COOKING: 0' | SERVES: 1 |

INGREDIENTS

- ¼ cup mixed berries (fresh or frozen)
- ½ kiwi (peeled)
- 2 cups full-fat coconut milk
- 2 scoops organic soy protein (vanilla flavor)
- ½ cup water
- Optional: 2 ice cubes

DIRECTIONS

1. Add all the ingredients to a blender, including the optional ice if desired, and blend for 1 minute.
2. Transfer the shake to a large cup or shaker and enjoy!
3. Alternatively, store the smoothie in an airtight container or a mason jar, keep it in the fridge, and consume within 2 days. Store for a maximum of 30 days in the freezer and thaw at room temperature.

NUTRITIONAL FACTS: Calories: 603 kcal Net Carbs: 11.5 g. Fat: 38.1 g. Protein: 52.9 g. Fiber: 4.5 g. Sugar: 9.9 g.

463. VANILLA MILKSHAKE (SOY, NUTS)

| PREPARATION: 5' | COOKING: 0' | SERVES: 1 |

INGREDIENTS

- 2 tbsp. cocoa butter
- 2 cups unsweetened almond milk
- ¼ cup hemp seeds
- 2 tbsp. coconut whipped cream
- 4-6 drops stevia sweetener
- 1 scoop organic soy protein (vanilla flavor)
- 4 ice cubes

DIRECTIONS

1. Add all the ingredients—except the coconut whipped cream—to a blender and blend for 2 minutes.
2. Transfer the shake to a large cup or shaker.
3. Serve with the coconut whipped cream on top, stir, and enjoy!
4. Alternatively, store the smoothie in an airtight container or a mason jar, keep it in the fridge, and consume within 3 days. Store for a maximum of 30 days in the freezer and thaw at room temperature.

NUTRITIONAL FACTS: Calories: 600 kcal Net Carbs: 5.3 g. Fat: 46.6 g. Protein: 39.3 g. Fiber: 4.3 g. Sugar: 3.3 g.

464. RASPBERRY LEMON PROTEIN SMOOTHIE (SOY)

| PREPARATION: 5' | COOKING: 0' | SERVES: 2 |

INGREDIENTS

- ¼ cup flaxseeds
- ½ cup water
- 2 cups full-fat coconut milk
- 1 organic lemon (with peel)
- ½ cup raspberries (fresh or frozen)
- 1 scoop organic soy protein (vanilla flavor)
- 4-6 drops stevia sweetener
- 2 ice cubes

DIRECTIONS

1. Mix the flaxseeds with the water in a medium-sized bowl. Allow the mixture to sit for up to 30 minutes.
2. Add the soaked flaxseeds and the other ingredients to a blender and blend for 2 minutes.
3. Transfer the smoothie to a large cup or shaker, and enjoy!
4. Alternatively, store the smoothie in an airtight container or a mason jar, keep it in the fridge, and consume within 3 days. Store for a maximum of 30 days in the freezer and thaw at room temperature.

NUTRITIONAL FACTS: Calories: 314 kcal Net Carbs: 6.7 g. Fat: 23.7 g. Protein: 17.8 g. Fiber: 6.3 g. Sugar: 4.2 g.

465. BREAKFAST BOOSTER (SOY)

| PREPARATION: 5' | COOKING: 0' | SERVES: 1 |

INGREDIENTS

- 1 cup coconut milk
- 2 tbsp. cocoa butter
- 1 scoop organic soy protein (vanilla flavor)
- 4 ice cubes
- Pinch of Himalayan salt
- 5 strawberries (fresh or frozen)
- 1 tsp. matcha powder
- 1 tsp. guarana powder
- 4-6 drops stevia sweetener

DIRECTIONS

1. Add all the required ingredients to a blender and blend for 1 minute.
2. Transfer the shake to a large cup or shaker, and enjoy!
3. Alternatively, store the smoothie in an airtight container or a mason jar, keep it in the fridge, and consume within 2 days. Store for a maximum of 30 days in the freezer and thaw at room temperature.

NUTRITIONAL FACTS: Calories: 357 kcal Net Carbs: 5.8 g. Fat: 25.8 g. Protein: 24.8 g. Fiber: 4.7 g. Sugar: 3.2 g.

466. CINNAMON PEAR PROTEIN SHAKE (SOY, NUTS)

PREPARATION: 5'   **COOKING:** 0'   **SERVES:** 1

INGREDIENTS

- 1 tsp. freeze-dried pear powder
- 1 medium Hass avocado (peeled, pitted, and halved)
- 2 cups unsweetened almond milk
- 1 scoop organic soy protein (vanilla flavor)
- ½ tsp. cinnamon
- 4-6 drops stevia sweetener
- 2 ice cubes

DIRECTIONS

1. Add all the required ingredients to a blender, including the optional ice cubes if desired, and blend for 1 minute.
2. Transfer to a large cup or shaker and enjoy!
3. Alternatively, store the smoothie in an airtight container or a mason jar, keep it in the fridge, and consume within 3 days. Store for a maximum of 30 days in the freezer and thaw at room temperature.

NUTRITIONAL FACTS: Calories: 398 kcal Net Carbs: 5.4 g. Fat: 28 g. Protein: 28.8 g. Fiber: 14.9 g. Sugar: 4.4 g.

467. RASPBERRY COCO SHAKE (SOY, NUTS)

PREPARATION: 5'   **COOKING:** 0'   **SERVES:** 2

INGREDIENTS

- 1 ½ cups unsweetened almond milk
- 1 scoop organic soy protein (chocolate flavor)
- ½ cup full-fat coconut milk
- ½ cup raspberries (fresh or frozen)
- 4 drops stevia sweetener
- 2 ice cubes

DIRECTIONS

1. Put all the ingredients in a blender and blend for about 1 minute, or until the shake reaches the desired consistency.
2. Transfer the shake to a large cup or shaker and enjoy!
3. Alternatively, store the smoothie in an airtight container or mason jar in the fridge, and consume within 3 days. Store for a maximum of 30 days in the freezer and thaw at room temperature before serving.

NUTRITIONAL FACTS: Calories: 383 kcal Net Carbs: 5.6 g. Fat: 28.6 g. Protein: 24.6 g. Fiber: 6.5 g. Sugar: 4.8 g.

468. BULLETPROOF PROTEIN SHAKE (SOY)

PREPARATION: 5'   **COOKING:** /   **SERVES:** 2

INGREDIENTS

- 4 tbsp. chia seeds
- ½ cup water
- 1 medium Hass avocado (pitted, peeled)
- 1 scoop organic soy protein (chocolate flavor)
- 1 cup full-fat coconut milk
- 2 tsp. vanilla extract
- Pinch of Himalayan salt
- 4 ice cubes

DIRECTIONS

1. Put the chia seeds and water in a blender and allow the seeds to soak at least 10 minutes.
2. Add all remaining ingredients to the blender and blend for about 1 minute, or until the shake reaches the desired consistency.
3. Transfer the shake to two large cups or shakers and enjoy!
4. Alternatively, store the smoothie in an airtight container or canning jar in the fridge, and consume within 2 days. Store for a maximum of 30 days in the freezer and thaw at room temperature before serving.

NUTRITIONAL FACTS: Calories: 448 kcal Net Carbs: 5 g. Fat: 39.55 g. Protein: 16 g. Fiber: 12.7 g. Sugar: 4.5 g.

469. ALMOND SMOOTHIE

PREPARATION: 10'   **COOKING:** 10'   **SERVES:** 2

INGREDIENTS

- ¾ cup almonds, chopped
- ½ cup heavy whipping cream
- 2 teaspoons butter, melted
- ¼ teaspoon organic vanilla extract
- 7–8 drops liquid stevia
- 1 cup unsweetened almond milk
- ¼ cup ice cubes

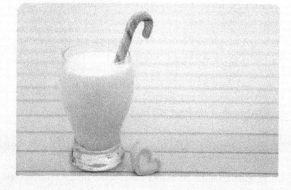

DIRECTIONS

1. In a blender, put all the listed Ingredients: and pulse until creamy.
2. Pour the smoothie into two glasses and serve immediately.

NUTRITIONAL FACTS: Calories 365 Net Carbs 4.5 g Total Fat 34.55 g Saturated Fat 10.8 g Cholesterol 51 mg Sodium 129 mg Total Carbs 9.5 g Fiber 5 g Sugar 1.6 g Protein 8.7 g

470. MOCHA SMOOTHIE

PREPARATION: 10'   **COOKING:** 10'   **SERVES:** 2

INGREDIENTS

- 2 teaspoons instant espresso powder
- 2-3 tablespoons granulated erythritol
- 2 teaspoons cacao powder
- ½ cup plain Greek yogurt
- 1 cup unsweetened almond milk
- 1 cup ice cubes

DIRECTIONS

1. In a blender, put all the listed Ingredients: and pulse until creamy.
2. Pour the smoothie into two glasses and serve immediately.

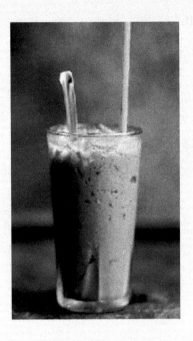

NUTRITIONAL FACTS: Calories 70 Net Carbs 5.5 g Total Fat 2.8 g Saturated Fat 1 g Cholesterol 4 mg Sodium 133 mg Total Carbs 6.5 g Fiber 1 g Sugar 4.3 g Protein 4.4 g

471. STRAWBERRY SMOOTHIE

PREPARATION: 10'   **COOKING:** 10'   **SERVES:** 2

INGREDIENTS

- 4 ounces frozen strawberries
- 2 teaspoons granulated erythritol
- ½ teaspoon organic vanilla extract
- 1/3 cup heavy whipping cream
- 1¼ cups unsweetened almond milk
- ½ cup ice cubes

DIRECTIONS

1. In a blender, put all the listed Ingredients: and pulse until creamy.
2. Pour the smoothie into two glasses and serve immediately.

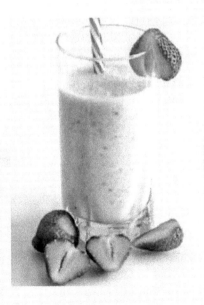

NUTRITIONAL FACTS: Calories 115 Net Carbs 4.5 g Total Fat 9.8 g Saturated Fat 4.8 g Cholesterol 27 mg Sodium 121 mg Total Carbs 6.3 g Fiber 1.8 g Sugar 2.9 g Protein 1.4 g

472. RASPBERRY SMOOTHIE

PREPARATION: 10'   COOKING: 10'   SERVES: 2

INGREDIENTS
- ¾ cup fresh raspberries
- 3 tablespoons heavy whipping cream
- 1/3 ounce cream cheese
- 1 cup unsweetened almond milk
- ½ cup ice, crushed

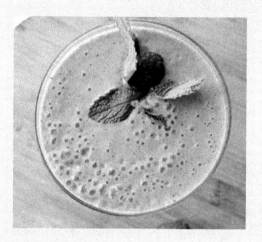

DIRECTIONS
1. In a blender, put all the listed Ingredients: and pulse until creamy.
2. Pour the smoothie into two glasses and serve immediately.

NUTRITIONAL FACTS: Calories 138 Net Carbs 3.8 g Total Fat 12 gSaturated Fat 6.4 g Cholesterol 36 mg Sodium 115 mg Total Carbs 7.3 g Fiber 3.5 g Sugar 2.1 g Protein 1.9 g

473. PUMPKIN SMOOTHIE

PREPARATION: 10'   COOKING: 10'   SERVES: 2

INGREDIENTS
- ½ cup homemade pumpkin puree
- 4 ounces cream cheese, softened
- ¼ cup heavy cream
- ½ teaspoon pumpkin pie spice
- ¼ teaspoon ground cinnamon
- 8 drops liquid stevia
- 1 teaspoon organic vanilla extract
- 1 cup unsweetened almond milk
- ¼ cup ice cubes

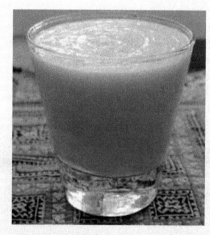

DIRECTIONS
1. In a blender, put all the listed Ingredients: and pulse until creamy.
2. Pour the smoothie into two glasses and serve immediately.

NUTRITIONAL FACTS: Calories 296 Net Carbs 5.4 g Total Fat 27.1 g Saturated Fat 16.1g Cholesterol 83 mg Sodium 266 mg Total Carbs 8 g Fiber 2.6 g Sugar 2.4 g Protein 5.6 g

474. SPINACH & AVOCADO SMOOTHIE

PREPARATION: 10' COOKING: 10' SERVES: 2

INGREDIENTS

- ½ large avocado, peeled, pitted, and roughly chopped
- 2 cups fresh spinach
- 1 tablespoon MCT oil
- 1 teaspoon organic vanilla extract
- 6–8 drops liquid stevia
- 1½ cups unsweetened almond milk
- ½ cup ice cubes

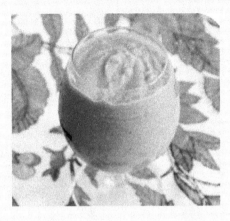

DIRECTIONS

1. In a blender, put all the listed Ingredients: and pulse until creamy.
2. Pour the smoothie into two glasses and serve immediately.

NUTRITIONAL FACTS: Calories 180 Net Carbs 0 g Total Fat 18 g Saturated Fat 9 g Cholesterol 0 mg Sodium 161 mg Total Carbs 6.5 g Fiber 4.3 g Sugar 0.6 g Protein 2.4 g

475. MATCHA SMOOTHIE

PREPARATION: 10' COOKING: 10' SERVES: 2

INGREDIENTS

- 2 tablespoons chia seeds
- 2 teaspoons matcha green tea powder
- ½ teaspoon fresh lemon juice
- ½ teaspoon xanthan gum
- 10 drops liquid stevia
- 4 tablespoons plain Greek yogurt
- 1½ cups unsweetened almond milk
- ¼ cup ice cubes

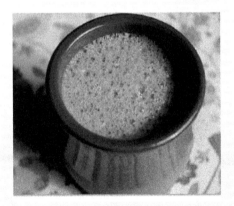

DIRECTIONS

1. In a blender, put all the listed Ingredients: and pulse until creamy.
2. Pour the smoothie into two glasses and serve immediately.

NUTRITIONAL FACTS: Calories 85 Net Carbs 3.5 g Total Fat 5.5 g Saturated Fat 0.8 g Cholesterol 2 mg Sodium 174 mg Total Carbs 7.6 g Fiber 4.1 g Sugar 2.2 g Protein 4 g

476. CREAMY SPINACH SMOOTHIE

PREPARATION: 10' **COOKING:** 10' **SERVES:** 2

INGREDIENTS

- 2 cups fresh baby spinach
- 1 tablespoon almond butter
- 1 tablespoon chia seeds
- 1/8 teaspoon ground cinnamon
- Pinch of ground cloves
- ½ cup heavy cream
- 1 cup unsweetened almond milk
- ½ cup ice cubes

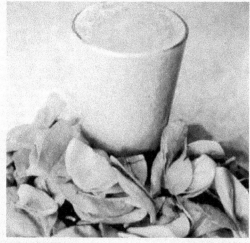

DIRECTIONS

1. In a blender, put all the listed Ingredients: and pulse until creamy.
2. Pour the smoothie into two glasses and serve immediately.

NUTRITIONAL FACTS: Calories 195 Net Carbs 2.8 g Total Fat 18.8 g Saturated Fat 7.5 g Cholesterol 41 mg Sodium 126 mg Total Carbs 6.1 g Fiber 3.3 g Sugar 0.5 g Protein 4.5 g

477. COCONUT MILK LATTE

PREPARATION: 5' **COOKING:** 5' **SERVES:** 2

INGREDIENTS

- 3 cups prepared hot coffee
- 1/2 cup coconut cream
- Dash of cinnamon

DIRECTIONS

1. Empty the espresso into a blender alongside the coconut milk.
2. Mix on medium-high for about a moment, or until the coconut milk is totally fused.
3. Fill a mug or serve over ice. You can spoon the foamed coconut milk on top for some "froth".
4. Change the measure of coconut milk to your taste buds... you may need pretty much.

NUTRITIONAL FACTS: Calories 114 Fat 12g Carbs 1g Sugar 2 Protein 1g

478. CHAMOMILE MINT TEA RECIPE

PREPARATION: 5' **COOKING:** 0' **SERVES:** 1

INGREDIENTS

- 1 tsp chamomile flowers
- 1 tsp peppermint leaves
- 1 cup (240 ml) boiling water

DIRECTIONS

1. Combine the chamomile and peppermint to a tea kettle
2. Mix for 4-5mins, discharges the herbs and drink.

NUTRITIONAL FACTS: Calories: 159 Fat 18g Carbs 9g Sugar 4g Protein 8g

479. KETO ICED APPLE GREEN TEA

PREPARATION: 5' **COOKING:** 0' **SERVES:** 2

INGREDIENTS

- 1 cup of brewed green tea
- 1 cup ice
- 1 tsp apple cider vinegar
- Stevie

DIRECTIONS

1. Mix the green tea with high temp water for 2-3 minutes.
2. Add every one of the Ingredients: to a blender and mix well.

NUTRITIONAL FACTS: Calories 190 Fat 17g Carbs 10g Sugar 1g Protein 3g

480. TURMERIC GINGER LIME TEA RECIPE

PREPARATION: 5'   COOKING: 0'   SERVES: 1

INGREDIENTS

- 1 lime
- 1 small turmeric root
- 1 piece of ginger

DIRECTIONS

1. Put 1 lime cut alongside all the turmeric and ginger pieces into a huge tea kettle.
2. Fill the tea kettle with bubbling high temp water.
3. Give the tea a chance to brew for 5 minutes.
4. Serve and enjoy hot or let it cool.

NUTRITIONAL FACTS: Calories: 500 Fat 40g Carbs 11g Sugar 1g Protein 25g

481. ZINGY SALTED LIME SODA

PREPARATION: 2'   COOKING: 0'   SERVES: 1

INGREDIENTS

- 1 lime
- 1 1/4 cups seltzer water
- 1/8 to 1/4 tsp salt

DIRECTIONS

1. Juice 1 lime and add the chilled seltzer water and salt to the lime juice.
2. Mix tenderly to disintegrate the salt.
3. Serve chilled.

NUTRITIONAL FACTS: Calories: 159 Fat 18g Carbs 9g Sugar 4g Protein 8g

482. CUCUMBER BASIL ICE CUBES RECIPE

PREPARATION: 5'   **COOKING:** 0'   **SERVES:** 3

INGREDIENTS
- 1 cucumber
- 5 small basil leaves
- Juice from 1/4 lime
- 1/4 cup water

DIRECTIONS
1. Put everything into the blender and mix well.
2. Strain the puree and empty the subsequent fluid into a huge ice shape plate or forms. Spare the subsequent cucumber solids to make this formula.
3. Leave to freeze for 4-5 hours.
4. Make beverages utilizing the ice 3D squares e.g., add them to water to enhance the taste or to vodka for a simple cucumber basil seasoned chilled vodka drink!

NUTRITIONAL FACTS: Calories: 45 Fat 0.5g Carbs 1g Sugar 0.3g Protein 9g

483. CUCUMBER LIME WATER

PREPARATION: 4'   **COOKING:** 0'   **SERVES:** 1

INGREDIENTS
- 1 cucumber
- 1 lime
- 50 fl oz. of water

DIRECTIONS
1. Strip the cucumber and afterward cut it up into 1/4-inch-thick cuts. Add to container
2. Press in juice from 1 lime.
3. Add the water and blend.
4. Sit in refrigerator medium-term.

NUTRITIONAL FACTS: Calories 140 Fat 12g Carbs 5g Sugar 2.1g Protein 8g

484. HONEYSUCKLE TEA

PREPARATION: 6H **COOKING:** 0' **SERVES:** 4

INGREDIENTS
- 1 part honeysuckle flowers
- 2 parts water
- Ice for serving

DIRECTIONS
1. Delicately break down your honeysuckle flowers. You can do that by hand or tenderly with a wooden spoon.
2. Add honeysuckle blossoms to a pitcher or cup.
3. Top with water and mix. Spread.
4. Put the pitcher in the cooler for about 6-15 hours.
5. Strain the blossoms out and make the most of your honeysuckle tea over ice.

An alternative Directions:
6. Add the broken-down honeysuckle blossoms to a pitcher or cup. Add water and blend. Spread.
7. Put the pitcher in full sun for 3-4 hours.
8. Strain the blooms out and serve and enjoy over ice.

NUTRITIONAL FACTS: Calories: 214 Fat 6g Carbs 4g Sugar 6g Protein 18g

485. KETO TURMERIC BONE BROTH

PREPARATION: 5' **COOKING:** 10' **SERVES:** 1

INGREDIENTS
- 1 cup of Keto bone broth
- 1 tsp turmeric powder
- 1 tsp ginger powder
- Dash of cumin powder
- Dash of pepper and salt to taste

DIRECTIONS
1. Heat up the bone soup and speed in different Ingredients:

NUTRITIONAL FACTS: Calories: 20 Fat 1g Carbs 0.1g Sugar 0.2g Protein 2g

486. KAMIKAZE SHOT SUGAR-FREE

PREPARATION: 1' **COOKING:** 0' **SERVES:** 2

INGREDIENTS

- 3/4 shaker Ice
- 2 tbsp. Lime Juice
- 2 g Granulated Stevia or Erythritol
- 1 shot Vodka

DIRECTIONS

1. Put ice in a shaker.
2. Add lime juice, sugar, and vodka.
3. Cover and shake.
4. Serve in a chilled rocks glass or short tumbler.

NUTRITIONAL FACTS: Calories: 109 Fat 3g Carbs 2g Sugar 1g Protein 12g

487. LOW CARB PINA COLADA

PREPARATION: 5' **COOKING:** 0' **SERVES:** 2

INGREDIENTS

- 3 ounces of rum
- 2/3 cup coconut milk
- 1/2 cup sugar-free pineapple syrup
- 2 cups crushed ice

DIRECTIONS

1. Add Ingredients: to a blender and blend until slushy. Makes two beverages
2. Check 5 grams of carb Nutrition.

NUTRITIONAL FACTS: Calories 215 Fat 10g Carbs 7g Sugar 3g Protein 23g

CHAPTER 24.
APPETIZERS

488. BACON PEPPERS

PREPARATION: 15' **COOKING:** 6' **SERVES:** 2

INGREDIENTS

- 2 jalapenos
- 1 oz. bacon, chopped, fried
- 1 teaspoon green onions, chopped
- 1 tablespoon coconut cream
- 2 oz. Cheddar cheese, shredded

DIRECTIONS

1. Trim the jalapenos and remove the seeds.
2. In the mixing bowl, mix up chopped bacon, green onions, coconut cream, and shredded cheese.
3. Fill the jalapenos with the bacon mixture.
4. Heat up the instant pot on saute mode for 5 minutes.
5. Put the jalapenos in the instant pot and cook them for 3 minutes from each side.

NUTRITIONAL FACTS: Calories 213 Fat 17.2 Fiber 0.6 Carbs 1.9 Protein 12.7

489. FAT BOMBS

PREPARATION: 10' **COOKING:** 10' **SERVES:** 3

INGREDIENTS

- 3 eggs
- 3 bacon slices
- ½ teaspoon cayenne pepper
- 2 tablespoons cream cheese
- ½ teaspoon salt

DIRECTIONS

1. Put the bacon in the instant pot and cook it on saute mode for 3 minutes from each side.
2. Then chop the bacon and put it in the bowl.
3. Crack the eggs in the instant pot and whisk gently.
4. Cook the eggs for 5 minutes on manual mode (high pressure). Make a quick pressure release.
5. Then transfer the cooked eggs in the bowl with bacon and shred.
6. Add cayenne pepper, cream cheese, and salt. Stir well.
7. Make the medium size bombs.

NUTRITIONAL FACTS: Calories 190 Fat 14.7 Fiber 0.Carbs 1 Protein 13.1

490. CHICKEN CELERY STICKS

PREPARATION: 15' **COOKING:** 15' **SERVES:** 4

INGREDIENTS
- 14 oz. chicken breast, skinless, boneless
- 1 cup of water
- 1 teaspoon salt
- ½ teaspoon onion powder
- 4 celery stalks
- 1 teaspoon Keto mayo

DIRECTIONS
1. Put the chicken breast in the instant pot.
2. Add water, salt, and onion powder.
3. Cook the chicken on manual mode (high pressure) for 15 minutes. Allow the natural pressure release for 6 minutes.
4. Remove the cooked chicken from the instant pot and shred it.
5. Add Keto mayo and stir well.
6. Fill the celery stalks with shredded chicken.

NUTRITIONAL FACTS: Calories 118 Fat 2.6 Fiber 0.3 Carbs 0.9 Protein 21.2

491. REUBEN PICKLES

PREPARATION: 20' **COOKING:** 2H **SERVES:** 6

INGREDIENTS
- 1-pound corned beef brisket
- 2 cups of water
- 1 cup pickled cucumbers
- 2 oz. provolone cheese, sliced

DIRECTIONS
1. Put corned beef brisket and water in the instant pot.
2. Cook the meat on manual mode (high pressure) for 2 hours. Allow the natural pressure release for 10 minutes.
3. Then remove the meat from water and slice it.
4. Make the Reuben pickles: pin the meat piece, pickled cucumber, and provolone cheese together to get the small bites.

NUTRITIONAL FACTS: Calories 164 Fat 12 Fiber 0.1 Carbs 0.8 Protein 12.7

492. PARMESAN BALLS WITH GREENS

PREPARATION: 10'   **COOKING:** 20'   **SERVES:** 4

INGREDIENTS

- 3 oz. Parmesan, grated
- 1 cup ground chicken
- 1 tablespoon chives, chopped
- 1 teaspoon cayenne pepper
- ¼ cup chicken broth
- 1 teaspoon coconut oil, softened

DIRECTIONS

1. Heat up coconut oil in the instant pot on saute mode.
2. Add ground chicken, cayenne pepper, chives, and chicken broth.
3. Close the lid and cook the chicken on manual mode (high pressure) for 15 minutes.
4. Then make a quick pressure release and open the lid.
5. Add Parmesan and stir the chicken mixture well.
6. Make the balls from the cooked mixture and cool them for 10 minutes before serving.

NUTRITIONAL FACTS: Calories 149 Fat 8.5 Fiber 0.1 Carbs 1.1 Protein 17.3

493. CHEESE STUFFED SHISHITO PEPPERS

PREPARATION: 20'   **COOKING:** 7'   **SERVES:** 4

INGREDIENTS

- 8 oz. shishito peppers
- 1 cup Cheddar cheese, shredded
- 4 tablespoons cream cheese
- 1 tablespoon fresh parsley, chopped
- ¼ teaspoon minced garlic
- 1 tablespoon butter, melted
- 1 cup water, for cooking

DIRECTIONS

1. Cut the ends of the peppers and remove the seeds.
2. After this, in the mixing bowl mix up shredded cheese, cream cheese, parsley, and minced garlic.
3. Then fill the peppers with cheese mixture and put in the baking mold.
4. Sprinkle the peppers with melted butter.
5. After this, pour water and insert the steamer rack.
6. Place the mold with peppers on the rack. Close and seal the lid.
7. Cook the meal on manual (high pressure) for 7 minutes. Allow the natural pressure release for 5 minutes

NUTRITIONAL FACTS: Calories 194 Fat 15. Fiber 2.6 Carbs 4.5 Protein 9.1

494. ROASTED TOMATILLOS

PREPARATION: 10'   COOKING: 10'   SERVES: 4

INGREDIENTS

- tablespoon Italian seasonings
- 4 tomatillos, sliced
- 4 teaspoons olive oil
- 4 tablespoons water

DIRECTIONS

1. Sprinkle the tomatillos with Italian seasoning.
2. Then pour the olive oil in the instant pot and heat it up on saute mode for 1 minute.
3. Put the tomatillos in the instant pot in one layer and cook them for 2 minutes from each side.
4. Then add water and close the lid.
5. Saute the vegetables for 3 minutes more.

NUTRITIONAL FACTS: Calories 51 Fat 5 Fiber 0.7 Carbs 2 Protein 0.3

495. CHICKEN&CHINESE CABBAGE SALAD

PREPARATION: 15'   COOKING: 10'   SERVES: 4

INGREDIENTS

- 12 oz. chicken fillet, chopped
- 1 teaspoon Cajun seasonings
- 1 tablespoon coconut oil
- 1 cup Chinese cabbage, chopped
- 1 tablespoon avocado oil
- 1 teaspoon sesame seeds

DIRECTIONS

1. Sprinkle the chopped chicken with Cajun seasonings and put in the instant pot.
2. Add coconut oil and cook the chicken on saute mode for 10 minutes. Stir it from time to time with the help of a spatula.
3. When the chicken is cooked, transfer it in the salad bowl.
4. Add Chinese cabbage, avocado oil, and sesame seeds.
5. Mix up the salad.

NUTRITIONAL FACTS: Calories 202 Fat 10.6 Fiber 0.4 Carbs 0.8 Protein 25

496. CAULIFLOWER FRITTERS

PREPARATION: 10' **COOKING:** 10' **SERVES:** 4

INGREDIENTS
- 1 cup cauliflower, boiled
- 2 oz. Cheddar cheese, shredded
- 2 tablespoons almond flour
- ½ teaspoon garlic powder
- 2 eggs, beaten
- 1 tablespoon avocado oil

DIRECTIONS
1. Mash the cauliflower and mix it up with Cheddar cheese, almond flour, garlic powder, and eggs.
2. Heat up the avocado oil on saute mode for 1 minute.
3. Meanwhile, make the fritters from the cauliflower mixture.
4. Put them in the hot oil and cook for 3 minutes from each side.

NUTRITIONAL FACTS: Calories 122 Fat 9 Fiber 1.2 Carbs 2.9 Protein 7.7

497. ZUCCHINI CHEESE TOTS

PREPARATION: 15' **COOKING:** 10' **SERVES:** 6

INGREDIENTS
- 4 oz. Parmesan, grated
- 4 oz. Cheddar cheese, grated
- 1 zucchini, grated
- 1 egg, beaten
- 1 teaspoon dried oregano
- 1 tablespoon coconut oil

DIRECTIONS
1. In the mixing bowl, mix up Parmesan, Cheddar cheese, zucchini, egg, and dried oregano.
2. Make the small tots with the help of the fingertips.
3. Then melt the coconut oil in the instant pot on saute mode.
4. Put the prepared zucchini tots in the hot coconut oil and cook them for 3 minutes from each side or until they are light brown.
5. Cool the zucchini tots for 5 minutes.

NUTRITIONAL FACTS: Calories 173 Fat 13.4 Fiber 0.5 Carbs 2.2 Protein 12.1

498. STEAMED SPINACH WITH GARLIC

PREPARATION: 5'   **COOKING:** 4'   **SERVES:** 4

INGREDIENTS
- 2 cups spinach, chopped
- 1 cup organic almond milk
- 1 teaspoon minced garlic
- 1 tablespoon butter
- ½ teaspoon salt
- 2 oz. Monterey Jack cheese, shredded

DIRECTIONS
1. Put all Ingredients: in the instant pot and stir gently.
2. Close and seal the lid.
3. Cook the meal on manual mode (high pressure) for 4 minutes. Make a quick pressure release.
4. After this, open the lid and stir the spinach well.

NUTRITIONAL FACTS: Calories 98 Fat 7.9 Fiber 0.3 Carbs 2.9 Protein 4.2

499. LEMON MUSHROOMS

PREPARATION: 10'   **COOKING:** 4'   **SERVES:** 2

INGREDIENTS
- 1 cup cremini mushrooms, sliced
- 1 teaspoon lemon zest, grated
- 1 tablespoon lemon juice
- ½ teaspoon salt
- ½ teaspoon dried thyme
- ½ cup of water
- 1 teaspoon almond butter

DIRECTIONS
1. Put all Ingredients: in the instant pot and stir them with the help of the spatula.
2. Then close and seal the instant pot lid.
3. Cook the mushrooms on manual mode (high pressure) for 4 minutes.
4. When the time of cooking is finished, allow the natural pressure release for 5 minutes.

NUTRITIONAL FACTS: Calories 62, Fat 4.6 Fiber 1.2 Carbs 3.5 Protein 2.7

500. FETA PSITI

PREPARATION: 10' **COOKING:** 6' **SERVES:** 6

INGREDIENTS

- 12 oz. Feta cheese
- ½ tomato, sliced
- 1 oz. bell pepper, sliced
- 1 teaspoon ground paprika
- 1 tablespoon olive oil
- 1 cup water, for cooking

DIRECTIONS

1. Sprinkle the cheese with olive oil and ground paprika and place it on the foil.
2. Then top Feta cheese with sliced tomato and bell pepper. Wrap it in the foil well.
3. After this, pour water and insert the steamer rack in the instant pot.
4. Put the wrapped cheese on the rack. Close and seal the lid.
5. Cook the cheese on manual mode (high pressure) for 6 minutes. Then make a quick pressure release.
6. Discard the foil and transfer the cheese on the serving plates.

NUTRITIONAL FACTS: calories 178, fat 14.5, fiber 0.5, carbs 4.2, protein 8.4

501. CAULIFLOWER QUESO

PREPARATION: 10' **COOKING:** 30' **SERVES:** 5

INGREDIENTS

- 2 cups cauliflower, chopped
- 1/3 cup cream cheese
- ½ cup Cheddar cheese
- 1 jalapeno, chopped
- 2 oz. scallions, diced
- 1 tablespoon nutritional yeast
- 1 tablespoon olive oil
- 2 garlic cloves, diced

DIRECTIONS

1. Put chopped cauliflower, cream cheese, Cheddar cheese, jalapeno, diced scallions, nutritional yeast, olive oil, and diced garlic clove.
2. Stir the mixture well with the help of the spoon and close the lid.
3. Cook the queso for 30 minutes on saute mode. Stir meal every 5 minutes to avoid burning.

NUTRITIONAL FACTS: Calories 146 Fat 12.1 Fiber 1.9 Carbs 5 Protein 6

502. SWEET SMOKIES

PREPARATION: 5' **COOKING:** 15' **SERVES:** 3

INGREDIENTS
- 1 teaspoon Erythritol
- ½ teaspoon sesame seeds
- 2 tablespoons keto BBQ sauce
- 8 oz. cocktail sausages
- 1/3 cup chicken broth

DIRECTIONS
1. Put Erythritol, sesame seeds, BBQ sauce, and chicken broth in the instant pot.
2. Preheat the mixture on saute mode for 2 minutes.
3. Then add cocktail sausages and stir the mixture well.
4. Cook the meal for 10 minutes on saute mode. Stir the sausages every 2 minutes.

NUTRITIONAL FACTS: Calories 49 Fat 2.5 Fiber 5.7 Carbs 0.1 Protein 2.3

503. ROSEMARY CHICKEN WINGS

PREPARATION: 10' **COOKING:** 16' **SERVES:** 4

INGREDIENTS
- 4 chicken wings, boneless
- 1 tablespoon olive oil
- 1 teaspoon dried rosemary
- ½ teaspoon garlic powder
- ¼ teaspoon salt

DIRECTIONS
1. In the mixing bowl, mix up olive oil, dried rosemary, garlic powder, and salt.
2. Then rub the chicken wings with the rosemary mixture and leave for 10 minutes to marinate.
3. After this, put the chicken wings in the instant pot, add the remaining rosemary marinade and cook them on saute mode for 8 minutes from each side.

NUTRITIONAL FACTS: Calories 222 Fat 11.1 Fiber 0.2 Carbs 1.8 Protein 27.5

504. CLASSIC MEATBALLS

PREPARATION: 20' COOKING: 15' SERVES: 6

INGREDIENTS

- 7 oz. ground beef
- 7 oz. ground pork
- 1 teaspoon minced garlic
- 3 tablespoons water
- 1 teaspoon chili flakes
- 1 teaspoon dried parsley
- 1 tablespoon coconut oil
- ¼ cup beef broth

DIRECTIONS

1. In the mixing bowl, mix up ground beef, ground pork, minced garlic, water, and chili flakes, and dried parsley.
2. Make the medium size meatballs from the mixture.
3. After this, heat up coconut oil in the instant pot on saute mode.
4. Put the meatballs in the hot coconut oil in one layer and cook them for 2 minutes from each side.
5. Then add beef broth and close the lid.
6. Cook the meatballs for 10 minutes on manual mode (high pressure).
7. Then make a quick pressure release and transfer the meatballs on the plate.

NUTRITIONAL FACTS: Calories 131 Fat 5.6 Fiber 0 Carbs 0.2 Protein 18.9

505. BACON DEVILED EGGS

PREPARATION: 10' COOKING: 15' SERVES: 4

INGREDIENTS

- 2 eggs
- 1 teaspoon cream cheese
- 1 oz. Parmesan, grated
- ¼ teaspoon red pepper
- 1 oz. bacon, chopped
- 1 cup of water

DIRECTIONS

1. Pour water in the instant pot.
2. Add eggs and cook them for 5 minutes on manual mode (high pressure).
3. Then make a quick pressure release. Cool and peel the eggs.
4. After this, clean the instant pot bowl and put the bacon inside.
5. Cook it on saute mode for 10 minutes. Stir it from time to time to avoid burning.
6. Cut the eggs into halves.
7. Put the egg yolks in the bowl and smash them with the help of the fork.
8. Add red pepper, cooked bacon, and cream cheese. Mix up the mixture.
9. Then fill the egg whites with the bacon mixture.

NUTRITIONAL FACTS: Calories 98 Fat 7 Fiber 0.1 Carbs 1.1 Protein 7.8

506. SPINACH DIP

PREPARATION: 10' **COOKING:** 6H **SERVES:** 4

INGREDIENTS

- 2 cups spinach, chopped
- 1 cup Mozzarella, shredded
- 2 artichoke hearts, chopped
- 1 teaspoon ground ginger
- 1 teaspoon butter
- ½ teaspoon white pepper
- ½ cup heavy cream

DIRECTIONS

1. Put the spinach, artichoke hearts, and butter in the instant pot bowl.
2. Add Mozzarella, ground ginger, white pepper, and heavy cream. Stir the mixture gently.
3. Cook it in manual mode (Low pressure) for 6 hours. Then stir well and transfer in the serving bowl.

NUTRITIONAL FACTS: Calories 124 Fat 8 Fiber 4.8 Carbs 10.2 Protein 5.5

507. SAUSAGE BALLS

PREPARATION: 10' **COOKING:** 16' **SERVES:** 10

INGREDIENTS

- 15 oz. ground pork sausage
- 1 teaspoon dried oregano
- 4 oz. Mozzarella, shredded
- 1 cup coconut flour
- 1 garlic clove, grated
- 1 teaspoon coconut oil, melted

DIRECTIONS

1. In the bowl mix up ground pork sausages, dried oregano, shredded Mozzarella, coconut flour, and garlic clove.
2. When the mixture is homogenous, make the balls.
3. After this, pour coconut oil in the instant pot.
4. Arrange the balls in the instant pot and cook them on saute mode for 8 minutes from each side.

NUTRITIONAL FACTS: Calories 310 Fat 23.2 Fiber 4.9 Carbs 10.1 Protein 16.8

508. BLT DIP

PREPARATION: 10' **COOKING:** 20' **SERVES:** 3

INGREDIENTS

- 2 teaspoons cream cheese
- 3 oz. bacon, chopped
- 2 tablespoons sour cream
- 2 oz. Cheddar cheese, shredded
- ¼ teaspoon minced garlic
- 1 teaspoon smoked paprika
- 1 tomato, chopped
- ¼ cup lettuce, chopped

DIRECTIONS

1. Preheat the instant pot on saute mode.
2. Put the chopped bacon in the instant pot and cook it for 5 minutes. Stir it from time to time.
3. Then add cream cheese, sour cream, Cheddar cheese, garlic, smoked paprika, and tomato.
4. Close the lid and cook the dip on saute mode for 15 minutes.
5. Then stir it well and mix up with lettuce.

NUTRITIONAL FACTS: Calories 261 Fat 20.7 Fiber 0.5 Carbs 2.5 Protein 15.9

CHAPTER 25.
SNACKS

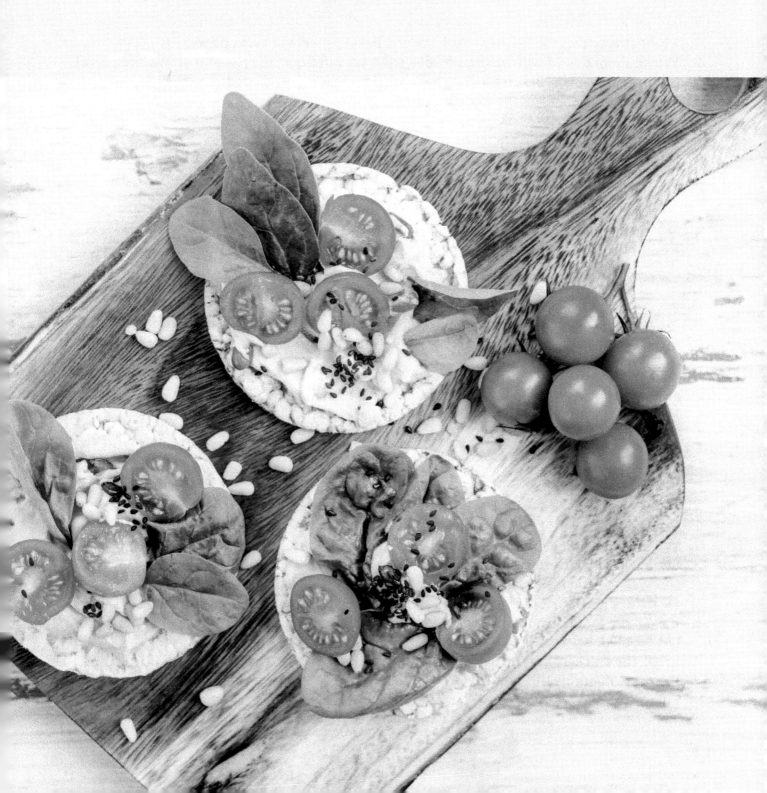

509. BLUEBERRY SCONES

PREPARATION: 15 **COOKING:** 25' **SERVES:** 2

INGREDIENTS

- 2 cups almond flour
- 1/3 cup Swerve sweetener
- ¼ cup coconut flour
- 1 tbsp. baking powder
- ¼ tsp salt
- 2 large eggs
- ¼ cup heavy whipping cream
- ½ tsp vanilla extract
- ¾ cup fresh blueberries

DIRECTIONS

1. Preheat your oven at 325 degrees F. Layer a baking sheet with wax paper.
2. Whisk almond flour with baking powder, salt, coconut flour, and sweetener in a large bowl.
3. Stir in eggs, vanilla, and cream then mix well until fully incorporated.
4. Add blueberries and mix gently.
5. Spread this dough on a baking sheet and form it into a 10x8-inch rectangle.
6. Bake these scones for 25 minutes until golden.
7. Allow them to cool then serve.

NUTRITIONAL FACTS: Calories: 266 Fat 25.7 g Saturated Fat 1.2 g Cholesterol 41 Sodium 18

510. HOMEMADE GRAHAM CRACKERS

PREPARATION: 5' **COOKING:** 30' **SERVES:** 12

INGREDIENTS

- 2 cups almond flour
- 1/3 cup Swerve Brown
- 2 tsp cinnamon
- 1 tsp baking powder
- Pinch salt
- 1 large egg
- 2 tbsp. butter, melted
- 1 tsp vanilla extract

DIRECTIONS

1. Preheat your oven at 300 degrees F.
2. Whisk almond flour, baking powder, salt, cinnamon, and sweetener in a large bowl.
3. Stir in melted butter, egg, and vanilla extract.
4. Mix well to form the dough then spread it out into a ¼-inch thick sheet.
5. Slice the sheet into 2x2-inch squares and place them on a baking sheet with wax paper.
6. Bake them for 30 minutes until golden then let them sit for 30 minutes at room temperature until cooled.
7. Break the crackers into smaller squares and put them back in the hot oven for 30 minutes. Keep the oven off during this time.
8. Enjoy.

NUTRITIONAL FACTS: Calories: 243 Fat: 21 g Cholesterol: 121 Sodium: 34 Carb0hydrates: 7.3 Protein: 4.3 g

511. BUFFALO CHICKEN SAUSAGE BALLS

PREPARATION: 5' COOKING: 25' SERVES: 2

INGREDIENTS

Sausage Balls:
- 2 14-ox sausages, casings removed
- 2 cups almond flour
- 1 ½ cups shredded cheddar cheese
- ½ cup crumbled bleu cheese
- 1 tsp salt
- ½ tsp pepper

Bleu Cheese Ranch Dipping Sauce:
- 1/3 cup mayonnaise
- 1/3 cup almond milk, unsweetened
- 2 cloves garlic, minced
- 1 tsp dried dill
- ½ tsp dried parsley
- ½ tsp salt
- ½ tsp pepper
- ¼ cup crumbled bleu cheese (or more, if desired)

DIRECTIONS

1. Preheat your oven at 350 degrees F.
2. Layer two baking sheets with wax paper and set them aside.
3. Mix sausage with cheddar cheese, almond flour, salt, pepper, and bleu cheese in a large bowl.
4. Make 1-inch balls out of this mixture and place them on the baking sheets.
5. Bake them for 25 minutes until golden brown.
6. Meanwhile, prepare the dipping sauce by whisking all of its ingredients in a bowl.
7. Serve the balls with this dipping sauce.

NUTRITIONAL FACTS: Calories: 183 Fat: 15 g Cholesterol 11 mg Sodium 31 mg Total carbohydrates 6.2 g Protein 4.5 g

512. BRUSSELS SPROUTS CHIPS

PREPARATION: 5' COOKING: 15' SERVES: 6

INGREDIENTS

- 1-pound Brussels sprouts, washed and dried
- 2 tbsp. extra virgin olive oil
- 1 tsp kosher salt

DIRECTIONS

1. Preheat your oven at 400 degrees F.
2. After peeling the sprouts off the stem, discard the outer leaves of the Brussel sprouts.
3. Separate all the leaves from one another and place them on a baking sheet.
4. Toss them with oil and salt thoroughly to coat them well.
5. Spread the leaves out on two greased baking sheets then bake them for 15 minutes until crispy.
6. Serve.

NUTRITIONAL FACTS: Calories: 188 Fat: 3 g Cholesterol: 101 Sodium: 54 mg Fiber 0.6 g Protein 5 g

513. KETO CHOCOLATE MOUSSE

PREPARATION: 5'   **COOKING:** 0'   **SERVES:** 2

INGREDIENTS

- 1 cup heavy whipping cream
- ¼ cup unsweetened cocoa powder, sifted
- ¼ cup Swerve powdered sweetener
- 1 tsp vanilla extract
- ¼ tsp kosher salt

DIRECTIONS

1. Add cream to the bowl of an electric stand mixture and beat it until it forms peaks.
2. Stir in cocoa powder, vanilla, sweetener, and salt.
3. Mix well until smooth.
4. Refrigerate for 4 hours.
5. Serve.

NUTRITIONAL FACTS: Calories: 153 Fat: 13 g Cholesterol: 6.5 mg Sodium: 81 mg Sugar 1.4 g Protein 5.8 g

514. KETO BERRY MOUSSE

PREPARATION: 5'   **COOKING:** 0'   **SERVES:** 2

INGREDIENTS

- 2 cups heavy whipping cream
- 3 oz. fresh raspberries
- 2 oz. chopped pecans
- ½ lemon, zested
- ¼ tsp vanilla extract

DIRECTIONS

1. Beat cream in a bowl using a hand mixer until it forms peaks.
2. Stir in vanilla and lemon zest and mix well until incorporated.
3. Fold in nuts and berries and mix well.
4. Cover the mixture with plastic wrap and refrigerate for 3 hours.
5. Serve fresh.

NUTRITIONAL FACTS: Calories: 254 Fat: 9 g Cholesterol: 13 mg Sodium: 179 mg Sugar 1.2 g Protein 7.5 g

515. PEANUT BUTTER MOUSSE

PREPARATION: 5' **COOKING:** 0' **SERVES:** 4

INGREDIENTS

- ½ cup heavy whipping cream
- 4 oz. cream cheese, softened
- ¼ cup natural peanut butter
- ¼ cup powdered Swerve sweetener
- ½ tsp vanilla extract

DIRECTIONS

1. Beat ½ cup cream in a medium bowl with a hand mixer until it forms peaks.
2. Beat cream cheese with peanut butter in another bowl until creamy.
3. Stir in vanilla, a pinch of salt, and sweetener to the peanut butter mix and combine until smooth.
4. Fold in the prepared whipped cream and mix well until fully incorporated.
5. Divide the mousse into 4 serving glasses.
6. Garnish as desired.
7. Enjoy.

NUTRITIONAL FACTS: Calories: 290 Fat: 21.5 Cholesterol: 12 Sodium: 9 Protein: 6

516. COOKIE ICE CREAM

PREPARATION: 10' **COOKING:** 120' **SERVES:** 2

INGREDIENTS

Cookie Crumbs
- ¾ cup almond flour
- ¼ cup cocoa powder
- ¼ tsp baking soda
- ¼ cup erythritol
- ½ tsp vanilla extract
- 1 ½ tbsp. coconut oil, softened
- 1 large egg, room temperature
- Pinch of salt

Ice Cream
- 2 ½ cups whipping cream
- 1 tbsp. vanilla extract
- ½ cup erythritol
- ½ cup almond milk, unsweetened

DIRECTIONS

1. Preheat your oven at 300 degrees F and layer a 9-inch baking pan with wax paper.
2. Whisk almond flour with baking soda, cocoa powder, salt, and erythritol in a medium bowl.
3. Stir in coconut oil and vanilla extract then mix well until crumbly.
4. Whisk in egg and mix well to form the dough.
5. Spread this dough in the prepared pan and bake for 20 minutes in the preheated oven.
6. Allow the crust to cool then crush it finely into crumbles.
7. Beat cream in a large bowl with a hand mixer until it forms a stiff peak.
8. Stir in erythritol and vanilla extract then mix well until fully incorporated.
9. Pour in milk and blend well until smooth.
10. Add this mixture to an ice cream machine and churn as per the machine's instructions.
11. Add cookie crumbles to the ice cream in the machine and churn again.
12. Place the ice cream in a sealable container and freeze for 2 hours.
13. Scoop out the ice cream and serve.
14. Enjoy.
15. Note: this recipe calls for an ice cream machine

NUTRITIONAL FACTS: Calories: 214 Fat: 19 Cholesterol: 15 Sodium: 12 Fiber: 2 Protein: 7

517. MOCHA ICE CREAM

PREPARATION: 10' **COOKING:** 0' **SERVES:** 2

INGREDIENTS

- 1 cup coconut milk
- ¼ cup heavy whipping cream
- 2 tbsp. erythritol
- 15 drops liquid stevia
- 2 tbsp. unsweetened cocoa powder
- 1 tbsp. instant coffee
- ¼ tsp xanthan gum

DIRECTIONS

1. Whisk everything except xanthan gum in a bowl using a hand mixer.
2. Slowly add xanthan gum and stir well to make a thick mixture.
3. Churn the mixture in an ice cream machine as per the machine's instructions.
4. Freeze it for 2 hours then garnish with mint and instant coffee.
5. Serve.
6. Note: this recipe calls for an ice cream machine

NUTRITIONAL FACTS: Calories: 267 Fat: 44.5 g Cholesterol: 153 mg Sodium: 217 mg

518. RASPBERRY CREAM FAT BOMBS

PREPARATION: 10' **COOKING:** 0' **SERVES:** 2

INGREDIENTS

- 1 packet raspberry Jello (sugar-free)
- 1 tsp gelatin powder
- ½ cup of boiling water
- ½ cup heavy cream

DIRECTIONS

1. Mix Jello and gelatin in boiling water in a medium bowl.
2. Stir in cream slowly and mix it for 1 minute.
3. Divide this mixture into candy molds.
4. Refrigerate them for 30 minutes.
5. Enjoy.

NUTRITIONAL FACTS: Calories: 197 Fat: 19.2 g Cholesterol: 11 mg Sodium: 78 mg

519. CAULIFLOWER TARTAR BREAD

PREPARATION: 10' **COOKING:** 50' **SERVES:** 4

INGREDIENTS

- 3 cup cauliflower rice
- 10 large eggs, yolks and egg whites separated
- ¼ tsp cream of tartar
- 1 ¼ cup coconut flour
- 1 ½ tbsp. gluten-free baking powder
- 1 tsp sea salt
- 6 tbsp. butter
- 6 cloves garlic, minced
- 1 tbsp. fresh rosemary, chopped
- 1 tbsp. fresh parsley, chopped

DIRECTIONS

1. Preheat your oven to 350 degrees F. Layer a 9x5-inch pan with wax paper.
2. Place the cauliflower rice in a suitable bowl and then cover it with plastic wrap.
3. Heat it for 4 minutes in the microwave. Heat more if the cauliflower isn't soft enough.
4. Place the cauliflower rice in a kitchen towel and squeeze it to drain excess water.
5. Transfer drained cauliflower rice to a food processor.
6. Add coconut flour, sea salt, baking powder, butter, egg yolks, and garlic. Blend until crumbly.
7. Beat egg whites with cream of tartar in a bowl until foamy.
8. Add egg white mixture to the cauliflower mixture and stir well with a spatula.
9. Fold in rosemary and parsley.
10. Spread this batter in the prepared baking pan evenly.
11. Bake it for 50 minutes until golden then allow it to cool.

NUTRITIONAL FACTS: Calories: 104 Fat: 8.9 g Cholesterol: 57 mg Sodium: 340 mg Carbohydrates: 4.7 g

520. BUTTERY SKILLET FLATBREAD

PREPARATION: 10' **COOKING:** 10' **SERVES:** 4

INGREDIENTS

- 1 cup almond flour
- 2 tbsp. coconut flour
- 2 tsp xanthan gum
- ½ tsp baking powder
- ½ tsp salt
- 1 whole egg + 1 egg white
- 1 tbsp. water (if needed)
- 1 tbsp. oil, for frying
- 1 tbsp. melted butter, for brushing

DIRECTIONS

1. Mix xanthan gum with flours, salt, and baking powder in a suitable bowl.
2. Beat egg and egg white in a separate bowl then stir in the flour mixture.
3. Mix well until smooth. Add a tablespoon of water if the dough is too thick.
4. Place a large skillet over medium heat and heat oil.

NUTRITIONAL FACTS: Calories: 272 Fat: 18 Cholesterol: 6.1

521. FLUFFY BITES

PREPARATION: 20' **COOKING:** 60' **SERVES:** 12

INGREDIENTS

- 2 Teaspoons Cinnamon
- 2/3 Cup Sour Cream
- 2 Cups Heavy Cream
- 1 Teaspoon Scraped Vanilla Bean
- ¼ Teaspoon Cardamom
- 4 Egg Yolks
- Stevia to Taste

DIRECTIONS

1. Start by whisking your egg yolks until creamy and smooth.
2. Get out a double boiler, and add your eggs with the rest of your ingredients. Mix well.
3. Remove from heat, allowing it to cool until it reaches room temperature.
4. Refrigerate for an hour before whisking well.
5. Pour into molds, and freeze for at least an hour before serving.

NUTRITIONAL FACTS: Calories: 363 Protein: 2 Fat: 40 Carbohydrates: 1

522. COCONUT FUDGE

PREPARATION: 20' **COOKING:** 60' **SERVES:** 12

INGREDIENTS

- 2 Cups Coconut Oil
- ½ Cup Dark Cocoa Powder
- ½ Cup Coconut Cream
- ¼ Cup Almonds, Chopped
- ¼ Cup Coconut, Shredded
- 1 Teaspoon Almond Extract
- Pinch of Salt
- Stevia to Taste

DIRECTIONS

1. Pour your coconut oil and coconut cream in a bowl, whisking with an electric beater until smooth. Once the mixture becomes smooth and glossy, do not continue.
2. Begin to add in your cocoa powder while mixing slowly, making sure that there aren't any lumps.
3. Add in the rest of your ingredients, and mix well.
4. Line a bread pan with parchment paper, and freeze until it sets.
5. Slice into squares before serving.

NUTRITIONAL FACTS: Calories: 172 Fat: 20 Carbohydrates: 3

523. NUTMEG NOUGAT

PREPARATION: 30' **COOKING:** 60' **SERVES:** 12

INGREDIENTS
- 1 Cup Heavy Cream
- 1 Cup Cashew Butter
- 1 Cup Coconut, Shredded
- ½ Teaspoon Nutmeg
- 1 Teaspoon Vanilla Extract, Pure
- Stevia to Taste

DIRECTIONS
1. Melt your cashew butter using a double boiler, and then stir in your vanilla extract, dairy cream, nutmeg and stevia. Make sure it's mixed well.
2. Remove from heat, allowing it to cooldown before refrigerating it for a half hour.
3. Shape into balls, and coat with shredded coconut. Chill for at least two hours before serving.

NUTRITIONAL FACTS: Calories: 341 Fat: 34 Carbohydrates: 5

524. SWEET ALMOND BITES

PREPARATION: 30' **COOKING:** 90' **SERVES:** 12

INGREDIENTS
- 18 Ounces Butter, Grass Fed
- 2 Ounces Heavy Cream
- ½ Cup Stevia
- 2/3 Cup Cocoa Powder
- 1 Teaspoon Vanilla Extract, Pure
- 4 Tablespoons Almond Butter

DIRECTIONS
1. Use a double boiler to melt your butter before adding in all of your remaining ingredients.
2. Place the mixture into molds, freezing for two hours before serving.

NUTRITIONAL FACTS: Calories: 350 Protein: 2 Fat: 38

525. STRAWBERRY CHEESECAKE MINIS

PREPARATION: 30' **COOKING:** 120' **SERVES:** 12

INGREDIENTS

- 1 Cup Coconut Oil
- 1 Cup Coconut Butter
- ½ Cup Strawberries, Sliced
- ½ Teaspoon Lime Juice
- 2 Tablespoons Cream Cheese, Full Fat
- Stevia to Taste

DIRECTIONS

1. Blend your strawberries together.
2. Soften your cream cheese, and then add in your coconut butter.
3. Combine all ingredients together, and then pour your mixture into silicone molds.
4. Freeze for at least two hours before serving.

NUTRITIONAL FACTS: Calories: 372 Protein: 1 Fat: 41 Carbohydrates: 2

526. COCOA BROWNIES

PREPARATION: 10' **COOKING:** 30' **SERVES:** 12

INGREDIENTS

- 1 Egg
- 2 Tablespoons Butter, Grass Fed
- 2 Teaspoons Vanilla Extract, Pure
- ¼ Teaspoon Baking Powder
- ¼ Cup Cocoa Powder
- 1/3 Cup Heavy Cream
- ¾ Cup Almond Butter
- Pinch Sea Salt

DIRECTIONS

1. Break your egg into a bowl, whisking until smooth.
2. Add in all of your wet ingredients, mixing well.
3. Mix all dry ingredients into a bowl.
4. Sift your dry ingredients into your wet ingredients, mixing to form a batter.
5. Get out a baking pan, greasing it before pouring in your mixture.
6. Heat your oven to 350 and bake for twenty-five minutes.
7. Allow it to cool before slicing and serve room temperature or warm.

NUTRITIONAL FACTS: Calories: 184 Protein: 1 Fat: 20 Carbohydrates: 1

527. CHOCOLATE ORANGE BITES

PREPARATION: 20' COOKING: 120' SERVES: 6

INGREDIENTS
- 10 Ounces Coconut Oil
- 4 Tablespoons Cocoa Powder
- ¼ Teaspoon Blood Orange Extract
- Stevia to Taste

DIRECTIONS
1. Melt half of your coconut oil using a double boiler, and then add in your stevia and orange extract.
2. Get out candy molds, pouring the mixture into it. Fill each mold halfway, and then place in the fridge until they set.
3. Melt the other half of your coconut oil, stirring in your cocoa powder and stevia, making sure that the mixture is smooth with no lumps.
4. Pour into your molds, filling them up all the way, and then allow it to set in the fridge before serving.

NUTRITIONAL FACTS: Calories: 188 Protein: 1 Fat: 21 Carbohydrates: 5

528. CARAMEL CONES

PREPARATION: 25' COOKING: 120' SERVES: 6

INGREDIENTS
- 2 Tablespoons Heavy Whipping Cream
- 2 Tablespoons Sour Cream
- 1 Tablespoon Caramel Sugar
- 1 Teaspoon Sea Salt, Fine
- 1/3 Cup Butter, Grass Fed
- 1/3 Cup Coconut Oil
- Stevia to Taste

DIRECTIONS
1. Soften your coconut oil and butter, mixing together.
2. Mix all ingredients together to form a batter, and ten place them in molds.
3. Top with a little salt, and keep refrigerated until serving.

NUTRITIONAL FACTS: Calories: 100 Fat: 12 Grams Carbohydrates: 1

529. CINNAMON BITES

PREPARATION: 20' **COOKING:** 95' **SERVES:** 6

INGREDIENTS

- 1/8 Teaspoon Nutmeg
- 1 Teaspoon Vanilla Extract
- ¼ Teaspoon Cinnamon
- 4 Tablespoons Coconut Oil
- ½ Cup Butter, Grass Fed
- 8 Ounces Cream Cheese
- Stevia to Taste

DIRECTIONS

1. Soften your coconut oil and butter, mixing in your cream cheese.
2. Add all of your remaining ingredients, and mix well.
3. Pour into molds, and freeze until set.

NUTRITIONAL FACTS: Calories: 178 Protein: 1 Fat: 19

530. SWEET CHAI BITES

PREPARATION: 20' **COOKING:** 45' **SERVES:** 6

INGREDIENTS

- 1 Cup Cream Cheese
- 1 Cup Coconut Oil
- 2 Ounces Butter, Grass Fed
- 2 Teaspoons Ginger
- 2 Teaspoons Cardamom
- 1 Teaspoon Nutmeg
- 1 Teaspoon Cloves
- 1 Teaspoon Vanilla Extract, Pure
- 1 Teaspoon Darjeeling Black Tea
- Stevia to Taste

DIRECTIONS

1. Melt your coconut oil and butter before adding in your black tea. Allow it to set for one to two minutes.
2. Add in your cream cheese, removing your mixture from heat.
3. Add in all of your spices, and stir to combine.
4. Pour into molds, and freeze before serving

NUTRITIONAL FACTS: Calories: 178 Protein: 1 Fat: 19

531. EASY VANILLA BOMBS

PREPARATION: 20' **COOKING:** 45' **SERVES:** 14

INGREDIENTS
- 1 Cup Macadamia Nuts, Unsalted
- ¼ Cup Coconut Oil / ¼ Cup Butter
- 2 Teaspoons Vanilla Extract, Sugar Free
- 20 Drops Liquid Stevia
- 2 Tablespoons Erythritol, Powdered

DIRECTIONS
1. Pulse your macadamia nuts in a blender, and then combine all of your ingredients together. Mix well.
2. Get out mini muffin tins with a tablespoon and a half of the mixture.
3. Refrigerate it for a half hour before serving.

NUTRITIONAL FACTS: Calories: 125 Fat: 5 Carbohydrates: 5

532. MARINATED EGGS.

PREPARATION: 2H 10' **COOKING:** 7' **SERVES:** 4

INGREDIENTS
- 6 eggs
- 1 and ¼ cups water
- ¼ cup unsweetened rice vinegar 2 tablespoons coconut aminos
- Salt and black pepper to the taste 2 garlic cloves, minced
- 1 teaspoon stevia 4 ounces cream cheese
- 1 tablespoon chives, chopped

DIRECTIONS
1. Put the eggs in a pot, add water to cover, bring to a boil over medium heat, cover and cook for 7 minutes.
2. Rinse eggs with cold water and leave them aside to cool down.
3. In a bowl, mix 1 cup water with coconut aminos, vinegar, stevia and garlic and whisk well.
4. Put the eggs in this mix, cover with a kitchen towel and leave them aside for 2 hours rotating from time to time.
5. Peel eggs, cut in halves and put egg yolks in a bowl.
6. Add ¼ cup water, cream cheese, salt, pepper and chives and stir well.
7. Stuff egg whites with this mix and serve them.
8. Enjoy!

NUTRITIONAL FACTS: Calories: 289 kcal Protein: 15.86 g Fat: 22.62 g Carbohydrates: 4.52 g Sodium: 288 mg

533. SAUSAGE AND CHEESE DIP.

PREPARATION: 10' **COOKING:** 130' **SERVES:** 28

INGREDIENTS

- 8 ounces cream cheese
- A pinch of salt and black pepper
- 16 ounces sour cream
- 8 ounces pepper jack cheese, chopped
- 15 ounces canned tomatoes mixed with habaneros
- 1 pound Italian sausage, ground
- ¼ cup green onions, chopped

DIRECTIONS

1. Heat up a pan over medium heat, add sausage, stir and cook until it browns.
2. Add tomatoes mix, stir and cook for 4 minutes more.
3. Add a pinch of salt, pepper and the green onions, stir and cook for 4 minutes.
4. Spread pepper jack cheese on the bottom of your slow cooker.
5. Add cream cheese, sausage mix and sour cream, cover and cook on High for 2 hours.
6. Uncover your slow cooker, stir dip, transfer to a bowl and serve.
7. Enjoy!

NUTRITIONAL FACTS: Calories: 132 kcal Protein: 6.79 g Fat: 9.58 g Carbohydrates: 6.22 g Sodium: 362 mg

534. TASTY ONION AND CAULIFLOWER DIP.

PREPARATION: 20' **COOKING:** 30' **SERVES:** 24

INGREDIENTS

- 1 and ½ cups chicken stock
- 1 cauliflower head, florets separated
- ¼ cup mayonnaise
- ½ cup yellow onion, chopped
- ¾ cup cream cheese
- ½ teaspoon chili powder
- ½ teaspoon cumin, ground
- ½ teaspoon garlic powder
- Salt and black pepper to the taste

DIRECTIONS

1. Put the stock in a pot, add cauliflower and onion, heat up over medium heat and cook for 30 minutes.
2. Add chili powder, salt, pepper, cumin and garlic powder and stir.
3. Also add cream cheese and stir a bit until it melts.
4. Blend using an immersion blender and mix with the mayo.
5. Transfer to a bowl and keep in the fridge for 2 hours before you serve it.
6. Enjoy!

NUTRITIONAL FACTS: Calories: 40 kcal Protein: 1.23 g Fat: 3.31 g Carbohydrates: 1.66 g Sodium: 72 mg

535. PESTO CRACKERS.

PREPARATION: 10'   COOKING: 17'   SERVES: 6

INGREDIENTS
- ½ teaspoon baking powder
- Salt and black pepper to the taste
- 1 and ¼ cups almond flour ¼ teaspoon basil, dried 1 garlic clove, minced
- 2 tablespoons basil pesto
- A pinch of cayenne pepper
- 3 tablespoons ghee

DIRECTIONS
1. In a bowl, mix salt, pepper, baking powder and almond flour.
2. Add garlic, cayenne and basil and stir.
3. Add pesto and whisk.
4. Also add ghee and mix your dough with your finger.
5. Spread this dough on a lined baking sheet, introduce in the oven at 325 degrees F and bake for 17 minutes.
6. Leave aside to cool down, cut your crackers and serve them as a snack.
7. Enjoy!

NUTRITIONAL FACTS: Calories: 9 kcal Protein: 0.41 g Fat: 0.14 g Carbohydrates: 1.86 g Sodium: 2 mg

536. PUMPKIN MUFFINS.

PREPARATION: 10'   COOKING: 15'   SERVES: 18

INGREDIENTS
- ¼ cup sunflower seed butter
- ¾ cup pumpkin puree 2 tablespoons flaxseed meal ¼ cup coconut flour
- ½ cup erythritol ½ teaspoon nutmeg, ground
- 1 teaspoon cinnamon, ground ½ teaspoon baking soda 1 egg ½ teaspoon baking powder
- A pinch of salt

DIRECTIONS
1. In a bowl, mix butter with pumpkin puree and egg and blend well.
2. Add flaxseed meal, coconut flour, erythritol, baking soda, baking powder, nutmeg, cinnamon and a pinch of salt and stir well.
3. Spoon this into a greased muffin pan, introduce in the oven at 350 degrees F and bake for 15 minutes.
4. Leave muffins to cool down and serve them as a snack.
5. Enjoy!

NUTRITIONAL FACTS: Calories: 65 kcal Protein: 2.82 g Fat: 5.42 g Carbohydrates: 2.27 g Sodium: 57 mg

537. KETO CORNBREAD

PREPARATION: 5' **COOKING:** 2' **SERVES:** 2

INGREDIENTS

- 1 ¾ oz. almond flour
- ¼ tsp baking powder
- 1/8 tsp salt
- 1 tbsp. melted butter
- 1 egg

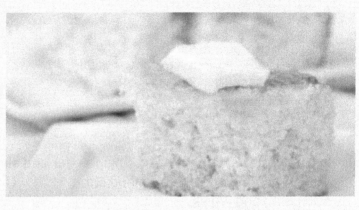

DIRECTIONS

1. Take a small bowl, place butter and egg in it, whisk until combined and then whisk in flour, baking powder, and salt until smooth batter comes together.
2. Take a small microwave proof container, spoon prepared batter in it, and then microwave for 1 minute and 45 seconds at high heat setting until cooked.
3. When done, cut bread into slices, then spread with butter and serve.

NUTRITIONAL FACTS: 116.2 Calories; 10.4 g Fats; 4.3 g Protein; 1.1 g Net Carb; 1.5 g Fiber;

538. FLAX SEED BREAD SANDWICH

PREPARATION: 10' **COOKING:** 10' **SERVES:** 2

INGREDIENTS

- 4 oz. ground flaxseed
- 2 tsp coconut flour
- ½ tsp baking soda
- 1 tsp apple cider vinegar
- 2 tbsp. almond milk, unsweetened

Seasoning:
- ¼ tsp sesame seeds
- ¼ tsp pumpkin seeds
- ¼ tsp sunflower seeds
- Peanut butter for serving

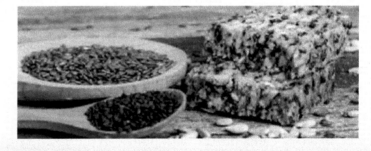

DIRECTIONS

1. Take a medium bowl, place flaxseed in it, add flour, baking soda, vinegar, and milk and mix by using hand until smooth dough ball comes together.
2. Take a shallow dish, place sesame seeds, pumpkin seeds and sunflower seeds in it and then stir until mixed.
3. Divide dough ball into two pieces, roll each piece into a loaf and then press into seed mixture until evenly coated on both sides.
4. Place dough onto a heatproof plate, microwave for 1 minute and then cool breads for 5 minutes.
5. Slice each bread into half, then spread with peanut butter and serve.

NUTRITIONAL FACTS: 191 Calories; 15.1 g Fats; 4.8 g Protein; 1.2 g Net Carb; 7.1 g Fiber

539. CHEESY JALAPENO CORNBREAD

PREPARATION: 5'   COOKING: 2'   SERVES: 2

INGREDIENTS
- 1 jalapeno pepper, chopped
- 1 ¾ oz. almond flour
- ¼ tsp baking powder
- 1 egg
- 1 tbsp. grated parmesan cheese

Seasoning:
- 1 tbsp. melted butter
- 1/8 tsp salt
- 1/8 tsp ground black pepper

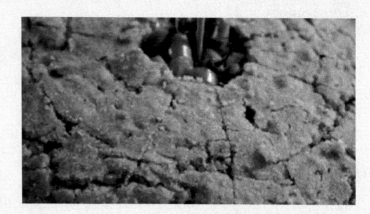

DIRECTIONS
1. Take a small bowl, place butter and egg in it, whisk until combined, and then whisk in remaining ingredients until smooth batter comes together.
2. Take a small microwave proof container, spoon prepared batter in it, and then microwave for 1 minute and 45 seconds at high heat setting until cooked.
3. When done, cut bread into slices, then spread with butter and serve.

NUTRITIONAL FACTS: 131 Calories; 11.1 g Fats; 4.8 g Protein; 1.1 g Net Carb; 0.9 g Fiber;

540. CHEESE CUP

PREPARATION: 5'   COOKING: 5'   SERVES: 2

INGREDIENTS
- 4 tsp coconut flour
- 1/16 tsp baking soda
- 1 tbsp. grated mozzarella cheese
- 1 tbsp. grated parmesan cheese
- 2 eggs

Seasoning:
- ¼ tsp salt
- ½ tsp dried basil
- ½ tsp dried parsley

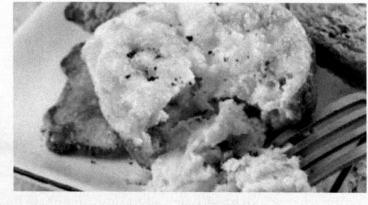

DIRECTIONS
1. Take a medium bowl, place all the ingredients in it, and whisk until well combined.
2. Take two ramekins, grease them with oil, distribute the prepared batter in it and then microwave for 1 minute and 45 seconds until done.
3. When done, take out muffin from the ramekin, cut in half, and then serve.

NUTRITIONAL FACTS: 125 Calories; 8.1 g Fats; 9.5 g Protein; 1.1 g Net Carb; 1.7 g Fiber;

541. CINNAMON MUG CAKE

PREPARATION: 5' **COOKING:** 5' **SERVES:** 2

INGREDIENTS
- 3 tbsp. almond flour
- 1 tbsp. erythritol sweetener
- 3 tbsp. butter, unsalted
- 2 tbsp. cream cheese
- 1 egg

Seasoning:
- 1 tsp baking soda
- ¾ tsp cinnamon

DIRECTIONS
1. Take a heatproof mug, place 2 tbsp. butter in it, and then microwave for 30 seconds or more until butter melts.
2. Then add remaining ingredients, reserving cream cheese and remaining butter, stir until mixed and microwave for 1 minute and 20 seconds until done.
3. Run a knife along the side of the mug and then take out the cake.
4. Melt the remaining butter, top it over the cake, then top with cream cheese, cut cake in half, and serve.

NUTRITIONAL FACTS: 298 Calories; 28.8 g Fats; 6.7 g Protein; 1.3 g Net Carb; 1.7 g Fiber;

542. SPICY DOSA

PREPARATION: 5' **COOKING:** 8' **SERVES:** 2

INGREDIENTS
- oz. almond flour
- ½ tsp ground cumin
- ½ tsp ground coriander
- oz. grated mozzarella cheese
- 4 oz. coconut milk, unsweetened

Seasoning:
- ¼ tsp salt
- 2 tsp avocado oil

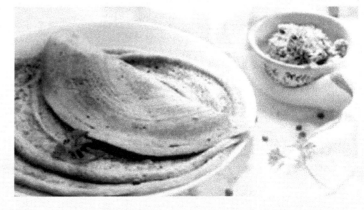

DIRECTIONS
1. Take a medium bowl, place all the ingredients in it except for oil, and stir until well combined and smooth batter comes together.
2. Take a medium skillet pan, place it over medium heat, add 1 tsp oil and when hot, pour in half of the prepared batter, spread it evenly in a circular shape, then switch heat to the low level and cook for 2 minutes per side until golden brown and cooked.
3. Transfer dosa to a plate, then repeat with the remaining batter and serve.

NUTRITIONAL FACTS: 181 Calories; 16.5 g Fats; 6 g Protein; 2 g Net Carb; 0 g Fiber;

543. GARLIC CHEESE BALLS

PREPARATION: 10' COOKING: 0' SERVES: 2

INGREDIENTS
- 2 bacon sliced, cooked, chopped
- ½ tsp minced garlic
- 2 oz. cream cheese, softened
- 2 tbsp. sour cream
- 3 tbsp. grated parmesan cheese

Seasoning:
- ½ tsp Italian seasoning

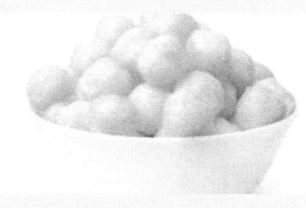

DIRECTIONS
1. Take a medium bowl, place cheese in it, then add remaining ingredients except for bacon and stir until mixed.
2. Cover the bowl, let it refrigerate for 1 hour until chilled, and then shape the mixture into four balls.
3. Roll the balls in chopped bacon until coated, refrigerate for 30 minutes until firm, and then serve.

NUTRITIONAL FACTS: 335 Calories; 28.7 g Fats; 12.4 g Protein; 5.8 g Net Carb; 0 g Fiber;

544. CHEDDAR AND GREEN ONION BISCUITS

PREPARATION: 5' COOKING: 8' SERVES: 2

INGREDIENTS
- 1 tsp chopped green onion
- 2 ½ tbsp. coconut flour
- 2 ½ tbsp. melted butter, unsalted
- 2 oz. grated cheddar cheese
- 1 egg
- ¼ tsp salt
- 1/8 tsp ground black pepper

Seasoning:
- 1/8 tsp baking powder
- ½ tsp garlic powder

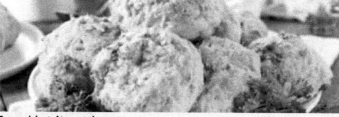

DIRECTIONS
1. Turn on the oven, then set it to 400 degrees F and let it preheat.
2. Take a medium bowl, place flour in it, and then stir in garlic powder, baking powder, salt, and black pepper.
3. Take a separate medium bowl, crack the egg in it, whisk in butter until blended, and then whisk this mixture into the flour until incorporated and smooth.
4. Fold in green onion and cheese, then drop the mixture in the form of mounds onto a cookie sheet greased with oil and bake for 8 minutes until lightly browned.
5. When done, brush biscuit with some more melted butter and then serve.

NUTRITIONAL FACTS: 272 Calories; 23 g Fats; 11.5 g Protein; 4.5 g Net Carb; 0.7 g Fiber;

545. BASIL WRAPPED CHEESE BALLS

PREPARATION: 10' COOKING: 0' SERVES: 2

INGREDIENTS
- 2 oz. grated cheddar cheese
- 3 oz. grated mozzarella cheese
- 3 oz. grated parmesan cheese
- ¼ tsp ground black pepper
- 8 basil leaves

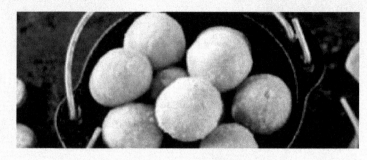

DIRECTIONS
1. Take a medium bowl, place all the cheeses in it, add black pepper, stir until blended, then cover the bowl and let it refrigerate for 30 minutes until firm.
2. Then shape the mixture into 1-inch long eight balls, then place each ball on the wide end of a basil leaf and roll it up.
3. Serve immediately.

NUTRITIONAL FACTS: 428 Calories; 31.4 g Fats; 28.9 g Protein; 7.5 g Net Carb; 0 g Fiber;

546. DOUBLE CHEESE CHIPS

PREPARATION: 10' COOKING: 10' SERVES: 2

INGREDIENTS
- 3 oz. grated cheddar cheese
- 5 oz. grated parmesan cheese
- 1/8 tsp onion powder
- 1/8 tsp ground cumin
- 1/8 tsp red chili powder

Seasoning:
- 1/8 tsp salt

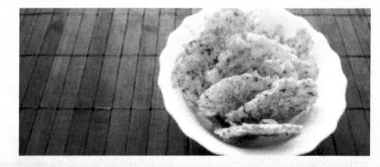

DIRECTIONS
1. Turn on the oven, then set it to 400 degrees F and let it preheat.
2. Take a medium bowl, place cheeses in it, add salt, onion powder, cumin, and red chili powder and stir until mixed.
3. Take a baking pan, line it with parchment paper, spread cheese mixture on it in an even layer, and then bake for 10 minutes until cheese has melted and begin to crisp.
4. When done, remove the baking pan from the oven, let it cool completely and then cut it into triangles.
5. Serve.

NUTRITIONAL FACTS: 468 Calories; 34.2 g Fats; 30.3 g Protein; 9.3 g Net Carb; 0 g Fiber;

547. BACON CAPRESE WITH PARMESAN

PREPARATION: 5' **COOKING:** 8' **SERVES:** 2

INGREDIENTS

- 2 slices of bacon
- 2 Roma tomato, sliced
- 1 tsp balsamic vinegar
- 2 tbsp. avocado oil
- 1 tbsp. grated parmesan cheese

Seasoning:
- ½ tsp salt
- ½ tsp ground black pepper

DIRECTIONS

1. Take a frying pan, place it over medium heat and when hot, add bacon and cook for 3 to 4 minutes until crispy.
2. Transfer bacon to a cutting board, let it cool for 5 minutes and then chop it.
3. Turn on the broiler and let it preheat.
4. Take a medium baking sheet, line it with aluminum foil, spray with oil, spread tomato slices on it, and then drizzle with vinegar and oil.
5. Season with salt and black pepper, sprinkle with cheese and bacon and then broil tomatoes for 1 to 2 minutes until cheese has melted.
6. Serve.

NUTRITIONAL FACTS: 355 Calories; 28 g Fats; 18.6 g Protein; 5.7 g Net Carb; 2.3 g Fiber;

548. EGG MCMUFFIN SANDWICH WITH AVOCADO AND BACON

PREPARATION: 10' **COOKING:** 15' **SERVES:** 62

INGREDIENTS

- 2 eggs, yolks and egg whites separated
- 1/3 cup grated parmesan cheese
- 2 oz. cream cheese, softened
- 2 slices of bacon
- ½ of avocado, sliced

Seasoning:
- 2/3 tsp salt
- 1 tsp avocado oil

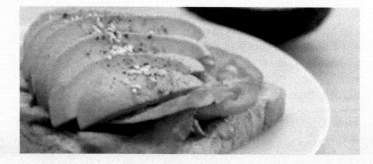

DIRECTIONS

1. Take a medium bowl, place egg yolks in it, add cream cheese, parmesan, and salt and whisk by using an electric blender until smooth.
2. Take another medium bowl, add egg whites, beat until stiff peaks form and then fold egg whites into egg yolk mixture until combined.
3. Take a skillet pan, place it over medium heat, add oil and when hot, add one-fourth of the batter, spread it into a 1-inch thick pancake, and then fry got 2 minutes per side until golden brown.
4. When done, let sandwiches cool for 5 minutes, top two muffins with bacon and avocado slices, cover the top with another muffin, and then serve as desired.

NUTRITIONAL FACTS: 355 Calories; 28 g Fats; 18.6 g Protein; 5.7 g Net Carb; 2.3 g Fiber;

549. HOT RED CHILI AND GARLIC CHUTNEY

PREPARATION: 25' **COOKING:** 15' **SERVES:** 1

INGREDIENTS
- Red chilies, dried – 14
- Minced garlic – 5 teaspoons
- Salt – 1/8 teaspoon
- Water – 1 and ¼ cups

DIRECTIONS
1. Place chilies in a bowl, pour in water and let rest for 20 minutes.
2. Then drain red chilies, chop them and add to a blender.
3. Add remaining ingredients into the blender and pulse for 1 to 2 minutes until smooth.
4. Tip the sauce into a bowl and serve straight away.

NUTRITIONAL FACTS: calories: 100, fat: 1, fiber: 2, carbs: 6, protein: 7

550. RED CHILIES AND ONION CHUTNEY

PREPARATION: 15' **COOKING:** 15' **SERVES:** 2

INGREDIENTS
- Medium white onion, peeled and chopped – 1
- Minced garlic – 1 teaspoon
- Red chilies, chopped – 2
- Salt – ¼ teaspoon
- Sweet paprika – 1 teaspoon
- Avocado oil – 2 teaspoons
- Water – ¼ cup

DIRECTIONS
1. Place a medium skillet pan over medium-high heat, add oil and when hot, add onion, garlic, and chilies.
2. Cook onions for 5 minutes or until softened, then season with salt and paprika and pour in water.
3. Stir well and cook for 5 minutes.
4. Then spoon the chutney into a bowl and serve.

NUTRITIONAL FACTS: calories: 121, fat: 2, fiber: 6, carbs: 9, protein: 5

551. FAST GUACAMOLE

PREPARATION: 10'   **COOKING:** 15'   **SERVES:** 2

INGREDIENTS

- Medium avocados, peeled, pitted and cubed – 3
- Medium tomato, cubed – 1
- Chopped cilantro – ¼ cup
- Medium red onion, peeled and chopped – 1
- Salt – ½ teaspoon
- Ground white pepper – ¼ teaspoon
- Lime juice – 3 tablespoons

DIRECTIONS

1. Place all the ingredients for the salad in a medium bowl and stir until combined.
2. Serve guacamole straightaway as an appetizer.

NUTRITIONAL FACTS: calories: 87, fat: 4, fiber: 4, carbs: 8, protein: 2

552. COCONUT DILL DIP

PREPARATION: 10'   **COOKING:** 15'   **SERVES:** 10

INGREDIENTS

- Chopped white onion – 1 tablespoon
- Parsley flakes – 2 teaspoons
- Chopped dill – 2 teaspoons
- Salt – ¼ teaspoon
- Coconut cream – 1 cup
- Avocado mayonnaise – ½ cup

DIRECTIONS

1. Place all the ingredients for the dip in a medium bowl and whisk until combined.
2. Serve the dip with vegetable sticks as a side dish.

NUTRITIONAL FACTS: Calories: 102, fat: 3, fiber: 1, carbs: 2, protein: 2

553. CREAMY MANGO AND MINT DIP

PREPARATION: 10' **COOKING:** 15' **SERVES:** 4

INGREDIENTS

- Medium green chili, chopped – 1
- Medium white onion, peeled and chopped – 1
- Grated ginger – 1 tablespoon
- Minced garlic – 1 teaspoon
- Salt – 1/8 teaspoon
- Ground black pepper – 1/8 teaspoon
- Cumin powder – 1 teaspoon
- Mango powder – 1 teaspoon
- Mint leaves – 2 cups
- Coriander leaves – 1 cup
- Cashew yogurt – 4 tablespoons

DIRECTIONS

1. Place all the ingredients for the dip in a blender and pulse for 1 to 2 minutes or until smooth.
2. Tip the dip into small cups and serve straightaway.

NUTRITIONAL FACTS: calories: 100, fat: 2, fiber: 3, carbs: 7, protein: 5

554. CREAMY CRAB DIP

PREPARATION: 5' **COOKING:** 10' **SERVES:** 12

INGREDIENTS

- Crab meat, chopped – 1 pound
- Chopped white onion – 2 tablespoons
- Minced garlic – 1 tablespoon
- Lemon juice – 2 tablespoons
- Cream cheese, cubed – 16 ounces
- Avocado mayonnaise – 1/3 cup
- Grape juice – 2 tablespoons

DIRECTIONS

1. Place all the ingredients for the dip in a medium bowl and stir until combined.
2. Divide dip evenly between small bowls and serve as a party dip.

NUTRITIONAL FACTS: Calories: 100, Fat: 4, Fiber: 1, Carbs: 4, Protein: 4

555. CREAMY CHEDDAR AND BACON SPREAD WITH ALMONDS

PREPARATION: 10'   **COOKING:** 10'   **SERVES:** 12

INGREDIENTS

- Bacon, cooked and chopped – 12 ounces
- Chopped sweet red pepper – 2 tablespoons
- Medium white onion, peeled and chopped – 1
- Salt – ¾ teaspoon
- Ground black pepper – ½ teaspoon
- Almonds, chopped – ½ cup
- Cheddar cheese, grated – 1 pound
- Avocado mayonnaise – 2 cups

DIRECTIONS

1. Place all the ingredients for the dip in a medium bowl and stir until combined.
2. Divide dip evenly between small bowls and serve as a party dip.

NUTRITIONAL FACTS: calories: 184, fat: 12, fiber: 1, carbs: 4, protein: 5

556. GREEN TABASCO DEVILLED EGGS

PREPARATION: 20'   **COOKING:** 10'   **SERVES:** 6

INGREDIENTS

- 6 Eggs
- 1/3 cup Mayonnaise
- 1 ½ tbsp. Green Tabasco
- Salt and Pepper, to taste

DIRECTIONS

1. Place the eggs in a saucepan over medium heat and pour boiling water over, enough to cover them.
2. Cook for 6-8 minutes.
3. Place in an ice bath to cool.
4. When safe to handle, peel the eggs and slice them in half.
5. Scoop out the yolks and place in a bowl.
6. Add the remaining ingredients.
7. Whisk to combine.
8. Fill the egg holes with the mixture.
9. Serve and enjoy!

NUTRITIONAL FACTS: Calories 175 Total Fats 17g Net Carbs: 5g Protein 6g Fiber: 1g

557. HERBED CHEESE BALLS

PREPARATION: 30' **COOKING:** 10' **SERVES:** 20

INGREDIENTS

- 1/3 cup grated Parmesan Cheese
- 3 tbsp. Heavy Cream
- 4 tbsp. Butter, melted
- ¼ tsp Pepper
- 2 Eggs
- 1 cup Almond Flour
- ¼ cup Basil Leaves
- ¼ cup Parsley Leaves
- 2 tbsp. chopped Cilantro Leaves
- 1/3 cup crumbled Feta Cheese

DIRECTIONS

1. Place the ingredients in your food processor.
2. Pulse until the mixture becomes smooth.
3. Transfer to a bowl and freeze for 20 minutes or so, to set.
4. Shale the mixture into 20 balls.
5. Meanwhile, preheat the oven to 350 degrees F.
6. Arrange the cheese balls on a lined baking sheet.
7. Place in the oven and bake for 10 minutes.
8. Serve and enjoy!

NUTRITIONAL FACTS: Calories 60 Total Fats 5g Net Carbs: 8g Protein 2g Fiber: 1g

558. CHEESY SALAMI SNACK

PREPARATION: 30' **COOKING:** 10' **SERVES:** 6

INGREDIENTS

- 4 ounces Cream Cheese
- 7 ounces dried Salami
- ¼ cup chopped Parsley

DIRECTIONS

1. Preheat the oven to 325 degrees F.
2. Slice the salami thinly (I got 30 slices).
3. Arrange the salami on a lined sheet and bake for 15 minutes.
4. Arrange on a serving platter and top each salami slice with a bit of cream cheese.
5. Serve and enjoy!

NUTRITIONAL FACTS: Calories 139 Total Fats 15g Net Carbs: 1g Protein 9g Fiber: 0g

559. PESTO & OLIVE FAT BOMBS

PREPARATION: 25' COOKING: 10' SERVES: 8

INGREDIENTS
- 1 cup Cream Cheese
- 10 Olives, sliced
- 2 tbsp. Pesto Sauce
- ½ cup grated Parmesan Cheese

DIRECTIONS
1. Place all of the ingredients in a bowl.
2. Stir well to combine.
3. Place in the freezer and freeze for 15-20 minutes, to set.
4. Shape into 8 balls.
5. Serve and enjoy!

NUTRITIONAL FACTS: Calories 123 Total Fats 13g Net Carbs: 3g Protein 4g Fiber: 3g

560. CHEESY BROCCOLI NUGGETS

PREPARATION: 25' COOKING: 10' SERVES: 4

INGREDIENTS
- 1 cup shredded Cheese
- ¼ cup Almond Flour
- 2 cups Broccoli Florets, steamed in the microwave for 5 minutes
- 2 Egg Whites
- Salt and Pepper, to taste

DIRECTIONS
1. Preheat the oven to 350 degrees F.
2. Place the broccoli florets in a bowl and mash them with a potato masher.
3. Add the remaining ingredients and mix well with your hands, until combined.
4. Line a baking sheet with parchment paper.
5. Drop 20 scoops of the mixture onto the sheet.
6. Place in the oven and bake for 20 minutes or until golden.
7. Serve and enjoy!

NUTRITIONAL FACTS: Calories 145 Total Fats 9g Net Carbs: 4g Protein 10g Fiber: 1g

561. SALMON FAT BOMBS

PREPARATION: 90' **COOKING:** 50' **SERVES:** 6

INGREDIENTS

- ½ cup Cream Cheese
- 1 ½ tbsp. chopped Dill
- 1 ¾ ounces Smoked Salmon, sliced
- 1 tbsp. Lemon Juice
- 1/3 cup Butter
- ¼ tsp Red Pepper Flakes
- ¼ tsp Garlic Powder
- Pinch of Salt
- ¼ tsp Pepper

DIRECTIONS

1. Place the butter, salmon, lemon juice, and cream cheese, in your food processor.
2. Add the seasonings.
3. Pulse until smooth.
4. Drop spoonfuls of the mixture onto a lined dish.
5. Sprinkle with the dill.
6. Place in the fridge for about 80 minutes.
7. Serve and enjoy!

NUTRITIONAL FACTS: Calories 145 Total Fats 16g Net Carbs: 7g Protein 3g Fiber: 1g

562. GUACAMOLE BACON BOMBS

PREPARATION: 30' **COOKING:** 10' **SERVES:** 6

INGREDIENTS

- 1 tsp minced Garlic
- ¼ cup Butter
- ½ Avocado, flesh scooped out
- 1 tbsp. Lime Juice
- 1 tbsp. chopped Cilantro
- 4 Bacon Slices, cooked and crumbled
- 3 tbsp. diced Shallots
- Salt and Pepper, to taste
- 1 tbsp. minced Jalapeno

DIRECTIONS

1. Place all of the ingredients, except the bacon, in your food processor.
2. Pulse until smooth. Alternatively, you can do this by whisking in a bowl. Just keep in mind that this way you will have chunks of garlic and jalapenos.
3. Transfer to a bowl and place in the freezer.
4. Freeze for 20 minutes, or until set.
5. Shape into 6 balls.
6. Coat them with bacon pieces.
7. Serve and enjoy!

NUTRITIONAL FACTS: Calories 155 Total Fats 15g Net Carbs: 4g Protein 4g Fiber: 3g

CHAPTER 26.
DESSERTS

563. SOUTHERN APPLE PIE

PREPARATION: 15' **COOKING:** 40' **SERVES:** 8

INGREDIENTS

Crust:
- 2 cups blanched almond flour
- ½ cup butter
- ½ cup powdered Erythritol
- 1 teaspoon allspice

Filling:
- 3 cups sliced apples
- ¼ cup melted butter
- ½ lemon, juiced
- ¼ cup powdered Erythritol
- ½ teaspoon allspice

Topping:
- Cinnamon, as desired
- Granulated Erythritol, as desired

DIRECTIONS

1. Prepare the crust; preheat oven to 375F.
2. Melt the butter in a microwave safe bowl.
3. Combine almond flour, melted butter, and remaining crust ingredients until the dough comes together.
4. Press the crust into 9-inch springform.
5. Cover the crust with parchment paper and baking balls (or rice) and bake 10 minutes.
6. In the meantime, make the filling; toss the sliced apples with juice.
7. Remove the crust from the oven. Fill with the apples in a circular pattern.
8. Combine butter, Erythritol, and allspice in a bowl.
9. Pour over the apples.
10. Bake the pie for 30 minutes.
11. Remove the pie from the oven and allow to cool.
12. Combine desired amounts of cinnamon and Erythritol.
13. Sprinkle the apples with the cinnamon mixture.
14. Slice and serve.

NUTRITIONAL FACTS: Calories 123, Fat 9.2g, Carbs 4.8g, Protein 8.3g

564. LEMON CHEESECAKE

PREPARATION: 15' **COOKING:** 25' **SERVES:** 12

INGREDIENTS

Crust:
- 2 teaspoons granulated Erythritol
- 2 cups almond flour
- ½ cup unsalted melted butter
- ¼ cup desiccated coconut

Filling:
- 1 tablespoon powdered gelatin
- 2 tablespoons granulated Erythritol
- ¾ cup boiling water
- ½ cup cold water
- 1lb. cream cheese
- 2 lemons, zested and juice

DIRECTIONS

1. Prepare the crust; combine the crust ingredients in a large mixing bowl.
2. Stir until the dough comes together.
3. Transfer the dough into 9-inch springform.
4. Place in a fridge while you make the filling.
5. Prepare the filling; pour the water in a bowl. Sprinkle over the gelatin powder. Pour in cold water and place aside for 5 minutes.
6. Beat cream cheese, gelatin mixture, Erythritol, lemon juice and zest in a mixing bowl.
7. Pour the filling over the crust.
8. Refrigerate for 2 hours.
9. Slice and serve.

NUTRITIONAL FACTS: Calories 143, Fat 9.2g, Carbs 4.8g, Protein 8.3g

565. NO-GUILT CHOCOLATE CAKE

PREPARATION: 15' + INACTIVE TIME **COOKING:** 25' **SERVES:** 8

INGREDIENTS

- ¾ cup butter
- 12oz. sugar-free quality dark chocolate, chopped or chocolate chips
- 1 teaspoon sugar-free vanilla extract
- 3 large eggs, room temperature
- 1 pinch salt
- ¼ cup granulated Erythritol
- 10 drops liquid Stevia

DIRECTIONS

1. Preheat oven to 350F.
2. Line 8-inch springform pan with baking paper. Additionally, grease with some coconut oil for easy removal.
3. Melt butter and chopped chocolate over a double boiler.
4. Remove from the heat and pour the mixture into a large bowl.
5. Beat in vanilla and salt.
6. Beat in the eggs, one at the time, and beating well after each addition.
7. Fold in the sweetener.
8. Strain the mixture through a fine sieve into the prepared springform.
9. Gently tap the springform onto the kitchen counter.
10. Bake the cake for 25 minutes.
11. Cool the cake to room temperature and refrigerate for at least 8 hours.
12. Slice and serve, with a dollop of whipped coconut cream.

NUTRITIONAL FACTS: Calories 103, Fat 9.2g, Carbs 4.8g, Protein 8.3g

566. CHEESE BERRY PIE

PREPARATION: 15' **COOKING:** 25' **SERVES:** 8

INGREDIENTS

Crust:
- 1 cup coconut oil, solid
- 4 large eggs
- 1 pinch salt
- 1 ½ cups softened coconut flour
- 1 tablespoon cold water
- ½ teaspoon baking powder

Filling:
- 1 ½ cups fresh blueberries
- 2 tablespoons granulated Erythritol
- 1 cup cream cheese

DIRECTIONS

1. Preheat oven to 350F.
2. Make the crust; combine coconut flour, salt, and baking powder in a bowl.
3. Work in coconut oil.
4. Add eggs, one at the time until incorporated.
5. Add water and stir until you have a smooth dough. Divide the dough into two equal parts.
6. Transfer the one part into 9-inch pie pan. Roll out the second and place aside.
7. Prepare the filling; spread cream cheese over the crust.
8. Toss the blueberries with the Erythritol and spread over the cheese.
9. Top the pie with the remaining dough.
10. Bake the pie for 25 minutes.
11. Cool the pie on a rack for 10 minutes.
12. Slice and serve.

NUTRITIONAL FACTS: Calories 143, Fat 9.2g, Carbs 4.8g, Protein 8.3g

567. THE BEST COOKIES

PREPARATION: 15' **COOKING:** 10' **SERVES:** 6

INGREDIENTS

- 1/3 cup coconut oil
- 1 ½ teaspoon sugar-free vanilla extract
- 1 medium egg
- 1 pinch salt
- 3 tablespoons granulated Erythritol
- 1 cup almond flour
- 2 tablespoons coconut flour
- ½ teaspoon cinnamon
- 1/3 cup sugar-free quality dark chocolate chips

DIRECTIONS

1. Preheat oven to 350F. Line baking sheet with a parchment paper.
2. In a mixing bowl, beat egg with vanilla and Erythritol.
3. Melt the coconut oil and fold into the egg mixture.
4. Fold in the remaining ingredients and stir until the dough comes together.
5. Let the dough stand for 5 minutes.
6. Scoop the dough with a cookie scoop, onto the baking sheet.
7. Press gently with the back of your spoon to flatten.
8. Bake the cookies for 10 minutes.
9. Cool briefly on a wire rack before serving.
10. Serve with a cup of almond milk and enjoy.

NUTRITIONAL FACTS: Calories 143, Fat 9.2g, Carbs 4.8g, Protein 8.3

568. SALTY CARAMEL CAKE

PREPARATION: 15' **COOKING:** 25' **SERVES:** 10

INGREDIENTS

- 2 cups blanched almond flour
- 3 tablespoons coconut flour
- 2 tablespoons vanilla whey protein powder
- ¾ tablespoon baking powder
- 1/3 cup unsalted butter
- 1 pinch salt
- ½ cup granulated Erythritol
- 3 large eggs, room temperature
- 1 teaspoon sugar-free vanilla extract
- ½ cup unsweetened almond milk
- 2 cups sugar-free caramel sauce
- Sea salt flakes, for sprinkle

DIRECTIONS

1. Preheat oven to 325F.
2. Line 2 8-inch spring form pans with baking paper.
3. In a mixing bowl, combine all the dry ingredients, except the sweetener.
4. In a separate bowl, cream butter, and Erythritol.
5. Beat in eggs, one at the time, followed by vanilla and almond milk
6. Fold the liquid ingredients into the dry ones.
7. Divide the batter between two spring form pans.
8. Bake the sponges for 25 minutes or until the inserted toothpick comes out clean.
9. Place the sponges aside to cool.
10. Spread 1 ½ cups of the caramel sauce over one sponge. Top with the second sponge.
11. Pour the remaining caramel over the top.
12. Sprinkle the caramel with salt flakes. Refrigerate the cake for 1 hour. Slice and serve.

NUTRITIONAL FACTS: Calories 143, Fat 9.2g, Carbs 4.8g, Protein 8.3g

569. LUSCIOUS RED VELVET CAKE

PREPARATION: 20' **COOKING:** 25' **SERVES:** 10

INGREDIENTS

Cake:
- 1 cup granulated Erythritol
- ½ cup coconut flour
- ½ cup Swerve
- 2 tablespoons raw cocoa powder
- 6 large eggs, separated
- ½ cup melted and cooled butter
- 2 tablespoons crème Fraiche
- 1 tablespoon powdered red food coloring
- 1 teaspoon white vinegar
- 1 teaspoon sugar-free vanilla

Frosting:
- 4oz. cream cheese
- 4 tablespoons softened unsalted butter
- 2 cups Swerve
- 1 tablespoon heavy cream
- ½ teaspoon sugar-free vanilla extract

DIRECTIONS

1. Preheat oven to 350F.
2. Line 9-inch springform with a baking paper and grease with some coconut oil.
3. Combine all the dry ingredients in a large mixing bowl.
4. In a separate bowl, beat eggs, butter, crème Fraiche, vinegar, and vanilla.
5. Fold the liquid ingredients into the dry ones and stir until smooth.
6. Pour the batter into the springform.
7. Bake the cake for 25-30 minutes or until the inserted toothpick comes out clean.
8. Make the frosting; beat cream cheese and butter in a bowl until fluffy.
9. Add sugar and heavy cream.
10. Beat until smooth.
11. Remove the cake from the springform once completely cold.
12. Top with the frosting.
13. Refrigerate the cake for 30 minutes.
14. Slice and serve.

NUTRITIONAL FACTS: Calories 143, Fat 9.2g, Carbs 4.8g, Protein 8.3g

570. SOUTHERN PECAN PIE

PREPARATION: 15' **COOKING:** 50' **SERVES:** 10

INGREDIENTS

Crust:
- 3 cups blanched almond flour
- 4 large eggs, room temperature
- ½ cup unsalted melted butter
- ½ cup Swerve
- 1 good pinch salt

Filling:
- 1 cup coconut oil or butter
- ¾ cup golden Swerve
- ½ cup granulated Erythritol
- 1 ½ tablespoon sugar-free maple syrup
- 4 large eggs, room temperature
- 1 ½ cup pecans, chopped
- ¾ cup pecan halves
- 2 teaspoon vanilla-bourbon extract

DIRECTIONS

1. Preheat oven to 325F.
2. Grease 10-inch cast iron skillet with butter.
3. In a large mixing bowl, combine the crust ingredients until the smooth dough is formed.
4. Transfer the dough into the skillet and press so you cover the bottom and sides.
5. Prepare the filling; melt butter in a saucepot and fold in sweeteners and sugar-free maple syrup. Stir until the sweeteners are dissolved. Place aside to cool.
6. Beat the eggs with cold syrup until fluffy. Fold in pecan pieces.
7. Pour the sauce into the crust.
8. Top with pecan halves.
9. Cover the pie with an aluminum foil. Bake the pie for 40 minutes.
10. Cool before slicing and serving.

NUTRITIONAL FACTS: Calories 143, Fat 9.2g, Carbs 4.8g, Protein 8.3g

571. PEPPERONI PIZZA CUPS

PREPARATION: 10' **COOKING:** 8' **SERVES:** 24

INGREDIENTS

- 24 mini mozzarella balls
- 24 small basil leaves
- 24 pepperoni slices in sandwich style
- sliced black olives, optional
- 1 small jar pizza sauce

DIRECTIONS

1. Preheat oven to 400°F, in the meantime take each pepperonis slice and make half inch cuts at the edges, giving it a shape of circular cross. Make sure that the center remains uncut.
2. Take the muffin pan, grease it with oil and adjust all the prepared pepperonis into it.
3. Place in the preheated oven and bake for 5 minutes or until the edges get crispy and the color is still red.
4. Remove from the oven and set aside to cool for 5 minutes, then transfer to the paper towel, so that the excess oil gets absorbed.
5. Clean the pan with a paper towel and place the cups again into the pan.
6. Put basil leaf in the center of each pepperoni, then add ½ tsp pizza sauce, mozzarella ball and olive slice in the end.
7. Bake in the oven for another 3 minutes or until the time when cheese starts melting.
8. Remove from the oven and set aside to cool for 5 minutes before transferring to the serving plate.

NUTRITIONAL FACTS: Calories: 70 Fat: 6 Carbohydrates: 1 Protein: 32

572. WHITE PIZZA FRITTATA

PREPARATION: 10' **COOKING:** 30' **SERVES:** 8

INGREDIENTS

- 5 ounces mozzarella cheese
- 9 ounces bag frozen spinach
- 12 large eggs
- 4 tablespoons olive oil
- 1 ounce pepperoni
- ¼ teaspoon nutmeg
- 1 teaspoon minced garlic
- ½ cup grated parmesan cheese
- ½ cup fresh ricotta cheese
- Salt and pepper

DIRECTIONS

1. Preheat oven to 375°F in the meantime you are getting things ready.
2. Take the frozen spinach and microwave it for 3 minutes or until defrosted.
3. Squeeze the spinach using your hands to drain the excess water.
4. Take a large bowl, crack all the eggs into it, and add the spices and olive oil. Whisk them together until well blended.
5. Add the spinach, parmesan cheese and ricotta cheese and make sure that the spinach is added in small pieces. Mix together all the ingredients to prepare a good mixture.
6. Transfer the mixture to the skillet, sprinkle cheese at the top, and then add the pepperoni.
7. Place in the preheated oven and bake for 30 minutes or until the time you are satisfied.
8. Remove from the oven once baked properly and serve with a keto sauce you love.

NUTRITIONAL FACTS: Calories: 301 Fat: 25 Carbohydrates: 3 Protein: 18

573. WALNUT COOKIES

PREPARATION: 10'   COOKING: 15'   SERVES: 6

INGREDIENTS

- 1/4 cup coconut flour
- 8 tablespoon butter
- 1/2 cup erythritol
- 1 cup walnuts
- 1 teaspoon ground nutmeg
- 1 teaspoon vanilla extract

DIRECTIONS

1. Preheat oven to 325°F, and in the meantime take the baking sheet and line it with parchment paper.
2. Grind the walnuts in a food processor and keep pulsing until they are well ground.
3. Add the vanilla extract, erythritol, nutmeg and coconut floor to the ground walnuts in the food processor. Pulse again until all the ingredients are blended.
4. Put butter in the food processor in the form of small pieces and pulse until you get a soft and smooth mixture.
5. Make 16 balls on the baking sheet with the help of a cookie scooper and use your hands to press them to give them a cookie shape.
6. Place in the preheated oven and bake for 15 minutes or until you find the cookies well baked.
7. Remove from the oven once baked, set them aside for 15-20 minutes to cool.
8. Sprinkle some additional nutmeg over the delicious walnut cookies if you like before you serve them.

NUTRITIONAL FACTS: Calories: 340 Fat: 26 Carbohydrates: 3 Protein: 19

574. FATHEAD SAUSAGE ROLLS

PREPARATION: 15'   COOKING: 30'   SERVES: 6

INGREDIENTS

- 1 egg
- Pre-shredded grated mozzarella cheese (170g)
- 6 sausages (500g)
- Almond flour (85g)
- 2 tablespoon cream cheese full fat
- 1 teaspoon onion flakes
- Pinch salt to taste
- Onion flakes to garnish

DIRECTIONS

1. Preheat oven to 350°F and in the meantime remove the casing of all sausages and discard them.
2. Transfer the sausages to the lined baking pan.
3. Place in the preheated oven and bake for around 10 minutes.
4. Take a medium size bowl, add almond flour and cheese to it. Mix them together completely.
5. Add the cream cheese to the mixture, whisk until fully blended.
6. Microwave the mixture for 60 seconds and remove, then stir a bit and microwave again for 30 seconds, remove and stir.
7. Crack the egg into the mixture, add the onion flakes and salt. Keep mixing and pressing with a spoon to prepare a soft dough.
8. Spread the dough over a parchment paper, place another parchment paper at the top, press with your hands and give it a shape of rectangle using a roller. Make sure that you roll evenly on all sides to prepare a good fat head pastry.
9. Cut a piece of the prepared fat head pastry and wrap it around a sausage. Repeat it with all the remaining sausages.
10. Cut the wrapped sausage rolls in your desired sizes, transfer them to the baking sheet and sprinkle the sesame seeds over the top if you prefer.
11. Heat the oven to 425°F, and bake for 15 minutes or until you get a golden brown look.
12. Remove from the oven once baked, and serve with your favorite keto sauce.

NUTRITIONAL FACTS: Calories: 470 Fat: 39 Carbohydrates: 5 Protein: 26

575. CHIA SEED CRACKERS

PREPARATION: 5' **COOKING:** 35' **SERVES:** 8

INGREDIENTS

- 1/2 cup ground chia seeds
- 1 1/2 cups water
- 1/4 teaspoon paprika
- 1/4 teaspoon black pepper
- 1/4 teaspoon dried oregano
- 3 oz. shredded cheddar cheese
- 2 tablespoon almond meal
- 1/4 teaspoon garlic powder
- 4 tablespoon olive oil
- 1/4 teaspoon salt

DIRECTIONS

1. Preheat oven to 375°F and in the meantime take a large bowl and mix oregano, garlic powder, almond meal, paprika, chia seeds, salt and pepper. Mix together until all the ingredients are well combined.
2. Take the olive oil and pour into the mixture. Whisk until fully blended.
3. Pour water into the mixture and keep mixing until you see the smoothness.
4. Add the shredded cheddar cheese, mix it well with the mixture using a spatula and then prepare the dough kneading with your hands.
5. Spread the dough on a parchment paper in the baking sheet, cover with another parchment paper from the top and make it 0.125 inch thin with the help of a roller.
6. Place in the preheated oven and bake for 30 minutes.
7. Cut into the shapes you like after removing from the oven and place in the oven again to bake for 5 minutes more or until the time you are satisfied.
8. Remove from the oven once properly baked and transfer to the wire rack to cool before you serve the delicious chia seed crackers.

NUTRITIONAL FACTS: Calories: 120 Fat: 13 Carbohydrates: 2 Protein: 4

576. CHEESY BISCUITS

PREPARATION: 20' **COOKING:** 20' **SERVES:** 9

INGREDIENTS

- 4 eggs
- 2 cups almond flour
- 2 ½ cups shredded cheddar cheese
- 1/4 cup half-and-half
- 1 tablespoon baking powder

DIRECTIONS

1. Preheat oven to 350°F and get the baking sheet ready by lining it with parchment paper.
2. Take a large bowl and mix the baking powder and almond flour in that.
3. Add cheddar cheese to the mixture and mix until well combined.
4. Take a small bowl, add half and half and also crack the eggs into it. Mix well until fully blended.
5. Add the eggs mixture to the flour mixture and keep whisking with the help of a spatula to prepare a smooth batter.
6. Take portions of the batter using a scoop and put them on the baking sheet. Make sure that you take the portions in even sizes and flatten them a bit from the top.
7. Place in the preheated oven and bake for 20 minutes or until the time you get a golden-brown look.
8. Remove from the oven once baked and transfer to the wire rack to cool before serving.

NUTRITIONAL FACTS: Calories: 320 Fat: 27 Carbohydrates: 8 Protein: 15

577. CHICKEN ROLLS WITH PESTO

PREPARATION: 20'   COOKING: 30'   SERVES: 1

INGREDIENTS
- Tablespoon pine nuts
- Yeast tablets
- Garlic cloves (chopped)
- Fresh basil
- Olive oil
- Chicken breast ready to slice:

DIRECTIONS
1. Season with salt and pepper.
2. Place each piece of the chicken breast between 2 pieces of plastic wrap. 7 Roll in a frying pan or pasta until the chicken breasts grow out.
3. 0.6 cm thick.
4. Remove the plastic wrap, then apply pesto to the chicken.
5. Roll up the chicken breast and tie it with the cocktail skewers.
6. Season with salt and pepper.
7. Dissolve the coconut oil in the pan and use a high temperature to brown all sides of the chicken skin.
8. Place the chicken rolls on a baking sheet, place in the oven, and bake for 15 to 20 minutes, until cooked.
9. Slice it diagonally and serve it with other pesto sauce.
10. It was served with tomato salad.

NUTRITIONAL FACTS: Calories: 150, Sodium: 33 mg, Dietary Fibre: 1.6 g, Total Fat: 4.3 g, Total Carbs: 15.4 g, Protein: 1.6 g.

578. SWEET AND SOUR SAUCE:

PREPARATION: 10'   COOKING: 10'   SERVES: 1

INGREDIENTS
- Apple cider vinegar
- 1/2 tablespoon tomato paste
- A teaspoon of coconut amino acid
- Bamboo spoon
- Water treatment
- Chopped vegetables.

DIRECTIONS
1. Mix kudzu powder with five tablespoons of cold water to make a paste.
2. Then put all the other spices in the pot, then add the kudzu paste.
3. Melt coconut oil in a pan and fry onions.
4. Add green pepper, cabbage, cabbage and bean sprouts, then cook until the vegetables are tender.
5. Add pineapple and cashew nuts and mix a few times.
6. Just pour a little spice into the pot.

NUTRITIONAL FACTS: Calories: 3495, Sodium: 33 mg, Dietary Fibre: 1.4 g, Total Fat: 4.5 g, Total Carbs: 16.5 g, Protein: 1.7 g.

579. COCONUT CURRY CAULIFLOWER SOUP

PREPARATION: 10' **COOKING:** 25' **SERVES:** 10

INGREDIENTS

- 2 tablespoons olive oil
- 1 onion, chopped
- 3 tablespoons yellow curry paste
- 2 heads cauliflower, sliced into florets
- 32 oz. vegetable broth
- 1 cup coconut milk
- Minced fresh cilantro

DIRECTIONS

1. In a pan over medium heat, add the oil.
2. Cook onion for 3 minutes.
3. Stir in the curry paste and cook for 2 minutes.
4. Add the cauliflower florets.
5. Pour in the broth.
6. Increase the heat to high and bring to a boil.
7. Lower the heat to medium.
8. Cook while covered for 20 minutes.
9. Add the coconut milk and cook for an additional minute.
10. Puree in a blender.
11. Garnish with fresh cilantro.

NUTRITIONAL FACTS: Calories 138 Total Fat 11.8g Saturated Fat 5.6g Cholesterol 0mg Sodium 430mg Total Carbohydrate 6.4g Dietary Fiber 3g Total Sugars 2.8g Protein 3.6g Potassium 318mg

580. CHOCOLATE CAKE WITH VANILLA GLAZE

PREPARATION: 20' **COOKING:** 40' **SERVES:** 6

INGREDIENTS

- ½ cup almond flour
- 4 tbsp butter
- 3 tbsp stevia powder
- 5 large egg yolks
- 1 tsp agar powder
- ½ tsp salt
- 2 tbsp cocoa powder
- 1 tsp chocolate extract, unsweetened

For the glaze:
- 1 cup Mascarpone cheese
- 5 large egg whites
- 2 tbsp swerve
- 2 tsp vanilla extract
- Dark chocolate chips, optional

DIRECTIONS

1. Plug in the instant pot and pour 1 cup of water in the stainless-steel insert. Line a fitting springform pan with some parchment paper and set aside.
2. In a large mixing bowl, combine egg yolks and butter. Beat with a hand mixer for 2-3 minutes, or until well combined. Add stevia, agar powder, salt, and cocoa, Beat again for 2 minutes. Finally, add almond flour and beat again until fully combined.
3. Pour the mixture in the springform pan and gently flatten the surface with a spatula.
4. Set the trivet on the bottom of your pot and place the pan on the top. Close the lid and adjust the steam release handle. Press the "Manual" button and set the timer for 40 minutes. Cook on "High" pressure.
5. Meanwhile, combine all glaze ingredients and remaining egg whites in a large mixing bowl. Beat until well combined and set aside.
6. When you hear the cooker's end signal, perform a quick pressure release and open the pot. Transfer the pan to a wire rack and let it cool for 10 minutes.
7. Top the cake with glaze and spread evenly. Add ½ cup of water to the pot and return the pan on top of the trivet. Close the lid and adjust the steam release handle. Cook for 1 minutes on the "Manual" mode.
8. When done, perform a quick pressure release and open the pot.
9. Chill to a room temperature and refrigerate for 20 minutes before serving.
10. Optionally, top with some dark chocolate chips for some extra flavor.

NUTRITIONAL FACTS: Calories 263 Total Fats: 21.5g Net Carbs: 3.6g Protein: 12.3g Fiber: 1.6g

581. RUM TRUFFLES

PREPARATION: 20' **COOKING:** 30' **SERVES:** 5

INGREDIENTS

- ½ cup dark chocolate chips, melted
- 1 cup heavy cream
- ¼ cup granulated stevia
- ¼ tsp xanthan gum
- 3 egg yolks
- ½ cup whipped cream

Spices:
- ½ tsp rum extract
- ¼ tsp cinnamon, ground
- ½ tsp stevia powder

DIRECTIONS

1. In a mixing bowl, combine egg yolks, granulated stevia, and xanthan gum. Using a hand mixer, beat until well incorporated. Add heavy cream, melted chocolate chips, rum extract, cinnamon, and stevia powder. Beat for 1 more minute and then pour into oven-safe ramekins. Wrap the top of each ramekin with aluminum foil and set aside.
2. Plug in your instant pot and pour 1 cup of water in the stainless-steel insert. Position a trivet on the bottom and place ramekins on top. Close the lid and adjust the steam release handle. Press the "Manual" button and set the timer for 30 minutes. Cook on "High" pressure.
3. When you hear the cooker's end signal, release the pressure naturally. Open the pot and top with whipped cream and powdered stevia before serving.

NUTRITIONAL FACTS: Calories 208 Total Fats: 18.5g Net Carbs: 9.4g Protein: 3.2g Fiber: 0.1g

582. MINT CAKE

PREPARATION: 15' **COOKING:** 45' **SERVES:** 8

INGREDIENTS

For the layers:
- 1 cup almond flour
- 1 cup coconut flour
- 1 tbsp stevia powder
- ¼ cup whole milk

- 3 tbsp butter
- 5 large eggs
- 1 tsp vanilla extract
- ½ tsp salt

For the filling:
- ¼ cup butter
- ½ cup cream cheese
- 2 tsp stevia powder
- 1 tsp mint extract

DIRECTIONS

1. In a large mixing bowl, combine almond flour, coconut flour, stevia powder, and salt. Mix until combined and set aside.
2. In a separate bowl, combine eggs, butter, milk, and vanilla extract. Using a hand mixer, beat until fluffy and then gradually add to dry ingredients. Mix until all well incorporated. Set aside.
3. In another bowl, combine all filling ingredients. With a paddle attachment on, beat until well combined and set aside.
4. Pour 1 cup of water in the stainless steel of your instant pot. Line a fitting springform pan with some parchment paper. Set the trivet on the bottom of the pot and place the pan on top. Pour half of the layer mixture in the pan and close the lid. Adjust the steam release handle and press the "Manual" button. Set the timer for 20 minutes and cook on "High" pressure,
5. When you hear the cooker's end signal, perform a quick pressure release and open the pot. Transfer the layer to a wire rack to cool. Repeat the process with the remaining mixture.
6. When the second layer is done, spread the filling over and top with the remaining layer. Close the lid of your pot and adjust the steam release handle. Press the "Manual" button and set the timer for 5 minutes on "High" pressure.
7. When done, perform a quick pressure release and open the pot.
8. Chill to a room temperature before serving and optionally, garnish with some fresh mint.

NUTRITIONAL FACTS: Calories 398 Total Fats: 33.8g Net Carbs: 6.6g Protein: 10.5g Fiber: 7.5g

583. VANILLA CHERRY PANNA COTTA

PREPARATION: 10' **COOKING:** 5' **SERVES:** 2

INGREDIENTS

For the vanilla layer:
- 1 cup heavy whipping cream
- 2 tbsp whole milk
- 1 tsp agar powder
- ½ tsp vanilla extract
- 1 tbsp walnuts, roughly chopped

For the cherry layer:
- 1 cup heavy whipping cream
- 1 tsp agar powder
- 1 tbsp almonds, roughly chopped
- 2 tsp cherry extract

DIRECTIONS

1. Plug in the instant pot and combine all vanilla layer ingredients in the stainless-steel insert. Press the "Saute" button and stir constantly. Bring it to a light simmer and then press "Cancel" button. Transfer to a large bowl and set aside.
2. Clean the pot and pat-dry with a kitchen paper. Now, add all cherry layer ingredients and stir well. Again, bring it to a light simmer, stirring constantly.
3. Pour about ½-inch thick vanilla layer in a medium-sized glass. Now, add the second layer of the cherry mixture. Repeat the process until you have used both mixtures.
4. Optionally, garnish with some fresh mint and refrigerate for at least 1 hour before serving.

NUTRITIONAL FACTS: Calories 467 Total Fats: 48.7g Net Carbs: 4.6g Protein: 4.5g Fiber: 0.8g

584. KETO BERRY PANCAKES

PREPARATION: 5' **COOKING:** 15' **SERVES:** 10

INGREDIENTS
- 1/2 cup almond flour
- 4 pieces large eggs
- 4 ounces cream cheese (softened)
- 1 teaspoon lemon zest
- 1 tablespoon butter (for frying)
- 1 tablespoon butter (for topping)
- 1/2 cup of frozen berries

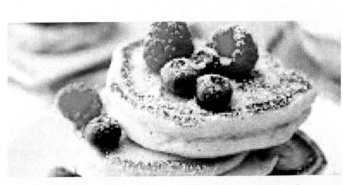

DIRECTIONS

1. In a mixing bowl, put in almond flour, eggs, cream cheese, and lemon zest. Whisk until the batter is well combined.
2. In a skillet over medium heat, melt the butter for frying.
3. Scoop about 3 tablespoons of batter and pour it on the skillet. Cook the pancake for about 2 minutes or until it turns golden.
4. Flip the pancake to its other side and cook it for another 2 minutes.
5. Transfer the cooked pancake to a plate. Continue cooking the rest of the batter.
6. Serve the pancakes topped with berries.

NUTRITIONAL FACTS: Calories: 110 Carbs: 2 g Fats: 10 g Proteins: 4 g Fiber: 1 g

585. MOCHA POTS DE CRÈME

PREPARATION: 10' **COOKING:** 15' **SERVES:** 4

INGREDIENTS

- 2 large eggs, separated
- 1 cup coconut milk, full-fat
- ¾ cup heavy cream
- 2 tbsp cocoa powder, unsweetened
- 3 tbsp brewed espresso
- 3 tbsp stevia powder

Spices:
- ¼ tsp salt
- 1 tsp vanilla extract

DIRECTIONS

1. In a small bowl, whisk together eggs, cocoa powder, espresso, stevia powder, vanilla, and salt. Set aside.
2. Plug in the instant pot and press the "Saute" button. Pour in the coconut milk and heavy cream. Give it a good stir and warm up.
3. Press the "Cancel" button and slowly pour the warm milk mixture over the egg mixture, whisking constantly.
4. Divide the mixture between 4 ramekins and loosely cover with aluminum foil.
5. Position a trivet at the bottom of your pot and pour in 2 cups of water. Gently place the ramekins on top and seal the lid.
6. Set the steam release handle to the "Sealing" position and press the "Manual" button.
7. Cook for 15 minutes.
8. When done, perform a quick pressure release and open the lid. Remove the ramekins and transfer to a wire rack. Cool to a room temperature and then refrigerate for about an hour.

NUTRITIONAL FACTS: Calories 257 Total Fats: 25.5g Net Carbs: 3.5g Protein: 5.5g Fiber: 2.1g

586. LEMON CAKE WITH BERRY SYRUP

PREPARATION: 15' **COOKING:** 30' **SERVES:** 8

INGREDIENTS

For the cake:
- 3 cups almond flour
- 3 tbsp stevia powder
- ¼ cup coconut milk, full-fat
- 1 tbsp coconut cream
- ¼ cup butter, softened
- 5 large eggs
- ¼ tsp salt
- 3 tsp baking powder
- 2 tsp lemon extract

For the syrup:
- ¼ cup raspberries
- ¼ cup blueberries
- 1 tbsp lemon juice, freshly squeeze
- ¼ cup granulated stevia

DIRECTIONS

1. In a large mixing bowl, combine together almond flour, stevia powder, baking powder, and salt.
2. Mix well and add eggs, one at the time, beating constantly.
3. Now add coconut milk, coconut cream, butter, and lemon extract. Using a paddle attachment beat for 3 minutes on medium speed.
4. Grease a small cake pan with some oil and line with parchment paper. Pour the mixture in it and tightly wrap with aluminum foil.
5. Plug in the instant pot and set the trivet at the bottom of the inner pot. Place the cake pan on top and pour in one cup of water.
6. Seal the lid and set the steam release handle to the "Sealing" position. Press the "Manual" button and cook for 25 minutes.
7. When done, perform a quick pressure release and open the lid. Carefully remove the pan and set aside.
8. Now press the "Saute" button. Add berries and pour in one cup of water and granulated stevia. Gently simmer for 5-6 minutes, stirring constantly.
9. Finally, add agar powder and give it a good stir. Cook until the mixture thickens.
10. Pour the syrup over chilled cake and refrigerate for 2 hours before serving.

NUTRITIONAL FACTS: Calories 186 Total Fats: 16g Net Carbs: 3.8g Protein: 6.4g Fiber: 1.3g

587. EASY RUM CHEESECAKE

PREPARATION: 15' **COOKING:** 15' **SERVES:** 10

INGREDIENTS

- 2 cups almond flour
- 4 large eggs, separated
- ¼ cup coconut cream
- 2 tbsp almond butter
- ¼ cup cocoa powder, unsweetened
- ¼ cup swerve
- 3 tsp baking powder
- 3 cups Mascarpone
- 1 cup plain Greek yogurt
- 2-3 drops stevia

Spices:
- 2 tsp rum extract
- ½ tsp cinnamon powder

DIRECTIONS

1. Plug in the instant pot and position a trivet. Pour in one cup of water in the stainless-steel insert and set aside.
2. Beat egg whites and swerve with a hand mixer until light foam appears. Add egg yolks, coconut cream, almond butter, baking powder, and cocoa powder, beating constantly.
3. Finally, add almond flour and continue to beat until completely combined.
4. Pour the mixture into lightly greased cake pan and cook for 15 minutes on the "Manual" mode.
5. When done, perform a quick pressure release and open the lid. Remove the cake from the pan and cool for a while.
6. Now combine Mascarpone and Greek yogurt. Add rum extract, cinnamon powder, and stevia. Using a hand mixer, mix well until completely combined.
7. Pour the mixture over the crust and refrigerate for a couple of hours before slicing.

NUTRITIONAL FACTS: Calories 247 Total Fats: 18.1g Net Carbs: 5.6g Protein: 15.6g Fiber: 1.7g

588. LEMON VEGAN CAKE

PREPARATION: 10' **COOKING:** 10' **SERVES:** 3

INGREDIENTS

- 1 cup of pitted dates
- 2-1/2 cups pecans
- 1-1/2 cup agave
- 3 avocados, halved & pitted
- 3 cups of cauliflower rice, prepared
- 1 lemon juice and zest
- ½ lemon extract
- 1-1/2 cups pineapple, crushed
- 1-1/2 teaspoon vanilla extract
- Pinch of cinnamon
- 1-1/2 cups of dairy-free yogurt

DIRECTIONS

1. Line your baking sheet with parchment paper.
2. Pulse the pecans in your food processor.
3. Add the agave and dates. Pulse for a minute.
4. Transfer this mix to the baking sheet. Wipe the bowl of your processor.
5. Bring together the pineapple, agave, avocados, cauliflower, lemon juice, and zest in your food processor. Get a smooth mixture.
6. Now add the lemon extract, cinnamon, and vanilla extract. Pulse.
7. Pour this mix into your pan, on the crust.
8. Refrigerate for 5 hours minimum.
9. Take out the cake and keep it at room temperature for 20 minutes.
10. Take out the cake's outer ring.
11. Whisk together the vanilla extract, agave, and yogurt in a bowl.
12. Pour on your cake.

NUTRITIONAL FACTS: Calories 688 Carbohydrates 100g Fat 28g Protein 9g Sugar 40g

589. DARK CHOCOLATE GRANOLA BARS

PREPARATION: 10' COOKING: 25' SERVES: 12

INGREDIENTS

- 1 cup tart cherries, dried
- 2 cups buckwheat
- ¼ cup of flaxseed
- 1 cup of walnuts
- 2 eggs
- 1 teaspoon of salt
- ¼ cup dark cocoa powder
- 2/3 cup honey
- ½ cup dark chocolate chips
- 1 teaspoon of vanilla

DIRECTIONS

1. Preheat your oven to 350 degrees F.
2. Apply cooking spray lightly on your baking pan.
3. Pulse together the walnuts, wheat, tart cherries, salt, and flaxseed in your food processor. Everything should be chopped fine.
4. Whisk together the honey, eggs, vanilla, and cocoa powder in a bowl.
5. Add the wheat mix to your bowl. Stir to combine well.
6. Include the chocolate chips. Stir again.
7. Now pour this mixture into your baking dish.
8. Sprinkle some chocolate chips and tart cherries.
9. Bake for 25 minutes. Set aside for cooling before serving.

NUTRITIONAL FACTS: Calories 364 Carbohydrates 37g Cholesterol 60mg Fat 20g Protein 6g Sugar 22g Fiber 4g Sodium 214mg

590. BLUEBERRY CRISP

PREPARATION: 5' COOKING: 30' SERVES: 4

INGREDIENTS

- ¼ cups pecans, chopped
- 1 cup buckwheat
- ½ teaspoon ginger
- 1 teaspoon of cinnamon
- 2 tablespoons olive oil
- ¼ teaspoon nutmeg
- 1 lb. blueberries
- 1 teaspoon of honey

DIRECTIONS

1. Preheat your oven to 350 degrees F.
2. Grease your baking dish.
3. Whisk together the pecans, wheat, oil, spices, and honey in a bowl.
4. Add the berries to your pan. Layer the topping on your berries.
5. Bake for 30 minutes at 350 F.

NUTRITIONAL FACTS: Calories 327 Carbohydrates 35g Fat 19g Protein 4g Sugar 14g Fiber 5g Sodium 2mg Potassium 197mg

591. CHOCOLATE CHIP QUINOA GRANOLA BARS

| PREPARATION: 5' | COOKING: 10' | SERVES: 16 |

INGREDIENTS

- ½ cup of chia seeds
- ½ cup walnuts, chopped
- 1 cup buckwheat
- 1 cup uncooked quinoa
- 2/3 cup dairy-free margarine
- ½ cup flax seed
- 1 teaspoon of cinnamon
- ½ cup of honey
- ½ cup of chocolate chips
- 1 teaspoon of vanilla
- ¼ teaspoon salt

DIRECTIONS

1. Preheat your oven to 350 degrees F.
2. Spread the walnuts, quinoa, wheat, flax, and chia on your baking sheet.
3. Bake for 10 minutes.
4. Line your baking dish with plastic wrap. Apply cooking spray. Keep aside.
5. Melt the margarine and honey in a saucepot.
6. Whisk together the vanilla, salt, and cinnamon into the margarine mix.
7. Keep the wheat mix and quinoa in a bowl. Pour the margarine sauce into it.
8. Stir the mixture. Coat well. Allow it to cool. Stir in the chocolate chips.
9. Spread your mixture into the baking dish. Press firmly into the pan.
10. Plastic wrap. Refrigerator overnight.
11. Slice into bars and serve.

NUTRITIONAL FACTS: Calories 408 Carbohydrates 31g Fat 28g Protein 8g Sugar 14g Fiber 6g Sodium 87mg

592. STRAWBERRY GRANITA

| PREPARATION: 10' | COOKING: 10' | SERVES: 8 |

INGREDIENTS

- 2 lb. strawberries, halved & hulled
- 1 cup of water
- Agave to taste
- ¼ teaspoon balsamic vinegar
- ½ teaspoon lemon juice
- Just a small pinch of salt

DIRECTIONS

1. Rinse the strawberries in water.
2. Keep in a blender. Add water, agave, balsamic vinegar, salt, and lemon juice.
3. Pulse many times so that the mixture moves. Blend to make it smooth.
4. Pour into a baking dish. The puree should be 3/8 inch deep only.
5. Refrigerate the dish uncovered till the edges start to freeze. The center should be slushy.
6. Stir crystals from the edges lightly into the center. Mix thoroughly.
7. Chill till the granite is almost completely frozen.
8. Scrape loose the crystals like before and mix.
9. Refrigerate again. Use a fork to stir 3-4 times till the granite has become light.

NUTRITIONAL FACTS: Calories 72 Carbohydrates 17g FAT 0G Sugar 14g Fiber 2g Protein 1g

593. APPLE FRITTERS

PREPARATION: 15' COOKING: 10' SERVES: 4

INGREDIENTS

- 1 apple, cored, peeled, and chopped
- 1 cup all-purpose flour
- 1 egg
- ½ cup cashew milk
- 1-1/2 teaspoons of baking powder
- 2 tablespoons of stevia sugar

DIRECTIONS

1. Preheat your air fryer to 175 degrees C or 350 degrees F.
2. Keep parchment paper at the bottom of your fryer.
3. Apply cooking spray.
4. Mix together ¼ cup sugar, flour, baking powder, egg, milk, and salt in a bowl.
5. Combine well by stirring.
6. Sprinkle 2 tablespoons of sugar on the apples. Coat well.
7. Combine the apples into your flour mixture.
8. Use a cookie scoop and drop the fritters with it to the air fryer basket's bottom.
9. Now air fry for 5 minutes.
10. Flip the fritters once and fry for another 3 minutes. They should be golden.

NUTRITIONAL FACTS: Calories 307 Carbohydrates 65g Cholesterol 48mg Total Fat 3g Protein 5g Sugar 39g Fiber 2g Sodium 248mg

594. ROASTED BANANAS

PREPARATION: 2' COOKING: 7' SERVES: 1

INGREDIENTS

- 1 banana, sliced into diagonal pieces
- Avocado oil cooking spray

DIRECTIONS

1. Take parchment paper and line the air fryer basket with it.
2. Preheat your air fryer to 190 degrees C or 375 degrees F.
3. Keep your slices of banana in the basket. They should not touch.
4. Apply avocado oil to mist the slices of banana.
5. Cook for 5 minutes.
6. Take out the basket. Flip the slices carefully.
7. Cook for 2 more minutes. The slices of banana should be caramelized and brown. Take them out from the basket.

NUTRITIONAL FACTS: Calories 121 Carbohydrates 27g Cholesterol 0mg Total Fat 1g Protein 1g Sugar 14g Fiber 3g Sodium 1mg

595. BERRY-BANANA YOGURT

PREPARATION: 10' **COOKING:** 0' **SERVES:** 1

INGREDIENTS

- ½ banana, frozen fresh
- 1 container 5.3ounes Greek yogurt, non-fat
- ¼ cup quick-cooking oats
- ½ cup blueberries, fresh and frozen
- 1 cup almond milk
- ¼ cup collard greens, chopped
- 5-6 ice cubes

DIRECTIONS

1. Take microwave-safe cup and add 1 cup almond milk and ¼ cup oats
2. Place the cups into your microwave on high for 2.5 minutes
3. When oats are cooked and 2 ice cubes to cool
4. Mix them well
5. Add all ingredients in your blender
6. Blend it until it gets a smooth and creamy mixture
7. Serve chilled and enjoy!

NUTRITIONAL FACTS: Calories: 379 Fat: 10g Carbohydrates: 63g Protein: 13g

596. AVOCADO CHOCOLATE MOUSSE

PREPARATION: 10' **COOKING:** 0' **SERVES:** 9

INGREDIENTS

- 3 ripe avocado, pitted and flesh scooped out
- 6 ounces plain Greek yogurt
- 1/8 cup almond milk, unsweetened
- ¼ cup espresso beans, ground
- ¼ cup of cocoa powder
- ½ teaspoon salt
- 2 tablespoons raw honey
- 1 bar dark chocolate
- 1 teaspoon vanilla extract

DIRECTIONS

1. Place all ingredients in your food processor
2. Pulse until smooth
3. Serve chilled and enjoy!

NUTRITIONAL FACTS: Calories: 208 Fat: 4g Carbohydrates: 17g Protein: 5g

597. APRICOT SQUARES

PREPARATION: 20' COOKING: 0' SERVES: 8

INGREDIENTS

- 1 cup shredded coconut, dried
- 1 teaspoon vanilla extract
- 1 cup apricot, dried
- 1 cup macadamia nuts, chopped
- 1 cup apricot, chopped
- 1/3 cup turmeric powder

DIRECTIONS

1. Place all ingredients in your food processor
2. Pulse until smooth
3. Place the mixture into a square pan and press evenly
4. Serve chilled and enjoy!

NUTRITIONAL FACTS: Calories: 201 Fat: 15g Carbohydrates: 17g Protein: 3g

598. RAW BLACK FOREST BROWNIES

PREPARATION: 2H 10 COOKING: 0' SERVES: 6

INGREDIENTS

- 1 and ½ cups cherries, pitted, dried and chopped
- 1 cup raw cacao powder
- ½ cup dates pitted
- 2 cups walnuts, chopped
- ½ cup almonds, chopped
- ¼ teaspoon salt

DIRECTIONS

1. Place all ingredients in your food processor
2. Pulse until small crumbs are formed
3. Press the brownie batter in a pan
4. Freeze for two hours
5. Slice before serving and enjoy!

NUTRITIONAL FACTS: Calories: 294 Fat: 18g Carbohydrates: 33g Protein: 7g

599. BERRY PARFAIT

PREPARATION: 10' **COOKING:** 10' **SERVES:** 5

INGREDIENTS

- 7oz / 200g almond butter
- 3.5oz / 100g Greek yogurt
- 14oz / 400g mixed berries
- 2 tsp honey
- 7oz / 200g mixed nuts

DIRECTIONS

1. Mix the Greek yogurt, butter, and honey until its smooth.
2. Add a layer of berries and a layer of the mixture in a glass until it's full.
3. Serve immediately with sprinkled nuts.

NUTRITIONAL FACTS: Calories: 250 Carbohydrates: 17 g Protein: 7.2 g Fat: 19.4 g Sugar: 42.3 g Fiber: 6.6 g Sodium: 21 mg

600. SHERBET PINEAPPLE

PREPARATION: 20' **COOKING:** 0' **SERVES:** 4

INGREDIENTS

- 1 can of 8-ounce pineapple chunks
- 1/3 cup of orange marmalade
- ¼ teaspoon of ground ginger
- ¼ teaspoon of vanilla extract
- 1 can of 11-ounce orange sections
- 2 cups of pineapple, lemon or lime sherbet

DIRECTIONS

1. Drain the pineapple, ensure you reserve the juice.
2. Take a medium-sized bowl and add pineapple juice, ginger, vanilla and marmalade to the bowl
3. Add pineapple chunks, drained mandarin oranges as well
4. Toss well and coat everything
5. Free them for 15 minutes and allow them to chill
6. Spoon the sherbet into 4 chilled stemmed sherbet dishes
7. Top each of them with fruit mixture
8. Enjoy!

NUTRITIONAL FACTS: Calories: 267 Cal Fat: 1 g Carbohydrates: 65 g Protein: 2 g

CONCLUSION

Whether you have met your weight loss goals, you cannot just suddenly start consuming carbs again for it will shock your system. Have an idea of what you want to allow back into your consumption slowly. Be familiar with portion sizes and stick to that amount of carbs for the first few times you eat post-keto.

Start with non-processed carbs like whole grain, beans, and fruits. Start slow and see how your body responds before resolving to add carbs one meal at a time.

The things to watch out for when coming off keto are weight gain, bloating, more energy, and feeling hungry. The weight gain is nothing to freak out over; perhaps, you might not even gain any. It all depends on your diet, how your body processes carbs, and, of course, water weight. The length of your keto diet is a significant factor in how much weight you have lost, which is caused by the reduction of carbs. The bloating will occur because of the reintroduction of fibrous foods and your body getting used to digesting them again. The bloating van lasts for a few days to a few weeks. You will feel like you have more energy because carbs break down into glucose, which is the body's primary source of fuel. You may also notice better brain function and the ability to work out more.

The ketogenic diet is the ultimate tool you can use to plan your future. Can you picture being more involved, more productive and efficient, and more relaxed and energetic? That future is possible for you, and it does not have to be a complicated process to achieve that vision. You can choose right now to be healthier and slimmer and more fulfilled tomorrow. It is possible with the ketogenic diet.

This is not a fancy diet that promises falsehoods of miracle weight loss. This diet is proven by years of science and research, which benefits not only your waistline, but your heart, skin, brain, and organs. It does not just improve your physical health but your mental and emotional health as well. This diet improves your health holistically.

Keto diet provides long term health benefits compare to other diet plans. During keto diet near about 75 to 90 percent of calories comes from fats, an adequate number of calories

5 to 20 percent comes from proteins and 5 percent of calories from carb intake.

What began as a simple spark of curiosity ended on a high note: keto, a term you constantly read and heard about. Now you have all the knowledge in the world to lead a lifestyle that is truly worthy of your time, energy, and effort.

Being 50 years old or more is not bad. It is how we handle ourselves in this age that matters. Most of us would have just moved on and dealt with things as they would have arrived. That is no longer the case. It is quite literally survival of the fittest.

Do not give up now as there will be quite a few days where you may think to yourself, "Why am I doing this?" and to answer that, simply focus on the goals you wish to achieve.

A good diet enriched with all the proper nutrients is our best shot of achieving an active metabolism and efficient lifestyle. A lot of people think that the Keto diet is simply for people who are interested in losing weight. You will find that it is quite the opposite. There are intense keto diets where only 5 percent of the diet comes from carbs, 20 percent is from protein, and 75 percent is from fat. But even a modified version of this which involves consciously choosing foods low in carbohydrate and high in healthy fats is good enough.

Thanks for reading this book. I hope it has provided you with enough insight to get you going. Don't put off getting started. The sooner you begin this diet, the sooner you'll start to notice an improvement in your health and well-being.

CPSIA information can be obtained
at www.ICGtesting.com
Printed in the USA
LVHW100602220221
679596LV00009B/414